39 ⁹⁵

T5-CPV-015

Pediatric Rehabilitation

A Team Approach
for Therapists

Pediatric Rehabilitation

A Team Approach for Therapists

Edited by

Martha K. Logigian, M.S., O.T.R.
Instructor, Department of Orthopedic Surgery,
Harvard Medical School; Director of
Rehabilitation Services, Brigham and Women's
Hospital, Boston

Judith D. Ward, M.O.E., O.T.R.
Associate Professor, Occupational Therapy
Department, University of New Hampshire,
Durham

Little, Brown and Company
Boston / Toronto / London

ST. PHILIP'S COLLEGE LIBRARY

Copyright © 1989 by Martha K. Logigian and
Judith D. Ward

First Edition

All rights reserved. No part of this book may be
reproduced in any form or by any electronic or
mechanical means, including information storage
and retrieval systems, without permission in
writing from the publisher, except by a reviewer
who may quote brief passages in a review.

Library of Congress Catalog Card No. 88-83985

ISBN 0-316-53084-0

Printed in the United States of America

MV

ST. PHILIP'S COLLEGE LIBRARY

In memory of
Joyce Connell,
Allied Health Editor,
Little, Brown and Company

Contents

Contributing Authors

Diane M. Erlandson, R.N., M.S.
Clinical Specialist in Rheumatology, Rheumatology Department, Brigham and Women's Hospital, Boston

Judith Falconer, Ph.D., O.T.R./L.
Assistant Professor of Physical Therapy and Medicine and Director of Graduate Studies, Programs in Physical Therapy, Northwestern University Medical School, Chicago

Joan M. Izen, M.A., CCC/SP
Private Practitioner and Regional Preschool Consultant, Southeastern Regional Education Service Center, Derry, New Hampshire

Karen Jacobs, M.S., O.T.R./L., F.A.O.T.A.
Adjunct Clinical Instructor, Boston University, Sargent College, Department of Occupational Therapy, Boston

Mary Louise Jani, M.S., P.T.
Pediatric Physical Therapist and Consultant in private practice, Winchester, Massachusetts

Debora D. Kent, M.A., CCC/SP
Speech-Language Pathologist, Visiting Nurse Associates, Dedham, Massachusetts

Patricia A. R. Laverdure, O.T.R.
Pediatric Developmental Consultant in private practice, Reston, Virginia

Martha K. Logigian, M.S., O.T.R.
Instructor, Department of Orthopedic Surgery, Harvard Medical School; Director of Rehabilitation Services, Brigham and Women's Hospital, Boston

Alice A. Sapienza, M.S., O.T.R.
Chief Occupational Therapist, St. Mary's Hospital for Children, Bayside, New York

Judith D. Ward, M.O.E., O.T.R.
Associate Professor, Occupational Therapy Department, University of New Hampshire, Durham

Preface

This book presents rehabilitation programs for children with physical or emotional problems. It is designed for students and entry level clinicians in allied health and special education, particularly in the disciplines of occupational therapy, physical therapy, and speech-language pathology.

The text begins with an introductory chapter on normal development and descriptions of the members of the health-care team. Chapter 2, Cerebral Palsy, includes discussions of neurodevelopmental treatment and self-care and feeding; Chapter 3, Mental Retardation, discusses educational issues and behavioral therapy; Chapter 4, Infantile Autism, covers the learning environment and language stimulation. Chapter 5, Learning Disabilities, describes work-related programs and sensory integration and is complemented by Chapter 6, Attention Deficit Disorders/Hyperactivity. Chapter 7, Communication Disorders, focuses on stuttering and disorders resulting from cleft palate and hearing loss; it also includes a section on nonverbal communication. A team approach to the care of children with arthritis is presented in Chapter 8, Juvenile Rheumatoid Arthritis. Chapter 9, Physical Disorders, covers birth defects and muscular diseases and includes an indepth section on visual disorders. Chapter 10, Medical Disorders, covers asthma, burns, cancer, cardiac disorders, cystic fibrosis, diabetes, hemophilia, and sickle cell anemia, including the emotional aspects of certain disorders. Chapter 11, Psychosocial Disorders, covers anxiety, anorexia nervosa, conduct disorders, and substance abuse, including discussions of the different treatment settings available.

Each chapter integrates information on specific treatment programs that are relevant to a given disorder. These disorders may be encountered at home, in day care, hospitals, schools, or special programs, and we have attempted to address problems unique to these environments. The design of each chapter includes relevant information on the disorder, particularly etiology, prevalence, prognosis, medical manifestations and tests, team assessment, and treatment with special emphasis on the role of the occupational therapist. Practical information for therapists and their patients, including two resource appendixes for adaptive equipment, lists of advocacy associations, and a chapter appendix on pediatric assessments, is also presented.

The authors wish to extend special thanks to our families, Ted, Anne, and Jeremy Ward, and Eric Logigian; to Shana Wagger, Development Editor at Little, Brown, for her assistance in seeing this manuscript to its completion; Barbara Ward for her support of the idea of this text; and Yvonne Wellington for her patience in typing.

M. K. L.
J. D. W.

Pediatric Rehabilitation

A Team Approach
for Therapists

1 Introduction

Martha K. Logigian

In recent years, numerous advances have been made in the identification of conditions that contribute to dysfunctional conditions in children. These advances include adequate prenatal care such as prenatal monitoring by amniocentesis and ultrasound, which assist in the identification and possible prevention of the birth of severely disabled children. Monitoring of the mother's exposure to radiation and to hazardous drugs such as Dilantin and alcohol is also an aid in prevention. Immunization programs for women have reduced the incidence of the sequelae of rubella. Fetal monitoring and neonate intensive care units have had significant impact on the health and well-being of the newborn and contribute to the expectation of a normal life for the high-risk infant.

Although the incidence of chronic childhood disorders has changed minimally in recent years (Table 1-1), survival estimates have improved considerably. Survival into adulthood for most children with chronic diseases is now a near normal expectation.

In developing intervention strategies for special needs children and their families, an ideal framework encompasses human development. This includes physical neurologic, and cognitive development, the human relationships involved, and the child's capacities for organizing and differentiating experience, that is, adaptive and coping skills. A framework such as this

1

TABLE 1-1. Estimated prevalence of chronic diseases and conditions in children, ages 0–20 in the United States—1980

Disorder	Prevalence estimates per 1000	Range of prevalance estimates per 1000
Arthritis	2.2	1.0–3.0
Asthma	38.0	20.0–53.0
Moderate to severe	10.0	8.0–15.0
Autism	.44	.40–.48
Central nervous system injury		
Traumatic brain injury	.05	
Paralysis	2.1	2.0–2.3
Cerebral palsy	2.5	1.4–5.1
Chronic renal failure	.080	
Terminal	.010	
Nonterminal	.070	
Cleft lip palate	1.5	1.3–2.0
Congenital heart disease	7.0	2.0–7.0
Severe congenital heart disease	.50	
Cystic fibrosis	.20	
Diabetes mellitus	1.8	1.2–2.0
Down's syndrome	1.1	
Hearing impairment	16.	
Deafness	.1	0.6–.15
Hemophilia	.15	
Leukemia		
Acute lymphocytic leukemia	.11	
Mental retardation	25.0	20.0–30.0
Muscular dystrophy	.06	
Neural tube defect	.45	
Spina bifida	.40	
Encephalocele	.05	
Phenylketonuria	.10	
Sickle cell disease	.46	
Sickle cell anemia	.28	
Seizure disorder	3.5	2.6–4.6
Visual impairment	30.0	20.0–35.0
Impaired visual acuity	20.0	
Blind	.6	.5–1.0

Source: From S. L. Gortmaker and W. Sappenfeld. Chronic childhood disorders: Prevalence and impact. *Pediatr. Clin. North Am.* 31(1):5, 1984. Reprinted with permission.

enhances understanding of the range and variation in human functioning [7].

At birth, the newborn responds to the environment in a reflexive manner. As the nervous system develops and successful learning experiences occur, the child progresses from total dependency to active participation. In normal development, these progressive changes in behavior occur in an orderly, sequential fashion. The child accomplishes tasks in a hierarchic and predictable manner, that is, subsequent skills are built on those that precede them. And all children presumably go through the same stages in the same order, which enables their predictability. Table 1-2 presents developmental milestones from birth to 18 years of age [1, 3, 6, 9].

Variations in the developmental process can occur because of variations in the child, the environment, or both. Physical or emotional illness may modify the expected developmental progression by affecting the child's interactions with the physical and social environment, whereas aspects of the child's environment, such as parents, peers, or school systems, may be altered as a result of the illness [13].

The concept of developmental hierarchy [14] is important in pediatric habilitation. Children are evaluated with scales that are based on developmental norms. The absence of age-appropriate skills is considered dysfunctional [11]. Developmental treatment consists of facilitating the acquisition of absent skills or the refinement of impaired age-appropriate skills. These skills are encouraged in the sequence in which they would normally develop.

Although developmental skills are divided into domains of function (movement, language, social/adaptive skills, cognition) in the child, they cannot be easily separated. Development in one area influences development in another. For example, speech is a physical function that is socially determined and its quality influenced by intelligence. In childhood, great spurts of energy are devoted to skill acquisition. There may be periods where it appears development has slowed. This plateau in developmental progression may reflect practice or refinement of a particular skill rather than acquisition of new skills. Development is qualitative (e.g., skills become more refined and complex over time) and quantitative (e.g., children grow taller and add words to their vocabulary) [15].

The therapist uses knowledge of human development to understand what skills the child needs at a particular time and what setting and treatment techniques will provide the appropriate stimulation for development. Moreover, every child is part of a family unit, and the support of parents is critical to the child's healthy development. If the child needs an intervention program, the parents may be asked to take on additional responsibilities as teacher, therapist, program reinforcer, or treatment manager. Professionals must recognize that families need information about their child's problems, time for adjustment to the problems, support for their grief, and respect for their efforts at coping.

MOVEMENT

The development of movement [2, 4] begins in the embryo following a set timetable. On the twenty-sixth day of gestation, two bulges seen on the sides of the embryo are the arms. On the twenty-eighth day the leg buds appear. During the second month the extremities (thighs, knees, lower legs, ankles, hands, fingers) develop into segments, which by the end of the second month have their characteristic shape. At this time the embryo is approximately 4 cm long, and the skeleton is cartilaginous in nature. By the third month there is calcification of the cartilage. During the sixth and seventh weeks the first connections between the nerves and muscles occur, and this fetal motor sequence continues to develop to the fourteenth week. There are no true movements until after the seventh week when the first movements are of the trunk. The upper trunk bends forward and backward in reflex motions triggered by pressure, sound, and contact stimuli (e.g., lips touched, upper body bends to side, and arms draw back). These are primitive, isolated reflexes, as isolated movements develop later.

By the eighth week, the palms are sensitive, and the hand closes when touched. During the ninth and tenth weeks there is an increase in the number of nerve and muscle connections. By the fourteenth week all of the body's basic movements have occurred (e.g., kick; move feet and toes; bend knees, elbows, and wrists; clench fists; turn head; wrinkle brow).

By the fifth month, the mother feels the movements of the fetus. There are complicated

ST. PHILIP'S COLLEGE LIBRARY

TABLE 1-2. Developmental milestones

Age	Gross motor	Fine motor	Self care	Language	Cognition	Social/emotional
1 mo	Partial head control; Primitive reflexes predominate	Grasp reflex; Clenched fist	Sucking and swallowing	Random vocalizations; Alert to sound	Fixates on objects and follows 90°	Quiets when picked up
2 mo	Good head control; Raises/maintains head 45° in prone	Follows object past midline	Hand to mouth	Social smile	Repeats random movements	Quiets to face or voice
3 mo	In prone head/chest to 90° with forearm support; Primitive reflexes less	Hands held open	Suck/swallow and bite reflexes less	Coos	Recognizes mother	Watches adult walk across room
4 mo	Pulls to sitting with assist	Hands come to midline; Mouths objects; Reaches	Recognizes bottle; Takes puréed foods	Spontaneous utterances; Combinations of random syllables	Shakes rattle; Regards hands	Responds to familiar people
5 mo	Pulls to sitting; Rolls to supine when prone	Uses palmar prehension	Integration of bite reflex	Orients toward sound; Differentiated crying	Looks at objects being held	Smiles spontaneously at image in mirror
6 mo	Rolls in both directions prone	Transfers toys	Closes lip on spoon to remove food	Vocalizes consonants	Follows path of dropped object	Recognizes self in mirror
7 mo	Sits unsupported 30 sec.; Bounces when standing; Sits without support	Reaches purposefully; Feeds self cookie	Drinks from cup with assist	Imitates noise; Responds to name	Plays peek-a-boo	Extends arms to be picked up; Reaches for image of self in mirror
8 mo	Crawls in prone	Rings bell	Chews with lateral tongue motion	Forms bisyllabic repetitions	Imitates hand movements in repertoire	Explores features of familiar persons

4

ST. PHILIP'S COLLEGE LIBRARY

Age	Gross Motor	Fine Motor	Self-help	Language	Cognitive	Social
9 mo	From sitting assists in pull to stand Creeps	Radial raking grasp Pokes with index finger	Finger feeds	Imitates consonant/vowel combinations	Finds hidden object	Performs for social attention
10 mo	From sitting pulls to stand Cruises along furniture	Removes blocks from container Begins pincer grasp Claps	Eats mashed table foods	Imitates non-speech sounds	Responds to simple commands Attempts to imitate movements	Imitates patty-cake
11 mo	Walks with one hand held	Uses pincer grasp	Swallows with mouth closed Stops drooling Assists with dressing	Looks at familiar objects/persons when named	Reacts to novel features of an object	Offers toy
12 mo	Stands alone Makes first steps	Rolls ball in imitation Throws objects	Feeds self from spoon with spills	Uses two to three specific words	Points to common objects	Responds differently to young children
15 mo	Walks with stability	Builds tower with blocks	Lifts, replaces, drinks from cup	Uses 10–12 words in one-word sentences	Follows one-step commands	Uses gestures
18 mo	Stops and starts Runs stiffly, jumps Seats self in small chair	Marks with pencils Scribbles, throws ball Puts pegs in hole	Spoon feeds Independent in feeding Takes off clothes	Uses jargon Knows body parts	Follows two-step commands Points to one picture	Begins parallel play
24 mo	Walks up/down stairs Jumps from bottom step	Imitates vertical lines Builds six-block tower Draws circle	Dons/doffs shoes	Three-word sentences Uses "I"	Points to four to five body parts Puts simple puzzles together Recognizes constancy of external objects Egocentricity central pattern	Plays near other children

TABLE 1-2 (CONTINUED)

Age	Gross motor	Fine motor	Self care	Language	Cognition	Social/emotional
30 mo	Walks up stairs with alternating feet	Builds eight-block tower	Puts on simple clothes	Uses three sentence types	Identifies objects by their use	"Terrible twos"
	Kicks ball	Imitates paper folding	Washes/dries hand with assist		Understands one	Plays with other children
					Matches colored cubes	Discriminates boys/girls
3 yr	Stands on one foot	Copies a circle	Removes/puts on all clothing	900–1000 words	Recognizes common objects	Begins imitative play
	Rides tricycle using pedals	Cuts with scissors	Unbuttons easy buttons	Short simple sentences	Tells simple story	Continues parallel play, some sharing
					Differentiates big/small	Explores materials
	Runs		Feeds self	Uses four grammatic constructions	Preoperational thought patterns	
4 yr	Hops on one foot	Copies a cross	Buttons large buttons, zips	1500 words	Understands function of common objects/body parts	Plays with peers/small groups
	Catches/throws ball	Does 12–16-piece puzzle	Begins laces	Uses complex sentences	Begins similarities	Curious, questioning
		Cuts line with scissors			Draws person with three parts	Begins sense of humor
5 yr	Walks downstairs with alternating feet	Copies a square	Completes self-care routines independently	2000 words	Draws person with five parts	Aware of social routines
	Skips	Shows hand preference		Articulation good		Begins to see self in relation to world
						Begins to understand time concepts
						Understands sharing

6

Age						
6 yr	Jumps from 12 in. Throws ball accurately	Copies diamond shape Cuts out picture with scissors	Cuts with knife Uses telephone Laces/ties shoes	Uses irregular verbs/comparative adjectives Tells imaginary stories	Draws person with clothes, neck, full body Understands number concepts 1–10 Can copy and begins to decode symbols and shapes Learns by concrete experiences and participation	Begins to leave family for school, friends Easily frustrated Enjoys dramatic play
7 yr					Can perform motor and self-care skills required of life situation Prelogical, perceptual reasoning (child sees relationships via trial and error). Things seen as having a single property at a time	
7–9 yr					Begins abstract thinking. Logical reasoning emerges, still concrete. Understands reversibility, constancy of physical objects	Learns to relate to adults and make ethical judgments. Role of peers important
9–11 yr					Use of abstraction grows	Increased awareness of opposite sex Peer influence very important
12–14 yr					Uses formal operational thought, deductive reasoning	Begins to assert independence Develops sense of identity
14–18 yr					Refines thinking process. Increases knowledge	Sex roles very important Begins to make career choices

reflex movements occurring, which are components of movement patterns. During the eighth month the head is down (head is the heaviest body part). The arms and legs are active, but the body is difficult to move due to the lack of space.

At birth, flexor musculature predominates. For example, the child is frequently seen with the knees flexed close to the stomach and the hands and arms near the face and chest when in a supine position. Many other reflexes are exhibited at birth, such as primitive grasp and asymmetric tonic neck, or develop shortly after birth [Table 2-1]. Each contributes to the child's development of movement and occurs in step with the development of sensation. For example, impulses from the eyes, ears, touch receptors in the skin, and proprioceptors in muscles and joints are fundamental in the development of locomotion.

During the first years of life, locomotor development is intense and rapid. Development takes place in a cephalocaudal direction, and from proximal to distal joints. The infant learns to stand then walk, allowing further environmental exploration, which contributes to the development of eye-hand coordination and visual/perceptual skills.

Gross movements develop first, then fine, manipulative movements, until age 6. As motor skills develop, the child is able to accomplish more developmental activities. For example, the child gains head control and thus, with support, can move from supine to sitting. Eye fixation and tracking enable the child to reach for objects in midline. Gross arm movements allow reaching to the midline, head, back, and toes.

Mastery is gained of new skills such as feeding (Table 1-3; see also Chapter 2). For example, the development of eye-hand coordination allows the child to use finger foods. With an increase in trunk control, more reaching can occur, and emerging grasp patterns allow for the use of utensils. Equilibrium reactions in sitting mean that the child can sit independently and reach for objects. With the refinement of grasp

patterns (Figure 1-1), dressing and manipulation of objects such as fasteners can occur.

Body proportions also develop, and by age 8, width develops. The latter occurs from 2 to 4 years of age as well. Adolescents experience another growth period, with a width increase during the latter half of puberty. An increase in weight and height accompanies this development. From age 6 to 20 strength increases, in males up to the twenties, in females up to age 14. Information on growth curves for children from birth to 18 years in the United States can be obtained form the U.S. Department of Health and Welfare [12].

LANGUAGE

The development of language begins at birth when the infant cries using vowel sounds and is alert to environmental sounds. Typical infant reactions to unexpected loud noises include a prominent startle, widening of the eyes, body jerk, or an attempt to search for the source. By 1 month a wail can be heard. At 2 months there are spontaneous vocalizations (babble). An intentional "listening" posture is observed by the third or fourth month. At this age the infant begins to visually scan the environment with purposeful attempts to localize sound sources. Improved motor skills of the head, neck, and upper trunk enable the deliberate search for the location of what was heard. The child becomes interested in sounds and may become totally absorbed in play with sound-producing toys.

Between 3 and 6 months of age the infant begins to engage in vocal play, babbling and cooing softly to self, imitating self vocalizations and eventually those of others. By 6 months there is structure to the babble. From 6 to 10 months the child begins to respond purposefully to sounds, meaningful or not. A call of the child's name will result in rapid eye contact with the speaker. When the telephone rings the baby may gaze at it and then to a parent in anticipation. When a parent says "bye bye," the baby will likely raise a hand in appropriate gesture.

At 9 months the infant can make bisyllabic

TABLE 1-3. Sequence of oral motor and feeding skill development

Age	Reflexes	Jaw	Lips	Gums/teeth
Newborn	Palmomental Babkin Rooting Gag Automatic phasic bite release			
1 mo		Opens jaw widely to grasp nipple. Vertical movement during suckling	Upper lip exerts more pressure on nipple. No lateral lip closure. Lips closed as rest. Touch of nipple on lips causes mouth to open	
2 mo	Palmomental Babkin Rooting Gag Automatic phasic bite release Suckle swallow			
3 mo	Palmomental disappearing Babkin disappearing Rooting present in breastfed Automatic phasic bite release disappearing		Lateral borders of lips close on nipple causing a dimpling of the upper lip	
4 mo	Rooting completely gone in bottle fed Gag Automatic phasic bite release disappearing		Continued increase in lateral lip closure. Lateral aspects of lower lip are active. Pouts lips to shift food. Cannot pull food from spoon. Smacks lips	

TABLE 1-3 (CONTINUED)

Age	Reflexes	Jaw	Lips	Gums/teeth
5 mo	Rooting disappearing in breast fed; Gag decreased in strength	Munching with suckling and sucking. Phasic bite pattern; may bite down on spoon to increase stability. Intrinsic jaw stability developing	Lower lip protrudes to provide stability for upper lip to move. Purses lips at corners. Lips active with jaw movement. Continued spillage from lips	
6 mo	Gag decreasing	Jaw does not yet have the stability for cup drinking, thus child may revert to lower patterns with suckling and tongue protrusion. Munching with gross tongue mobility	Lower lip protrudes under utensil to increase stability. Passive upper lip closure but cannot put food from spoon. Lips increase activity in chewing. Lower lips roll out slightly and lips separate. On the chewing side, the lips are drawn up and in. Lips drawing when food is on them, but they do not clean food off	0–1 tooth
7 mo	Adultlike gag reflex	Munching patterns with a horizontal shift with tongue. Jaws close on a solid and then tongue sucks or suckles it	Forward and downward motion of upper lip to remove food from spoon. Lower lip draws in during removal of spoon	
8 mo		Holds jaw closed while a piece of a soft solid is broken off	Upper lip active in removing food from spoon	0–4 teeth
9 mo		Munches with diagonal-circular movement when food is transferred from side to side. When food is between the central incisors, a phasic bite release pattern is used with lateral tongue mobility. When food in center of tongue, tongue moves in vertical orientation in unison with jaw munching	Lips active with jaw movement	4–8 teeth
10 mo			Lower lip draws in to remove food completely. Incisors actively clean lower lip	
11 mo				
12 mo		Jaw is gaining control over gross vertical and lateral movement. Controlled munch on soft solid; phasic bite release on hard	Upper lip closure with no food or liquid loss	
15 mo			Upper lip draws in to clean food from it. Lower lip moves over upper lip	6–10 teeth
18 mo		Rotary chew	Lateral lip flexibility	8–12 teeth
24 mo				16–20 teeth

Age	Buccal cavity	Tongue	Swallow	Drooling	Self feeding
Newborn		0–2 weeks, sucking motion 2–4 weeks, suckle-swallow with tongue protrusion		Little in supine, increased in other positions	
1 mo	Cheeks cause air swallowing. No excess space in cavity. Sucking pads present	Suckle with some suck: two sucks to one breath. Protrudes during swallowing. Fills mouth, presses against palate, cheeks; tip on lower lip. Limited mobility. Limited curling around nipple, cupping during crying and mouthing	Tongue protrusion		
2 mo		Suckling pattern. Spoon: suckle-swallow with tongue protrusion; difficulty moving food to back of mouth; some food pushed out of mouth	Suckle-swallow with tongue protrusion		
3 mo	Decreased sucking pads	Suckling predominant with longer sequences. Tongue protrusion as nipple touches lip. Tongue protrusion in anticipation	Decreased choking		Increased body activity when visualizes bottle
4 mo	Cavity increases	Suckling predominant but more intrinsic musculature use resulting in increased sucking and negative pressure. Tongue protrusion in anticipation. Decrease in			Pats bottle

11

TABLE 1-3 (CONTINUED)

Age	Buccal cavity	Tongue	Swallow	Drooling	Self feeding
		nonnutritive sucking. Tongue quivers with fatigue at end of feeding. May thrust out solid foods			
5 mo	Elongation of oralpha-ryngeal area. Buccal cavity developed	Suckling/sucking patterns continue. Tongue quiet in mouth in anticipation	Increased control of suck-swallow mechanism but coughing and gagging are still present. Tongue protrusion in swallow	Decreased in stable positions; increased with cutting teeth	
6 mo	Inner cheeks draw in during eating	Suck with occasional suckling	No pause in suck to swallow, may cough or choke. Swallowing produces tight lip closure. Tongue may protrude between gums. Swallowing puréed and semisolid foods is very controlled. Swallowing ground foods elicits a gag or choke	Increased when cutting teeth, babbling, or using hands for reaching	Plays with spoon; pushes it away or brings to mouth
7 mo			Tongue elevation to swallow. Pulls away from cup after two or three sucks to control swallowing		
8 mo			Sucking, swallowing, and breathing patterns are coordinated and controlled		Feeds self finger foods; holds own bottle
9 mo	Cheek musculature gaining coordination	Sucking with no liquid loss	Swallows with vertical tongue movement	Increased when cutting teeth and acquiring motor skills	

12

TABLE 1-3 (CONTINUED)

Age	Buccal cavity	Tongue	Swallow	Drooling	Self feeding
10 mo		Sucking. Tongue transfers food horizontally			
11 mo		Lateral tongue movement matured. Tongue protrusion may appear voluntarily as exploration occurs. Tongue retracted in anticipation			Holds own bottle well. Holds and lifts cup with spillage
12 mo		Tongue transfers laterally with control. Increased awareness of tongue	Infrequent coughing or gagging		
15 mo		Tongue licks lower lip			Finger feeds part of meal. Grasps spoon and puts into dish, filling it with difficulty. Turns spoon over as it is brought to mouth
18 mo					Uses two hands on cup with little spillage. Uses fingers to fill spoon. Brings spoon to mouth and turns it over while in mouth
24 mo	Cheek musculature draws in and cooperates with lateral tongue movement in chew. Cheeks provide exterior stability to jaw	Tongue licks upper lip			Uses one hand to hold onto cup with no spillage. Fills spoon without the use of fingers. Brings spoon to mouth without turning

13

	Age (weeks)	Description	Stimulation
	12	Reflexive, ulnar side strongest, no reaching before eye contact	Place objects in hand; hang toys in crib to stimulate eye contact and tracking
	16	Mouthing of fingers and mutual fingering; retains object placed in hand; no visually directed grasp until both hand and object in field of vision	Toys hanging within swiping reach; toys on floor within visual field and hand reach
	20	Primitive squeeze, raking; fingers only, no thumb or palm involved; immediate approach and grasp on sight	Toys of varied textures, colors, sizes shapes, and weights
	24	Palmar or squeeze grasp; still no thumb participation; eyes and hands combine in joint action	Place toys in different positions and distances so eyes and hands must search
	28	Radial-palmar or whole-hand grasp; radial side stronger; thumb begins to adduct; unilateral approach; transfer from one hand to the other	Toys that can be picked up and transferred by one hand, must be washable and safe (mouthing)
	32	Inferior scissors or superior-palm grasp; known as monkey grasp because thumb is adducted, not opposed	Toys with smaller and thinner circumferences, to strengthen thumb adductor
	36	Radial-digital or inferior forefinger grasp; fingers on radial side provide pressure on object; thumb begins to move toward opposition by pressing toward PIP joint of forefinger; finer adjustment of digits	More pliable materials, including sand, clay, yarn, tissue paper, tape and many types of finger food for self-feeding and exploration
	40	Inferior-pincer grasp; thumb moves toward DIP joint of forefinger; poking finger, inhibition of other four digits, beginning of voluntary release	Many small objects with a variety of shapes to examine and palpate, toys with holes and indentations to poke and explore
	44	Neat pincer or forefinger grasp with slight extension of wrist	Tiny objects to pick up and drop, such as dry cereal
	52	Opposition or superior-forefinger grasp, wrist extended and deviated to ulnar side for efficient prehension, release smooth for large objects, clumsy for small objects	Toys that provide repeat motions of release, such as blocks and container, both becoming gradually smaller

FIG. 1-1. Sequential development of prehension. (From R. P. Erhardt. Sequential levels in development of prehension. *Am. J. Occup. Ther.* 28:592, 1974. Copyright © 1974 by the American Occupational Therapy Association, Inc. Reprinted with permission.)

repetitions, such as "dada" and "baba." The 10- to 15-month-old child points to people and labeled objects, gets what a parent asks for, and imitates sounds and simple words. From 12 to 18 months real words develop, such as "mommy" or "gimme."

The 15- to 18-month old responds consistently to verbal commands and uses them in the form of one- to two-word utterances to satisfy needs and wants. The child's rapidly increasing receptive and expressive language skills result from the solid auditory foundation that has taken a minimum of 18 months to establish.

From 18 to 24 months several words together can be heard, such as "more milk." The child has 18 words by 18 months and 240 words by age 24 months [17]. From 24 to 36 months the child develops sentence structure (e.g., "Where mommy go?"). From 36 to 48 months, during operational changes, the child has accomplished hundreds of words.

After the simple-sentence stage, there is great variability in language development. From the 48-month point the child learns to apply language rules. For example, adding "ed" on the end of a word to signify past tense. From 84 to 90 months all parts of speech are learned, and there is normal articulation. By age 7 or 8 years there is good syntax (see Chapter 7).

SOCIAL/ADAPTIVE SKILLS

Skills developed to achieve successful mastery of the environment are referred to as developmental tasks, and such tasks arise at specific times in life. Successful achievement of these tasks should lead to happiness and success with later tasks, whereas failure can lead to unhappiness, disapproval by society, or difficulty with later tasks [8]. To develop a specific skill, the individual must have the physical and emotional maturity for the performance of the task. In addition, as the child develops, the importance of the task within the child's sociocultural environment and the child's personal motivation take on greater significance in the accomplishment of the task.

From a general state of excitement at birth, the infant undergoes rapid change. Within a few weeks the child's emotional responses become differentiated and signs of pleasure and displeasure identifiable. Cries of hunger, pain, and discomfort can be differentiated by 1 month [17]. By 2 months signs of pleasure can be detected through sounds and movements. Eye tracking begins when the infant is only a few weeks old. By the age of 10 weeks the infant gives signs of recognition of parents and at 14 weeks can differentiate between strangers and familiar people.

During the first year of life, the mother-child relationship is the key to the social world of the child. Through this relationship the child begins to develop an awareness of self and the environment. A healthy mother-child relationship focuses on the needs of the infant. By the sixth month the child is spending more time with people in social interaction, manipulating toys, and exploring the environment.

As the child grows, attention span and interest in the environment expand, allowing the child to focus and manipulate several objects at a time. By 16 months the child reflects the impact of the social group and has a repertoire of emotions that can be expressed. At 18 months, the child is socially resistant to change in routine and exhibits egocentric behavior. These lessen as the child grows and has additional successful experiences alone and with others. The child shows affection spontaneously and obeys simple requests by the age of 2 years. The child will dramatize adult behavior, yet is slow to realize social requirements and has not yet made a complete distinction between self and others. The 3-year-old continues to develop these skills as well as a sense of time. Emotional outbursts occur but are typically brief. There is additional success in tasks such as self feeding and dressing. By 4 years of age, the child is independent in self care. Assertiveness is apparent by this age, with the child spending more time in social play and talking. Play is the way the child learns appropriate skills in preparation for school and ultimately employment (Table 1-4) [16].

TABLE 1-4 Age-appropriate toys

Toys	0–6 Mo	6–12 Mo	12–23 Mo	24–36 Mo
Mobiles (8–12 in. away is best vision)	a			
Crib gym	a			
Balls, textures, clutch and chime	a	b	b	b
Rattles	a	b		
Teethers	a	b		
Crib activity toy or activity center	a	b	b	
Mirror (nonbreakable)	a	b	b	b
Squeeze and squeak toys	a	b	b	b
Simple colorful pictures and happy-face pictures	a	b	b	b
Music box	a	b	b	b
Puppets	a	b	b	b
Soft dolls and stuffed animals	a	b	b	b
Peek-a-boo game	a	b	b	b
Floating water toys	a	b	b	b
Animal grabbers	a	b	b	b
Large snap-lock beads	a	b	b	b
Soft-stuffed animals (check for safety features)	a	b	b	b
Large rattles that children can grasp	a	b	b	b
Large soft blocks with pictures	a	b	b	
Picture books with stiff pages (cloth or cardboard)		a	b	b
Simple nesting toys		a	b	b
Plastic picture cards		a	b	b
Soft rubber balls; large plastic ball		a	b	b
Records of nursery rhymes, fingerplays, animal sounds		a	b	b
Ticking clock or large wristwatch		a	b	b
Happy- and sad-face puppets		a	b	b
Baby doll		a	b	b
Rubber squeeze toys		a	b	b
Simple shape sorters (three to four shapes) or large plastic container with geometric blocks, large beads		a	b	b
Flat surface suction toys		a	b	
Walker		a	b	
Noisemakers, such as pots and pans			a	b
Crayon and paper			a	b
Soft plastic car or vehicle with wheels; toys with wheels			a	b
Small wooden blocks			a	b
Stacking (rings)			a	b
Balls and beanbags			a	b
Zippers and buttons attached to cloth (check for safety features)			a	b
Blocks—building or sorting			a	b
Peg and hole activities			a	b
Bead stringing—large			a	b
Clay			a	b

TABLE 1-4 (CONTINUED)

Toys	Age			
	0–6 Mo	6–12 Mo	12–23 Mo	24–36 Mo
Foot to floor vehicles			a	b
Textured objects			a	b
Activities that show small to large			a	b
Rocking horse			a	b
Doll carriage			a	b
Rocking chair (child sized)			a	b
Slide			a	b
Sand toys			a	b

[a] Toy can be introduced sometime in this period according to child's developmental readiness.
[b] Age-span toy is likely to continue to be used.
Source: Adapted from *Toys: When to Introduce What*. East Aurora, NY: Fisher-Price, 1980.

Organized education begins at age 5, and the role of peers and school are of primary importance. (See Chapter 5 for a further discussion of public education for disabled children). From this point, school-aged children begin a separation from the family and develop a sense of belonging to a peer group and larger society. There is acquisition of social skills and values necessary for effective interaction with others and development of a sense of accomplishment, crucial to late middle childhood. School is the work of school-aged children. The school-aged child must learn to effectively cope with stress, anxiety, and other emotions in a socially acceptable fashion. Finally, the child adjusts to a work setting and acquires the skills and attitudes that lead to self-sufficiency [18].

COGNITION
Using Piaget's theory of cognitive development, intelligence also develops through a sequence of progressively more complex patterns of action and thinking, beginning with reflexive action present at birth and culminating in abstract thinking. The child assimilates or fits a perception of the environment to a personal system and then adapts or modifies to accommodate this to external reality.

Periods of cognitive development [15] begin with the sensorimotor period from birth to about 2 years of age. The child exhibits primarily overt acts, moving from a purely reflex level to awareness and responsiveness to the immediate environment, and acts at a perceptual level. At birth to 1 month the infant is practicing reflexes, that is, the infant "knows" nothing. From 1 to 4 months there is a beginning of repetition of responses to the environment, exploration of the infant's own body, and attempts to reproduce encounters with something new connected with the infant's own body (e.g., grasps, sucks, listens, looks, touches). From 4 to 8 months the infant is more oriented to the world about and begins to recognize familiar objects and intentionality of own behavior (e.g., rubs, strikes, shakes objects). From 8 to 12 months there is increased orientation to the "outside-self" world. The child begins to anticipate events on the basis of observed stimuli and behaves in a goal-directed manner. At 12 to 18 months the child begins to explore the world about, getting into things, and seeks new accommodations. From 18 to 24 months the child begins to move into the conceptual-symbolic realm. The child starts to represent symbolically events not present, that is, knowing the "not-here." A simple plan in actions under consideration begins.

The next period is called "preoperational thought period," incorporating 2 through 7 years of age. The child learns to understand and use simple symbols as representations. Piaget describes this as learning signifiers, internal representations, (word, image) that stand for some aspect of reality differentiated from significates, which are the child's understanding of that aspect of reality. Two to four years of age present the beginnings of representational thought. Four- to five-and-one-half-year-olds exhibit simple representations or intuitions, while five-and-one-half to seven-year-olds exhibit articulated representations or intuitions.

The concrete operations period is from 7 to 11 years. At this time the child begins to show stable and orderly adaptations to the environment. Simple cognitive structures are recognized and organized into a coherent series (for example, arithmetic operations), if not rote. The child has the concept of hierarchic classifications and comprehends relations among levels of hierarchy. Although still experience bound, the child can produce classes of objects and use overall guiding principles of class inclusion, that is, relations of parts to wholes and parts to parts, to answer questions involving tasks of conservation of volume or mass, such as When the shape of the clay ball is changed to make it taller, is it more clay? The child also understands notions of past and future.

The formal operations period is from 11 years to adulthood. The older child is no longer reality bound and begins to learn to conceptualize the purely abstract world of hypothetical possibility. The child can reason deductively, develop propositions, hypothesize, and check hypotheses.

THE TEAM

Due to the complexity of the problems faced by children with physical and emotional handicaps, a team approach is needed to provide optimum care. The rehabilitation team [14] is a group of multidisciplinary professionals who share the responsibility for the diagnosis and treatment of their clients/patients. Typically, the members include a pediatrician, nurse, psychologist, physical therapist, occupational therapist, speech-language pathologist, and social worker. A variety of consultants may also be involved at different times with the child's care, such as a psychiatrist, surgeon, dentist, clinical nurse specialist, dietician, respiratory therapist, audiologist, orthotist, bioengineer, and educator. Members of the rehabilitation, or health care team, often follow these children for many years. Initially, they are involved in the diagnosis and treatment of the child in the hospital, outpatient, or clinic setting. Subsequently, they assess the child's progress on a timely basis and provide additional therapy when needed. When the child reaches school age, the team members may be asked to participate in the educational assessment of the child and help establish goals and a treatment plan, that is, an individualized education plan (IEP). Typically, once the child is in a school program, therapists from the school provide the ongoing treatment and classroom consultation. In difficult situations rehabilitation team members may be asked to provide additional information in the form of a consultation.

The role of the team members is determined in part by their profession, composition of the team, and needs of the client. Given the nature of the team, roles of the members may change or vary relative to other team members [10]. For example, the child may have more language problems, thus requiring more input from the speech-language pathologist. The team member most actively involved in the case may act as team leader during discussions about the child. Another model of the team approach is the transdisciplinary team discussed in the section on Early Intervention in Chapter 2.

REHABILITATION TEAM
The pediatrician is board certified with experience in the field of developmental disorders.

This individual has working knowledge of child development, techniques in parent counseling, and knowledge of the use of the multidisciplinary method for diagnosis and habilitative prescription. In many centers, the pediatrician is the team leader.

The nurse is a board-certified R.N. with experience in pediatrics. This person has training in child development and parent counseling and is responsible for vital signs, distribution of medications, developmental screening, as well as the health and nutrition of the children cared for by the team.

When a child is discharged from a hospital, a home health nurse may be asked to provide follow-up care, thus having close contact with the family. The visiting nurse may implement medical procedures in the home and teach the family child management skills. Thus the nurse can monitor the child's development and family relationships, including their attitude toward the child, and home management needs. The home health nurse provides the family with information about community resources and may determine the need for medical consultation and referral for physical therapy, occupational therapy, speech-langugage pathology, family counseling, and social services.

The psychologist has a Ph.D. in clinical psychology with experience in developmental disabilities and the multidisciplinary team. The psychologist has knowledge of cognitive assessment, interpretation of pediatrict psychometric tests, educational remediation, and parent counseling techniques. Tests typically provided and interpreted are standard congitive batteries, for example, Stanford-Binet or WISC. This individual also makes observations about the affective behavior of the child and may provide direct service to the child and family in the form of counseling or training in behavioral management.

The physical therapist (PT) is a licensed professional with knowledge of child development and developmental disabilities. This person is responsible for the assessment of motor development and therapeutic programs that address motor development with particular emphasis on ambulation skills.

The occupational therapist (OT) is a licensed professional with knowledge of child development and developmental disabilities. This person is responsible for the assessment of fine motor and self-care skills and provision of developmental programs in self care, fine and gross motor skills, and feeding. In collaboration with the psychologist, the OT assesses perceptual/motor skills and designs programs to facilitate the development of deficit areas. The OT is the team member who provides splints and adaptive devices for positioning the child and activity or environmental adaption.

With the neonate, the roles of the OT and PT are quite similar, as both assess the developmental level of the infant and work to encourage age-appropriate sensorimotor skills. These therapists have specialized training in child development and neurodevelopmental treatment techniques, which include special handling and positioning of the infant. They begin working with the child in the neonate intensive care unit of the hospital and are part of the team at child development clinics, home health services, physical rehabilitation centers, and schools. Both are active participants in parent education.

The speech-language pathologist has a masters degree in speech-language pathology and may be licensed in certain states. This person has experience in the multidisciplinary team, as well as knowledge of audiology, language stimulation, and therapy. Language development and audiologic assessments and training are provided by this individual as well as family and team counseling in speech, language, and audiology treatment strategies.

The social worker (MSW) has a master's degree in social work and experience in the field of developmental disabilities and parent counseling. The MSW conducts the initial parent interview, assessing family coping skills and resource allocation, and provides information on attitude and emotional development of the child. Psychosocial support and resource management are typically provided by the social worker who often serves as an advocate for the child and family, helping to locate resources and support services. In addition, this team member is often responsible for leading family/educational programs and discharge planning.

EDUCATIONAL TEAM

Members of the educational team are similar to the rehabilitation team, but the role of the teacher is more pivotal. There may be special educators involved, such as resource room teachers. The school-based team recommends the optimal form of school placement for the child with a handicap. There is a spectrum of services offered children in the educational setting including those of a special school, special classes, or mainstreaming. The decision to place a child in one of these programs is based on the student's medical, educational, and psychological needs.

The school nurse can serve as a bridge between the educational and medical system. This may include monitoring the child's medication taken at school, interpreting medical data for teachers and parents, and taking part in student, parent, and teacher health education.

THE FAMILY

The birth of a handicapped child has a great impact on the family. Denial, anxiety, guilt, projection of blame, and grief are common parental reactions to the situation. Denial is likely to be the initial reaction, and professionals can become frustrated by it, as the parents may not acknowledge the need for treatment. However, denial is a psychological defense mechanism that can soften the blow of reality and requires patience and understanding of the team.

Anxiety about the child's management, future, and cost of care can be expected. There may also be anxiety about the unknown, as parents do not know what to expect from their child. Providing adequate information about the condition and teaching parents child care skills help ease some of this anxiety. However, in infancy it is difficult to predict the extent of the problem, so when the child reaches an early intervention program or special classroom, there may still be questions that have not and possibly cannot be answered. Sensitivity is required by those who inform parents about their child's condition. Too little information creates anxiety whereas too much information, too soon, can be overwhelming.

Parents need support, information, and time to adjust to the impact of a handicapped child on their lives. When things go wrong, some parents blame the professionals. They blame the physician for poor prenatal care or criticize therapists when the child is not progressing quickly. The professional must be certain to address the needs of the parents who may be projecting their fears and inadequacies on team members.

Some parents feel guilty about their child, for example a mother feeling that she was not attentive enough to prenatal care or that the handicapped child is punishment for some past wrong. Helping parents work through guilt feelings is necessary to give them the energy they will need for the present situation.

The parent's mourning may be a sign that they acknowledge the child's handicap and may be a prelude to adjustment. Team members should help parents to develop coping skills and adaptive behavior, so that they can regain their self-esteem.

The family has the criticial role in decision making, as ultimately they become the advocate for the most appropriate services for the child. When the parents are involved in the child's program, there is greater understanding of the issues involved and more likelihood of compliance with recommendations. For their part, team members need to recognize that they are working with parents who are physically, socially, and emotionally involved in their child's care. Professionals need to be clear in their explanations (using a minimum of jargon), help parents formulate questions, and allow time for acceptance and adjustment. Parents should be encouraged to read medical and school records and comment on them. All options for treatment should be discussed with them. Information on the child's condition must be made available, and they should have access to parent education meetings and appropriate literature. Feedback to the team from the family is always encouraged. Additionally, the assessment, individualized program plan of goals and measurable objectives, and periodic progress reports are reviewed and signed by the parents.

REFERENCES
1. Batshaw, M. L. and Perret, Y. M. *Children with Handicaps: A Medical Primer* (2nd ed.). Baltimore: Brookes, 1986.
2. Carlsoo, S. *How Man Moves.* London: Heinemann, 1972.
3. Coley, I. L. *Pediatric Assessment of Self-Care Activities.* St. Louis: Mosby, 1978.
4. Crelin, E. S. Development of the musculoskeletal system. *Clin. Symp.* 33(1): 1981.
5. Daub, M. M. The Human Development Process. In H. L. Hopkins and H. D. Smith (eds.), *Willard and Spackman's Occupational Therapy* (6th ed.). Philadelphia: Lippincott, 1983.
6. D'Eugenio, D. B., and Moersch, M. S. *Developmental Programming for Infants and Young Children.* Ann Arbor: University of Michigan Press, 1981.
7. Greenspan, S. I. Adaptive and psychopathologic patterns in infancy and early childhood: an overview. *Child. Today* 21, July–Aug., 1981.
8. Havinghurst, R. J. *Developmental Tasks and Education* (3rd ed.). New York: McKay, 1974.
9. Kleinberg, S. B. *Educating the Chronically Ill Child.* Rockville, MD: Aspen, 1982.
10. Monahan, J. *Management of Behavioral Problems in the Physically Disabled Child.* Boston: Tufts Research and Training Center, 1982.
11. Mosey, A. C. *Three Frames of Reference for Mental Health.* Thorofare, N.J.: Slack, 1970.
12. *NCHS Growth Curves for Children.* U.S. Department of Health and Welfare. Ser. 11, No. 165. DHEW No. (PHS) 78-1650.
13. Perrin, E. C., and Gerrity, P. S. Development of children with a chronic illness. *Pediatr. Clin. North Am.* 31(1):19, 1984.
14. Scheinar, A. P. *The Allied Professionals: An Alternative Model of the Multiple Disciplinary Team.* Rochester, N.Y.: Monroe Developmental Center, 1973.
15. Stevens-Long, J. *Adult Life: Developmental Processes.* Palo Alto: Mayfield, 1979.
16. Toys: When to Introduce What. East Aurora, N.Y.: Fisher-Price Toys, 1980.
17. Warren, S. Notes from course in Special Education. Boston: Boston University, 1979.
18. Weitzman, M. School and peer relations. *Pediatr. Clin. North Am.* 31(1):59, 1984.

SUGGESTED READING
Boehm, H. *The Right Toys.* Toronto: Bantam, 1986.
Cloherty, J. P., and Stark, A. R. *Manual of Neonatal Care.* Boston: Little, Brown, 1980.
Dubowitz, L. M. S., Dubowitz, V., and Olber, C. Clinical assessment of gestational age in the newborn infant. *J. Pediatr.* 77:1, 1970.
Piaget, J. *The Essential Piaget.* New York: Basic, 1977.
Piaget, J. *The Language and Thought of the Child.* Cleveland: Meridian, 1955.
Piaget, J. *The Origins of Intelligence in Children.* New York: Norton, 1952.

Cerebral Palsy

Martha K. Logigian

Cerebral palsy (CP) is a nonprogressive disorder of brain function manifested by abnormalities of movement and posture and may be accompanied by intellectual and language deficits. First described by Little [35] in 1861, it is not a disease per se, but rather a group of symptoms resulting from damage to a child's brain before it has matured. It occurs in 2 in every 1000 live births, affecting 500,000 persons in the United States, males more than females. The incidence appears to be influenced by the birth weight of the infant and is on the rise because of an increase in the survival rate of premature and high-risk infants. A fetus that was not considered viable in past years now has a chance for survival due to pediatric intensive care units and advances made in perinatology such as the incubator, pediatric respirators (for the treatment of respiratory distress syndrome), antibiotics, treatment for Rh blood disorders, and fetal monitoring.

Prenatal circumstances associated with CP include adverse intrauterine development such as placental insufficiency and brain malformations; exposure to congenital infection such as rubella, toxoplasmosis, and syphilis; chromosomal defects; exposure to toxins such as alcohol and Dilantin; and Rh incompatibility. Paranatal circumstances include birth trauma, hypoxia due to anesthetic or analgesic drugs, infection such as meningitis and encephalitis, respiratory distress syndrome, intraventricular hemorrhage, and hyperbilirubinemia. Postnatal circumstances include head trauma, infection, degenerative diseases, and cerebrovascular disease.

TYPES OF CEREBRAL PALSY

CP can be classified physiologically according to the type of motor dysfunction and the limbs affected. Mixed types are frequently seen as well as changes in physical findings that occur with age.

Spastic CP is characterized by hyperactive reflexes, exaggerated stretch reflexes, and augmented responses with clonus. There is a tendency toward greater involvement of the antigravity muscles and contractures affecting these muscles [33].

Spastic CP is commonly subdivided according to the distribution of involvement.

1. Spastic hemiplegia refers to involvement of the arm and leg on one side of the body. The upper extremity is usually more involved than the lower extremity. This type of CP may be the result of early childhood head trauma or stroke. Sensory deficits are usually not involved. Low [36] recommends specific techniques to be used when evaluating the child to elicit abnormalities in mild cases of hemiparesis. These include heel walking, running instead of walking, and supination of the forearm, which results in slight elbow flexion on the spastic side.

2. Spastic diplegia refers to involvement of all four extremities, with the lower extremities more involved than the upper extremities. This type of deficit is commonly associated with the premature infant. In prematurity, a fragile area exists in the superior section of the motor strip. If, for example, the premature infant experiences hypoxia due to respiratory distress syndrome, this part of the brain is the first to experience damage. This area of the motor strip controls movements of the lower extremities. Thus, they are affected more than the upper extremities in the child with spastic diplegia [3].

3. Spastic paraplegia refers to involvement of only the lower extremities, with no involvement of the upper extremities. Often this condition turns out to be diplegia or the result of a spinal cord lesion rather than a cerebral lesion. The principal physical findings are hip and knee flexion, adductor spasticity leading to scissoring of the lower extremities, and heel cord tightness [36].

4. Spastic monoplegia and triplegia are uncommon and refer to involvement of one extremity (former) and three extremities (latter).

5. Spastic quadriplegia refers to involvement of all four extremities. The terms bilateral hemiplegia and tetraplegia are also used to describe this syndrome, although they often are used to describe involvement of all four extremities with the upper extremities more involved than the lower. This is often the result of severe anoxia, hemorrhage, and developmental malformations [30]. The prognosis in this type of CP is poor for survival, intellectual functioning, and seizure activity.

Dyskinetic CPs are characterized by abnormal, involuntary, and uncoordinated movements that disappear during sleep. The most common is athetosis, which is characterized by slow, writhing, rotary movements, which vary in degree depending on the state of relaxation of the patient and are commonly aggravated by emotional tension. Usually all extremities are involved as well as the face, neck, and paravertebral muscles. Continuous movement causes hypertrophy especially around the neck and shoulders. More severely involved children may have sudden, sharp movements resembling dystonia. Neonatal jaundice (kernicterus) and anoxia are the precursor of athetosis. When jaundice is the cause there is a high risk of nerve deafness and paresis of upward gaze [30, 36].

Ataxic cerebral palsy is characterized by a

lack of coordination of fine and gross motor movements, which is manifested as an awkwardness of posture, balance, and orientation in space. It is probably the result of lesions in the cerebellum or cerebellar pathways.

Rigid CP is characterized by "lead pipe" muscle resistance that is continuous to slow passive movement. If the muscle resistance is discontinuous it is often referred to as "cog-wheel" rigidity. "The resistance is greater to slow than to rapid motion, whereas, in spasticity, there is greater resistance to rapid motion" [33]. There is no involuntary motion associated with this type of CP. Intelligence, however, is often impaired with this type.

Tremor CP is characterized by involuntary rhythmic muscle contraction and relaxation. Both rigid and tremor types of CP are rare.

Atonic CP is a rare type characterized by lack of muscle tone, often referred to as "floppy" muscle tone. There is delay in developmental milestones and increased deep tendon reflexes, which are commonly seen only in young children due to an increase in muscle tone with age. A characteristic finding is flexion of both hips when the child is suspended under the arm (Förster's sign) [36].

Mixed types of CP involve several types of CP occurring in one child resulting from pyramidal and extrapyramidal involvement. The most common combination is athetosis and spasticity [36], but other combinations can be observed such as rigidity and ataxia or spasticity and tremor. Mental retardation and other associated features are common due to the extent of the brain damage.

ASSOCIATED PROBLEMS

Initially, the neonate's clinical picture is subject to change due to the immaturity of the nervous system. As the nervous system matures, clinical manifestations become delineated and classification occurs.

Infants who have suffered perinatal trauma experience various sequential changes of muscle tone and an abnormal evolution of postural reflexes. Most often there is a gradual change from generalized hypotonia of the newborn period to spasticity of later life. In the hypotonic infant there is often a depression of the respiratory reflex, resulting in breathing abnormalities. Sucking and swallowing reflexes may be weak or absent, resulting in feeding difficulties. Palmar and plantar grasps may be weak, the Moro reflex may be absent, and placing and stepping reactions may be difficult to elicit. Mild degrees of hypotonia can be documented by a head lag and a lack of normal biceps flexor tone in the traction response from the supine position. The Landau reflex is often abnormal [52]. After 12 to 48 hours the hypotonic infant often becomes "jittery," with a shrill and monotonous cry, the Moro reflex becomes exaggerated, there is an increased startle response to sound, and the face assumes a staring or "worried" appearance. The deep tendon reflexes become hyperactive, and an increased extensor tone develops. Seizures may appear at this time [39].

Often the earliest sign of spasticity is the presence of increased resistance on passive supination of the forearm, or on flexion and extension of the ankle and knee. A more reliable sign of the presence of spasticity is a sustained tonic neck reflex [39].

Abnormalities in muscle tone (for example, spasticity or hypotonicity and reduced postural control) are comon in the child with CP. Delayed or abnormal motor development and decreased voluntary motor control are also noticeable.

With a normally developing child, primitive postural reflexes observed as an infant are inhibited and integrated into voluntary movement as the central nervous system (CNS) matures (Table 2-1). With the CP child, primitive reflexes tend to be stronger and retained and can lead to movement abnormalities that persist into adulthood. For example, the asymmetrical tonic neck reflex (ATNR) and the tonic labyrinthine reflex (TLR) are particularly obvi-

TABLE 2-1. Postural reactions

Postural reflex	Stimulus	Origin of afferent impulses	Age reflex appears	Age reflex disappears
Local static reactions	Gravitation	Muscles		
Stretch reflex			Any age	
Positive supporting action			Well-developed in 50% of the newborn	Indistinguishable from normal standing
Placing reaction			Newborn	Covered up by voluntary action
Segmental static reactions	Movement	Contralateral muscles		
Crossed extensor reflex			Newborn	7–12 mo
Crossed adductor reflex to quadriceps jerk			3 mo	8 mo
General static reactions	Position of head in space	Otolith Neck muscles Trunk muscles		
Tonic neck reflex			Never sustained and complete	
Neck-righting reflex			4–8 mo	Covered up by voluntary action
Grasp reflex: Palmar			Fifth intrauterine mo	4–5 mo
Plantar			Newborn	9–12 mo
Moro reflex			Third intrauterine mo	4–5 mo
Labyrinthine accelerating reactions	Change in rate of movement	Semicircular canals		
Linear acceleration: Parachute reaction			7–9 mo	Covered up by voluntary action
Angular acceleration: Postrotational nystagmus			Any age	

Source: From Menkes, J. H. The Neuromotor Mechanism. In R. E. Cooke (ed.), *The Biologic Basis of Pediatric Practice*. New York: McGraw-Hill, 1968. Reproduced with permission.

ous and are retained long after these reflexes should normally be integrated by the CNS. "Scissors gait" (adduction and internal rotation of the hips) and "toewalking" (positive supporting reaction, equinus varus of the feet) are examples of motor abnormalities commonly associated with the growing child with CP.

Among other primitive motor behavior retained beyond normal development are flexor withdrawal, extensor thrust, crossed extension, positive supporting reaction, associated reactions [25], symmetrical tonic neck reflex, neck-righting reaction, and the Moro reflex. It should be noted that Gans [25] believes that the presence of protective extension reactions is considered a good indicator of ambulation potential.

In addition to motor deficits, a number of medical and rehabilitation problems become more apparent as the child develops, including seizure disorders, gastrointestinal problems, mental retardation, and communication disorders.

Seizures occur in one third to one half of all children with CP as either an isolated incident or as recurrent seizures [58]. Medication for control of seizure activity is often necessary. Emotional support of the child and family is critical as they face an adjustment process relative to the social and physical complications associated with seizures and their control. Table 2-2 provides further information on the types of seizures commonly seen in children and the medication usually recommended for the control of seizures [3, 23]. Table 2-3 provides information on what to do in the event of a seizure.

Intellectual deficits may be demonstrated in children with CP. Mental retardation is more commonly seen in children with bilateral, widespread cerebral lesions and is less common in children with extrapyramidal forms of CP and spastic diplegia [58]. Nevertheless, the cognitive development of these children demands careful and continuous assessment of their capabilities so that their capacity for learning and performance is not underestimated. Often influenced by motor deficits, sensorimotor disorders may also be identified. For example, the child may have difficulty developing eye-hand coordination, body scheme, and visual and auditory perception. Unusual environmental and sensory stimulation may be poorly tolerated, or the child may lack the ability to experience such stimuli. These problems can affect learning and thus emphasize the need for remedial educational and therapeutic programs.

Gastrointestinal disorders seen in children with CP include difficulties with swallowing, feeding, and drooling, including the presence of a gastroesophageal reflux seen in up to 50 percent of the severely involved children. The latter presents a particularly difficult problem as it may result in further complications, such as failure to thrive and aspiration pneumonia. Unfortunately, children with these problems do not tolerate clear liquids well, which contributes to the problem of constipation.

Growth and development can also be affected in children with CP, including a delay in attaining developmental milestones and abnormal bone growth that may result in skeletal abnormalities. Dentition can also be affected and may result in problems such as abnormal tooth development, overgrowth of gums due to the use of Dilantin, abnormal muscle pull, and oral motor deficits that make it difficult for a dentist to provide adequate periodontal care. Parents must pay particular attention to proper nutrition, well-baby care, and proper dental care to ensure good physical and oral health of the child.

Visual problems associated with CP include diplopia, strabismus, amblyopia, lack of upward gaze (as a result of kernicterus), retrolental fibroplasia (from excessive oxygen therapy), and hemianopia (in those with hemiplegia). Black [4] estimates that 40 percent of CP individuals have visual defects (see discussion in Chapter 9).

Hearing impairments are less common: Approximately 10 percent exhibit hearing loss [49]. An example of the type of problem seen is in children with kernicterus who often have a high-frequency hearing loss (see discussion in Chapter 2).

Communication disorders can result from cerebral damage to language centers in the dominant hemisphere or motor deficits that lead to articulation disorders, for example, pseudobulbar palsy. Nonvocal communication systems play a critical role in the development of communication skills in children with significant language impairment. They also help prevent an underestimation of the child's intellectual capabilities (see Chapter 7).

Due to limitations in gross and fine motor control complicated by some or all of the afore-

TABLE 2-2. Seizures common in children

Type	Occurrence	Clinical manifestations	Treatment	Side effects	
				Neurologic	Systemic
Grand mal seizure (tonic-clonic)	Most common disorder, except in infancy	Usually an aura of sensory phenomena precedes tonic-clonic movements of the extremities and a sudden loss of consciousness. May experience tongue biting or incontinence. Lasts 2–4 min after which child may be somnolent, confused, fatigued, and may complain of headache.	Phenobarbital (Luminal)	Sedation, ataxia, confusion, dizziness	Skin rash
			Phenytoin (Dilantin)	Ataxia, confusion, incoordination	Lymphadenopathy, gum hyperplasia, hirsutism, osteomalacia, skin rash, altered folate metabolism
			Primidone (Mysoline) Carbamazepine (Tegretol)	Same as Phenobarbital Ataxia, dizziness, diplopia, vertigo	Bone marrow suppression, gastrointestinal irritation, hepatotoxicity
Psychomotor seizures (temporal lobe, complex partial)	Throughout childhood and early adolescence	Automatisms: lip-smacking, staring, grimacing, hand posturing, laughing, grasping. Some experience an aura of bewilderment, alteration of consciousness, complex sensory experiences, hallucinations/illusions, involvement of affect. Lasts 5–15 min	Phenytoin Carbamazepine		
Focal motor	Childhood and early	Simple motor or sensory phenomena, so-	Phenobarbital Phenytoin		

Seizure type	Age	Characteristics	Treatment	Side effects	Side effects
seizures (simple partial)	adolescence	matosensory changes, vertiginous symptoms. Jacksonian march, speech/language changes	Primidone Carbamazepine	Ataxia, lethargy	Gastrointestinal irritation, skin rash, bone marrow suppression
Petit mal seizures (true, absence)	Onset 5–8 yr of age	Brief lapse (10–15 sec) of consciousness. May experience other phenomena (staring, blinking, lip smacking). Note: May recommend ketogenic diet as part of treatment (high fat, low carbohydrate)	Ethosuximide (Zarontin)	Ataxia, sedation	Hepatotoxicity, bone marrow suppression, irritation, weight gain, transient alopecia
			Sodium valproate (Depakene)		Anorexia
			Clonazepam (Clonopin)	Ataxia, sedation, lethargy	Skin rash, bone marrow suppression
			Trimethadione	Sedation, blurred vision	Same as ethosuximide
			Methsuximide (Celontin)	Ataxia, lethargy	
Infantile spasms	Seen during first 6 mo of life	Flexion of the head and extremities, or both, akinesia and reduced responsiveness may follow spasms or are only manifestations	ACTH followed by prednisone in 1 mo		Weakening of bone structure, increased blood pressure, cataracts, infection risk, gastrointestinal abnormalities
Febrile seizures	Febrile child 5 mo–3-yr old	Generalized tonic-clonic seizure lasting 2–5 min	Limited role for anticonvulsants in single febrile seizure, unless second febrile seizure then anticonvulsant therapy indicated. Phenobarbital for 2–3 yr is indicated if febrile seizure occurs after age 4		

TABLE 2-3. Response to seizure activity

1. Lay the child down in a safe place (e.g., bed, mat, floor).
2. Do not try to restrain the child in any way.
3. Loosen tight clothing.
4. Turn the child's head to the side to allow secretions to drain.
5. Keep the child's mouth clear. Do not insert a tongue blade.
6. Perform mouth-to-mouth resuscitation if breathing stops.
7. Observe and record the following:
   Behavioral changes prior to the episode (e.g., staring, falling)
   Length of seizure
   Body parts involved
   Types of movements noted (e.g., twitching, jerking, thrashing)
   Loss of consciousness
   Loss of bowel and bladder control
   Events following seizure (e.g., headache, confusion)
8. Report the seizure to the school nurse, child's physician, and parents as soon as possible.
If seizure activity lasts more than 3–4 min, emergency medical care is necessary, and the child should be taken to a hospital emergency room, as the seizure may become status epilepticus.

mentioned associated problems, the CP child faces a variety of functional problems throughout life. Difficulties in self care, mobility, and hand function have an impact on the child's educational and vocational activities and may affect independent living.

The psychological and social adjustment to a life-long disability can place significant demands on the individual and may lead to behavior problems intensified during adolescence. The ability of the family and community to accept the child with CP greatly affects the resolution of these problems [3].

DIAGNOSTIC PROCEDURES

Physicians use a variety of diagnostic procedures to assist in the understanding of the neurologic deficits of the child. These include

Computerized axial tomography (CAT scan)
Cortical and brainstem evoked potentials
Electroencephalography (EEG)
Radionuclide brain scans

In addition, a careful pediatric neurologic examination helps the physician detect neurologic abnormalities that may not have been apparent from the diagnostic procedures. This examination includes careful observation of reflex maturation and postural reactions.

Levine [34] suggests grouping clinical abnormalities into six major motor categories for diagnosing CP in children over the age of 1. The categories are (1) postures and movement patterns, (2) oral motor patterns, (3) strabismus, (4) tone of muscles, (5) evolution of postural reactions and landmarks, and (6) deep tendon, plantar, and infantile reflexes. When abnormalities were found in four or more of these categories, the diagnosis of CP was likely.

During the early phases of development, the quality of the child's adaptive behavior may also demonstrate significant abnormalities. The child's tolerance for stimulation, variability of behavior, mental responsiveness, and social interaction can indicate an immaturity and dysfunction of the CNS. The astute therapist will be watching for abnormal adaptive behavior during the assessment and treatment program. Scherzer and Tscharnuter [54] suggest that further assessment by the therapist may be indicated to clarify the diagnosis of CNS dysfunction in infants. Symptoms indicative of the need for further investigation include

1. Stereotyped behavior, paucity of movement, excessive and disorganized movement
2. Poor control and alignment of the head, the face not in the vertical plane, hyperextension of the head and neck
3. Consistent elevation of the shoulder girdle, scapular protraction or retraction
4. Pronounced anterior or posterior pelvic tilt, incomplete hip extension
5. Hypotonicity with "frog" posture of the limbs

6. Hypotonicity when pulled into gravity
7. Low proximal tonus combined with high distal tonus, consistent fisting of the hands with pronation, and internal rotation of the arms
8. Pronounced extensor patterns of the legs with adduction of the hips and clawing of the toes
9. Feeding problems

DEVELOPMENTAL ASSESSMENT

A complete assessment typically includes gross and fine motor development; oral motor function; self-care skills; and perceptual, language, cognitive, and social/emotional development.

Standardized tests are often used (Tables 2-4 and 2-5); however, due to the physical limitations of the child, all sections of these tests may not be completed in the standardized fashion. The therapist often uses several assessment tools and clinical observations to obtain an accurate picture of the child's functional ability (Fig. 2-1; Table 2-6).

The assessment usually follows the arena method described under Early Intervention. Following this assessment, team members may recommend further evaluations to address specific problem areas such as hearing, with the recommendation of a comprehensive evaluation by an audiologist. Likewise vision may

TABLE 2-4. Developmental assessments

Test	Age	Items
Alpern-Boll Developmental Profile	Birth–12½ yr	Physical, self-help, social, academic, communication scales
Brazelton Neonatal Assessment Scale	Neonate	25 maneuvers to elicit infant's best performance
Bayley Scales of Infant Development	2–30 mo	Mental, motor scales; infant behavior record
Callier-Azuza Scales	Birth–9 yr	Motor language, social/emotional perception, cognition for multihandicapped children
Denver Developmental Screening Test	1 mo–6 yr	Fine motor/adaptive, gross motor, personal/social, language
Developmental Programming for Infants and Young Children	Birth–6 yr	Perceptual/fine motor, cognition, language, social/emotional, self care, gross motor
Gesell Developmental Schedules	4 wk–6 yr	Motor, adaptive, language, personal/social
Griffiths Mental Development Scale	Birth–2 yr 2–8 yr	Locomotion, personal/social skills, language/speech, eye-hand coordination, performance
Learning Accomplishment Profile	Birth–36 mo 36–72 mo	Gross and fine motor, cognitive, language, self-help, social/emotional
Milani-Comparetti Motor Developmental Screening Test	Birth–2 yr	Spontaneous behaviors (gross motor), evoked responses (reflexes)
Sewall Early Education Developmental (SEED) Profile	1 mo–4 yr	Gross/fine motor, perception, self care, language, social/emotional, cognition
Stycar Sequences	Birth–5 yr	Posture and large movements, vision and fine movements, hearing and speech, social behavior and play

TABLE 2-5. Publishers of assessment materials (United States)

American Association of Mental Deficiency, 5201 Connecticut Ave., N.W., Washington, DC 20015
American Guidance Service, Publishers Building, Circle Pines, MN 55014
American Printing House for the Blind, 1839 Frankfort Ave., Louisville, KY 40206
American Psychological Association, 1200 17th St., N. W., Washington, DC 20036
Bobbs-Merrill Co., 4300 West 62nd St., Indianapolis, IN 46268
California Test Bureau/McGraw-Hill, Del Monte Research Park, Monterey, CA 93940
Callier Center for Communication Disorders, University of Texas at Dallas, 1966 Inwood Rd., Dallas, TX 75235
Carolina Institute for Research on Early Education of the Handicapped, University of North Carolina, Chapel Hill, NC 27514
Council for Exceptional Children, 1920 Association St., Reston, VA 22091
Consulting Psychologists Press, 755 College Ave., Palo Alto, CA 94306
Counselor Recordings and Tests, Box 6184, Acklen Station, Nashville, TN 37212
The Devereux Foundation Press, Devon, PA 19333
Educational and Industrial Testing Service, Princeton, NJ 08540
Follett Educational Corp., 1010 West Washington Blvd., Chicago, IL 60607
Gallaudet College Book Store, Kendall Green, Washington, DC 20002
Grune & Stratton (Harcourt Brace Jovanovich), 757 Third Ave., New York, NY 10017
Harvard University Press, 79 Garden St., Cambridge, MA 02138
Houghton Mifflin Co., Test Editorial Offices, P. O. Box 1970, Iowa City, IA 52240
Humanities Press, Hillary House, Atlantic Highland, NJ 07716
Kaplan School Supply, 600 Jonestown Rd., Winston-Salem, NC 27103
Ladoca Project and Publishing Foundation, East 51st Ave. and Lincoln St., Denver, CO 80216
Language Research Associations, 450 East 59th St., Chicago, IL 60621
J. B. Lippincott Co., East Washington Square, Philadelphia, PA 19105
Charles E. Merrill Publishing Co., 1300 Alom Creek Dr., Columbus, OH 43216
Prentice-Hall International, Englewood Cliffs, NJ 07632
The Psychological Corporation, 304 East 45th St., New York, NY 10017
Psychologists and Educators Press, 419 Pendik, Jacksonville, IL 62650
Random House, 201 East 50th St., New York, NY 10022
Ramsco Publishing Co., P. O. Box N, 414 Main St., Laurel, MD 20707
Russell Sage Foundation, 230 Park Ave., New York, NY 10017
Science Research Associates, 250 East Erie St., Chicago, IL 60611
Sewall Rehabilitation Center, 1360 Vine, Denver, CO 80206
Slosson Educational Publications, 140 Pine St., East Aurora, NY 14052
Sboelting Co., 424 North Homan Ave., Chicago, IL 60624
Teachers College Press, 502 West 121st. St., New York, NY 10027
The University of Illinois Press, Urbana, IL 61801
The University of Michigan Press, Sales Department, P. O. Box 1104, Ann Arbor, MI 48106
The University of Nebraska Medical Center Print Shop, Ohama, NE 68105
University Park Press, Chamber of Commerce Building, Baltimore, MD 21202
Western Psychological Services, 12081 Wilshire Blvd., Los Angeles, CA 90025

need to be assessed by an ophthalmologist and feeding by an occupational therapist.

Due to the extent of the motor involvement in CP, a thorough evaluation of tone, sensori-motor development, reflex maturation, posture, and movement must be completed in addition to the investigation of functional limitations.

A home visit is typically made by the social

TABLE 2-6. Initial developmental evaluation: developmental history

Date Completed
    Informant
    Reliability

I.   Reason for referral
     Age disability recognized and symptoms
     noted
II. Family and genetic history
III. Pregnancy history
IV. Labor and delivery
V. Perinatal and neonatal events
    A. Condition at birth
    B. Neonatal history
VI. Developmental milestones
    A. Head balance and control
    B. Smiling
    C. Grasping
    D. Transferring
    E. Rolling
    F. Sitting
    G. Crawling
    H. Walking
    I. Hand preference
    J. Oral development
      1. Feeding and sucking
      2. Tongue and mouth problems
      3. Speech
      4. Dental development
    K. Hearing
    L. Vision
VII. Other developmental features
    A. Social
    B. Emotional
    C. Play interests
    D. Self care
      1. Feeding
      2. Dressing
      3. Toileting
    E. School
VIII. Review of systems
IX. Past medical history
    A. Previous evaluations
    B. Medication
    C. Therapy
    D. Braces/equipment
    E. Surgery
X.   Parental attitude and information

Source: From A. L. Scherzer and I. Tscharnuter. *Early Diagnosis and Therapy in Cerebral Palsy.* New York: Dekker, 1982. P. 49. Reprinted by courtesy of Marcel Dekker, Inc.

worker. This visit allows time for a parent interview and gives the professional an opportunity to gain insight into the child's behavior at home, difficulties the parents may have with caring for the child, and concerns and expectations the family may have about the child. It is useful if the home visit can be accomplished prior to the team assessment, so that relevant issues can be addressed at the time of the team evaluation. It is important for the team to understand how the child is managed at home and to gauge family resources and availability when recommending an intervention program to enable appropriate assistance and guidance of the parents in meeting the child's needs.

On completion of the assessment and development of goals and objectives, the team meets with the parents to review the findings. Parents need to understand that the child's developmental age and skill acquisition may not reflect the chronologic age of the child. Moreover, although the child may achieve early developmental milestones, these may not be indicative of normal development due to the quality of the motor pattern observed [54]. Long- and short-range program goals and measurable objectives are reviewed with the parents, and they are given an opportunity to comment on the assessment findings and program goals. They are also encouraged to discuss other needs and make recommendations they feel should be addressed in the therapeutic program.

As a practical matter, formal reevaluations are completed by the team at least yearly, although 6-month follow-up evaluations are most appropriate. Program plans including goals and measurable objectives are updated quarterly. Frequent informal reevaluations by the therapists should occur throughout the treatment program.

Early Intervention
Alice Sapienza

The term *early intervention* encompasses a range of stimulation and training activities for infants and young children at risk for delayed or

DATE: _____

PHYSICIAN: _____

AGE: _____

REFLEX/REACTION	AGE SPAN		PRESENT		COMMENTS
PRIMITIVE REFLEXES	ONSET	INTEG.	YES	NO	
Rooting	28 wk*	3 mo			
Sucking-swallowing	28 wk*	2–5 mo			
Traction	28 wk*	2–5 mo			
Moro	28 wk*	5–6 mo			
Flexor withdrawal	28 wk*	1–2 mo			
Extensor thrust		1–2 mo			
Crossed extension	28 wk*	1–2 mo			
Plantar grasp	28 wk*	9 mo			
Galant	32 wk*	2 mo			
Neonatal neck righting	34 wk*	4–5 mo			
Neonatal body righting	34 wk*	4–5 mo			
Neonatal lower extremity Positive supporting	35 wk*	1–2 mo			
Proprioceptive placing (LE)	35 wk*	2 mo			
Primary walking	37 wk*	2 mo			
Proprioceptive placing (UE)	Birth	2 mo			
Asymmetric tonic neck	Birth	4–6 mo			
Palmar grasp	Birth	4–6 mo			
Tonic labyrinthine prone	Birth	6 mo			
Tonic labyrinthine supine	Birth	6 mo			
Symmetric tonic neck	4–6 mo	8–12 mo			
Associated reactions	Birth–3 mo	8–9 yr			
Finger extension and sequencing		3–4 wk			
PREHENSILE REACTIONS					
Avoidance	Birth	6–7 yr			
Instinctive grasp	4–11 mo	Persists			
RIGHTING REACTIONS	ONSET	INTEG.	YES	NO	
Labyrinthine head righting	Birth–2 mo	Persists			
Optical righting	Birth–2 mo	Persists			
Body righting acting on the head	Birth–2 mo	Persists			
Neck righting acting on the body	4–6 mo	5 yr			
Body righting acting on the body	4–6 mo	5 yr			
Landau	3–4 mo	12–24 mo			
Positive supporting UE elbows	3 mo	Persists			

*Gestational age

FIG. 2-1 (CONTINUED)

REFLEX/REACTION	AGE SPAN		PRESENT	COMMENTS
Positive supporting UE hands	4–6 mo	Persists		
Amphibian	6 mo	Persists		
EQUILIBRIUM REACTIONS				
Visual placing (UE)	3–4 mo	Persists		
Visual placing (LE)	3–5 mo	Persists		
Protective extension downward (LE)	4 mo	Persists		
Protective extension forward (UE)	6–7 mo	Persists		
Protective extension sideward (UE)	7 mo	Persists		
Protective extension backward (UE)	9–10 mo	Persists		
Protective staggering (LE)	15–18 mo	Persists		
Hopping reaction (LE)	15–18 mo	Persists		
Dorsiflexion reaction (LE)	15–18 mo	Persists		
Protective shifting (LE)	15–18 mo	Persists		
TOTAL BODY FUNCTIONS				
Prone	6 mo	Persists		
Supine	7–8 mo	Persists		
Sitting	7–8 mo	Persists		
4-Point	9–12 mo	Persists		

FIG. 2-1. Reflex evaluation chart. (Adapted from M. R. Barnes, C. A. Crutchfield, and Heriza. *Neurophysiological Basis of Patient Treatment: Reflexes in Motor Development.* Atlanta: Stokesville, 1978.)

abnormal development. The type of intervention provided is based on the perceived needs of the children served and the philosophic orientation of the disciplines involved, such as motor and cognitive development and transdisciplinary therapy [56]. The former is the more traditional, interdisciplinary approach involving a variety of specialists, each working invidually with the child within their own area of expertise and training. The latter similarly has a multidisciplinary representation, but one team member is assigned to carry out all aspects of the child's program with input from other team members as needed.

The transdisciplinary approach has been viewed by many as the preferred approach particularly with infants who require multiple therapies. It eliminates fragmentation of the child and parents among several specialists and reinforces the parent as primary caregiver. However, it assumes a high degree of self-confidence of each team member in his or her own practice. The professional role must be relinquished to another, while remaining accountable for the child [21, 29].

The specialist team may vary in composition depending on funding, the population served, and the needs of the community. Usually the team includes a pediatrician, nurse, social worker, occupational therapist, physical therapist, special educator, speech-language pathologist, and psychologist.

Intervention programs are further characterized as home based, in which all or most of the therapeutic intervention is provided in the home, or centerbased, where the intervention is available at a facility, necessitating transportation of the child to a clinic or center for therapy. Some programs try to provide both types, recognizing the strengths and limitations of each.

Organized early intervention programs (EIP) have been in existence since the 1950s in CP centers. The origins of EIP can be traced to sensory stimulation experiments carried out in the 1930s and 1940s that demonstrated an improvement in IQ scores among institutionalized children [31].

The initial emphasis of early intervention was focused on motor development. This type of program gradually expanded to include social and language development. With the shift from institutionalization, parent involvement became a critical program component.

In the 1970s, guidelines [55] for intervention programs were established as a result of investigations carried out by the United Cerebral Palsy Association and the Bureau of the Handicapped of the U.S. Department of Health, Education, and Welfare. Their findings included recommendations for parents as primary care providers with care being provided in the home, parent tutoring by specially trained educators, and the availability of the multidisciplinary team and supportive services [22] to the family and educator. Influenced by these guidelines and the view that home programs are in context and allow parents the ease of generalizing the skills learned, center-based programs gave way to systematic home visiting [51]. However, due to the cost of home programs and limitations within some home-based environments, the trend is again shifting back to center-based programs.

Tjossem [61] states that three types of vulnerable, "at risk" infants have been identified needing early intervention. Each type has distinctive requirements for diagnosis, indentification, and intervention:

1. *Established risk:* Infants whose early appearing abnormal development is related to diagnosed medical disorders of known etiology and whose outcome has ranges of expected developmental delay, for example, Down's syndrome

2. *Environmental risk:* Infants who appear biologically intact but are deprived of normal life experiences and stimulation, such as family, health care, physical and social stimulation, and opportunities for expression of adaptive behaviors. Without intervention, these children are a high risk for delayed development

3. *Biologic risk:* Infants who have a history of prenatal, perinatal, or neonatal biologic problems suggestive of damage to the developing central nervous system, thus increasing the probability of abnormal development as the child grows. Although often difficult to diagnose, these children require careful follow-up and early intervention to enable optimal development

Moreover, these groups of risk are not mutually exclusive, and the determining elements of each can occur in interaction, resulting in a greater degree of probability for delayed or abnormal behavior.

Early intervention programs are designed to prevent or reduce the problems resulting from these risk conditions that may impair or interfere with the child's emotional, perceptual, cognitive, language, or motor development and to maximize the child's potential capabilities in these areas. In addition, they provide support and education for the child's parents, thus increasing their understanding and acceptance of their child's problems, enabling an ease of learning new skills necessary for an optimal environment of their special-needs child.

Entry into an intervention program begins with a referral, which is generally made by a health care provider or health service agency such as a visiting nursing association, a pediatrician, or self-referral by a parent. In some instances, interviews are set up with the parents to obtain further information about their child and the type of program they are seeking and to explain the program available to them. Admission of the child into a program is usually based on admission criteria established by the program and on the needs of the child and parents. Subsequently, an initial evaluation is conducted by individual team members or by the team as a whole, either at the center or in the child's home.

An increasingly popular method of initial evaluation used by early intervention programs is that of the "arena" method. This consists of the parents, child, and professional staff all in attendance for the evaluation. One team member is designated as the "primary facilitator" for the evaluation. The facilitator has direct contact with the child and conducts the entire assessment while suggestions and questions from the parents or the staff who are observing and recording the child's performance are directed to the facilitator. This procedure enables the parents to interact with the entire staff and allows the team the opportunity to observe the child's behavior in one testing session without each team member handling the child. However, this method can also present an overwhelming situation for the parents, and care must be taken to make it as comfortable as possible for them [21].

The initial assessment may include general behavioral observations including the social-emotional state of the child, motor/adaptive behavior, language and cognitive abilities, and self-help skills. The type of testing employed by early intervention programs varies widely. Some of the more commonly used developmental assessments include Bayley Scales of Infant Development, Gesell Developmental Schedules, Early Intervention Developmental Profile, Uzgiris-Hunt Ordinal Scales of Psychological Development, Sewall Early Education Developmental Profile, Denver Developmental Screening Test, Brazelton Neonatal Assessment Scale, and Learning Accomplishment Profile. More specific tests may also be used to gain supplemental information relative to areas of concern, for example, language and postural reflexes. Table 2-4 provides general information on developmental assessments.

Results of the assessment form the basis for the team's overall recommendations and individual program plan for the child. The program plan typically addresses those areas of development that are of concern to the team and parents. The systematic plan contains common team goals and measurable objectives, such as is illustrated in Figure 2-2. Both the program plan and assessment findings are reviewed by the team with the parents. Additionally periodic reassessments are undertaken to ascertain progress and to ensure that program projections for an individual child are met. Program goals not met as predicted would be revised at this time. Figure 2-3 displays a model developed by Simeonsson and Wiegerink [57] of a systemic, objective procedure to coordinate programs for handicapped children. Simeonsson and co-workers [56] also suggest the use of Goal Attainment Scaling and the Progress Oriented Family Record as means of empirical and clinical accountability in early intervention.

Parent involvement in the child's program is encouraged and may include a home program, participation in treatment sessions, and parent support meetings or counseling.

Acknowledged [22] benefits of early intervention programs include

Enabling the infant and parents to develop to their full potential

Strengthening good family development

Lessening of parent guilt, anger, and frustration

Reinforcing positive developmental patterns

Refocusing the traditional medical mode

Encouraging collaboration of health care providers

Name: _____	DOB: _____	Dates:	Initial _____
			1st Quarter _____
			2nd Quarter _____
			3rd Quarter _____
			4th Quarter _____

Priority (I, II, III)	General goal	Approach, methodology, equipment
I	Improve attending skills	Relaxation techniques
II	Increase receptive and expressive language skills	Language stimulation equipment

Goal (I, II, III)	Objective (1, 2, 3)	Specific objectives	Progress / Quarter emphasis			
			1	2	3	4
I	1	Utilizing relaxation techniques, Walter will relax for 10 or more minutes 80% of the time.			IP	
			X	X	X	X
	2	In a quiet area and with 1 : 1 therapy setting, Walter will attend to a task for 7 minutes or more 80% of the time.			IP	
			X	X	X	X
II	1	Walter will code all content categories at Stage I level of development: with echoic modeling 80% of the time,	X	X		
		spontaneously 80%			A	
				X	X	X
	2	Walter will code content categories at Stage II level of development: with echoic modeling 70% of the time,		A		
			X	X		
		spontaneously 50%			A	
				X	X	X
	3	Given two and three word commands, along with visual cues and physical prompts, Walter will follow through 75% of the time.			A	
			X	X	X	X

Progress key: B = beginning; IP = in progress; I = improved; A = achieved; G = generalized; M = maintained; NA = not achieved

FIG. 2-2. An individual program plan.

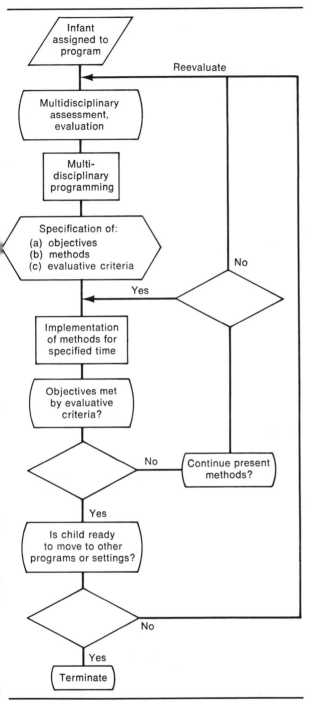

FIG. 2-3. An infant program model. (From R. J. Simeonsson and R. Wiegerink. Accountability: A dilemma in infant intervention. *Except. Child.* 41:474, 1975. Copyright 1975 by The Council For Exceptional Children. Reprinted with permission.)

CONTRACTURES AND DEFORMITIES

Due to abnormalities in motor control and muscle tone, the child with CP often develops contractures as a result of muscle shortening. This phenomenon can increase the child's susceptibility to joint deformities and limit joint mobility. Orthopedic surgery may be recommended to increase mobility through the release, lengthening, or transfer of affected muscles. Table 2-7 presents commonly performed orthopedic procedures. Surgical intervention for upper extremity deformities is uncommon, although spinal fusion may be recommended for children with severe scoliosis (more than a 45-degree angle). Braces may be used following surgery or may be recommended particularly for the lower extremities prior to surgery in an attempt to prevent contractures, stabilize joints, and facilitate ambulation.

Bryce [19], who recommends neurodevelopmental treatment (NDT) approach to spasticity, points out that "any distal stretch of spastic muscles will produce a shift of spasticity to the nearest joint." She uses the example of bracing the ankle into dorsiflexion, causing an increase in flexion of the knees and hips. Bryce further comments that although surgery may be necessary where structural changes have occurred in the tendon or joints, the surgical release of one group of muscles will not affect the pattern itself but will allow a stronger spastic response in opposing muscle groups. Thus, in a heel cord lengthening, the child risks an increase in flexion at the hip and knee unless sufficient normal active extension is available to counteract it.

Management of abnormal muscle tone poses difficult problems for the child, family, and team. In addition to a NDT program, the therapist may find that medication has been prescribed for the child to aid in the control of muscle tone. Among the medications commonly used are diazepam (Valium), dantrolene (Dantrium), and baclofen (Lioresal). The common side effects of all of these medications are sedation and increased drooling.

TABLE 2-7. Common musculoskeletal deformities and orthopedic surgery

Location	Deformity	Surgery	Splint
Shoulder	*Adduction	Subscapularis release	
	*Internal rotation	Rotational osteotomy	
Elbow/forearm	*Flexion	Elbow flexor release	
	*Pronation	Pronator teres release	
	Subluxation/dislocation of radial head	Radial head resection or oblique osteotomy of radial shaft and 180° forearm rotation	
Wrist	*Flexion	Lengthening or release of wrist flexors; wrist fusion	Cock-up splint
Hand/thumb	*"Thumb-in-palm" (flexion and adduction)	Matev's procedure: elongation of flexor pollicis longus, thenar muscles release, abduction/extension tendon shortening or transfer	
	"Clenched fingers" (flexion)	Flexor tendon lengthening	
Spine	Kyphoscoliosis	Spinal fusion	Back brace
Hip	Scissors gait *Adduction	Adductor tenotomy and obturator neurectomy (ATON)	Spica for 3 wk; cast bivalved after 3 wk then wear posterior shell after 6 wk; wear shell only at night; therapy after 3 wk
	Internal rotation	Derotational osteotomy	Unilateral spica for 6 wk; ROM after 6 wk; A-frame splint at night
	*Flexion	Iliopsoas tenotomy	Spica for 3–6 wk; posterior shell; weight bearing after 6 wk
	Subluxation/dislocation	ATON	
Knee	*Flexion	Hamstring release	Long leg cast 3 wk; long leg splint with bar at night; weight bearing after 3–6 wk
Ankle/foot	*Equinus/"toe walking": foot in plantar flexion so that only ball of foot rests on the ground; commonly combined with pes varus	Heel cord lengthening (TAL)	Short leg cast 6 wk; short leg braces in dorsiflexion at night; weight bearing in casts after 3 wk

TABLE 2-7. (CONTINUED)

Location	Deformity	Surgery	Splint
	Pes valgus (may lead to "rocker bottom foot"): eversion of the foot with the inner side of foot touching the ground	Grice-Green procedure (subtalar arthrodesis)	Long leg cast 4–6 wk then short leg cast 4–6 wk; weight bearing after in short leg cast
		Cavalier-Judet procedure	8 wk in cast; weight bearing after 4 wk
Other deformities of the foot	Hammer toes: flexion of the PIPs of the toes Hallux valgus: adduction of the great toe Metatarsus adductus: forefoot is angled away from the longitudinal axis toward the midline Pes planus ("flatfoot"): arches are flattened Calcaneus valgus: foot in dorsiflexion and eversion; weight of foot rests on the heel Prominent navicular and head of talus Pes varus: inversion of the foot with the outer side of the foot touching the ground		
Other deformities of the knee	Internal tibial torsion Tibial-femoral subluxation Chondromalacia patellae Patella alta		

TAL = tends Achille's lengthening; PIPs = proximal interphalangeal joints.
*Most common deformities.
Source: From E. E. Bleck. *Cerebral Palsy: Orthopedic Aspects.* Boston: Pediatric Rehabilitation; Tufts Research and Training Center, 1982.

Other modalities used in the control of spasticity are nerve blocks, inhibitive casting, and biofeedback.

Neurodevelopmental Treatment
Mary Louise Jani and Alice Sapienza

Because CP is primarily a motor syndrome [13], therapeutic intervention focuses on motor control, posture, and movement. Over the years, various therapeutic methods have been used, although NDT as developed by the Bobaths [8, 9] is the therapy of choice in many centers for CP children. NDT originated in England, as a result of years of treatment by the Bobaths of patients with CNS disorders, primarily children with CP. This approach is based on the view that CP results from a brain lesion that affects an immature brain, disrupting normal growth and development of the child [14]. As a result, the child's development appears delayed and has an abnormal course, which results in abnormal patterns of posture and movement. Many of the basic patterns of normal motor development, which provide the foundation for more complex functional skills, are unable to develop. The CP child is left with abnormal motor patterns that are used repeatedly and adapted for all-purpose activity.

Treatment is therefore primarily directed toward inhibiting the patterns of abnormal reflex activity and facilitating normal patterns of movement. This is done through techniques of handling. The techniques enable the child to learn the sensations of normal movements and to develop sensorimotor patterns that can be expanded for use in later skilled activities [9].

The treatment is not a "method," as a method is a rigid and standardized approach. Rather, NDT is a flexible approach to the multiple problems of the individual child with CP [11]. There are no prescribed exercises or patterns of movement for all children. However, on the basis of the individual child's abilities and disabilities, specific treatment is used for specific problems. Assessment and ongoing reassessment constitute an integral part of the treatment.

Many respected scientists have contributed to the theory and principles of NDT. The work of Magnus [37], Schaltenbrand [53], and Walshe [63] on posture, reflexes, and movement provided the theoretic framework for the Bobaths' development of reflex-inhibiting postures. These postures were used to break up the abnormal postures caused by tonic reflex activity associated with hypertonus. The continued presence of tonic reflex activity prevented the normal development of postural reflexes, which include protective, righting, and equilibrium reactions [9]. The studies by Rademaker [47] and Weisz [64] contributed to the Bobaths' concept of postural reflex mechanism as the basis of voluntary movements. Gesell and Amatruda [27], Illingworth [32], Thomas, Chesni, and Saint-Anne Dargassies [2], and McGraw [38] have described the gradual development or righting and equilibrium reactions, which underlie the sequence of development of the growing child's spontaneous motor abilities at various stages.

The end result has evolved into an approach that strongly uses assessment and treatment planning, facilitation of movements against gravity, and transition into functional skills [11]. Passive reflex-inhibiting postures are no longer used in treatment. Rather, NDT emphasizes facilitation of patterns of movement to improve coordination in posture and movement and to obtain more normal postural tone.

Following its beginnings in England, NDT became an acceptable treatment approach in the United States in the late 1960s for those with CP and adult hemiplegia. As it became increasingly more popular, the basic concepts of the Bobaths' approach modified and expanded to address the treatment of a wide variety of disabilities including neuromotor deficits and developmental and learning disabilities. Many physical and occupational therapists, speech-language pathologists, educators, and physicians have participated in the intensive training developed by the Neuro-Developmental Treatment Association, which certifies professionals as proficient in neurodevelopmental treatment.

PRINCIPLES OF TREATMENT

The inhibition of abnormal postural patterns and facilitation of normal motor patterns are key principles in NDT. They are based on the premise that the CP child exhibits abnormal coordination of muscle function in posture and movement, rather than a weakness or paralysis of muscles. Therefore, the focus of treatment is to improve muscle coordination in posture and movement, rather than strengthen weak muscles. This is accomplished by handling the child in specific ways to help acquire normal sensorimotor patterns of postural adjustment, much as the normal baby does in the first 3 years through continuous handling by the mother [9].

Motor development is dependent on sensory input, although the term *sensory-motor* more accurately describes the process of motor development. The early movements of the normal baby are spontaneous, accidental, and automatic. As the baby learns to control movements against gravity, voluntary initiation and control of movement develops. The child learns to move through the sensation of movement. All of the sensory systems are involved in this process: tactile, proprioceptive, kinesthetic, visual, and vestibular [6].

The baby with CP lacks many of these early movement experiences. The presence of abnormal postural tone limits the ability to move as well as limiting future abilities. Movement develops with the use of abnormal postural patterns.

The goal of NDT is to prepare the child for functional movement. The emphasis is placed on the development of patterns of coordination rather than the acquisition of motor milestones or following the normal sequence of developmental skills.

From the study of normal child development, several important concepts are relevant to NDT. Among them is the overlap in the development of motor activities. At any given stage of development, the child is practicing established patterns and is experimenting with the combination of different movements to develop new skills. Strict adherence to the normal sequence of motor development in treatment of the CP child is not advisable. Normal children sometimes omit stages or achieve skills in a different sequence. In addition, it takes CP children longer to develop some of the most important movements needed. Working to perfect one particular skill in the child before advancing to the next is not indicated as normal children perform a variety of activities all at the same time. In order to progress to a new skill, they rely on a number of other related skills that make the new one achievable.

In striving to attain a more difficult skill, the child often perfects the preceding one. However, it is important to realize that in the normal child, previously formed skills may be abandoned or may break down temporarily until the new skill becomes refined. By contrast, in the CP child, it takes more time to reach an advanced skill, and in doing so, the child may lose other skills previously acquired. Therefore, instead of concentrating on isolated activities, the therapist should work toward promoting "sequence of movement" [9].

Certain normal movements should not be encouraged in treatment, as they reinforce abnormal patterns of movement in the child with abnormal postural tone. It is necessary to assess what each child needs most at any stage or age, and then choose what is absolutely necessary in preparing for future functional skills, or improving those skills that have developed abnormally.

Of equal importance is the need to counteract abnormal motor patterns that prevent the child's functional activity. Thus, in treatment, inhibition of abnormal patterns occurs along with facilitation of more normal patterns.

The basis of all motor development is dynamic postural control against gravity. Righting and equilibrium reactions and use of the arms and hands for support, reach, grasp, and hold are the basic components that form skilled and voluntary movements. They remain automatic throughout adult life [10]. In NDT, the therapist uses these reactions in the child to achieve functional motor skills.

Righting reactions maintain the position of the head in space and the alignment of the head with the body and the body with the extremities [6]. These reflexes arise from sensory input from visual, tactile, proprioceptive, and vestibular receptors. They are present from birth in the normal full-term baby. The equilibrium reactions are automatic, compensatory reactions that provide adaptation of the whole body when the center of gravity is changed. They are elicited through vestibular stimulation and begin to develop in the normal baby from about the fifth month [16].

Handling the child allows the therapist to change the postural tone and guide the child's movement responses. It is very much an active and dynamic process, using automatic movement responses of the child rather than movements obtained by request. The child is handled from "key points of control" of the body. These key points may be proximal or distal body parts (head, shoulder girdle, trunk, pelvis or thenar eminence, calcaneus, and knees), which are carefully selected by the therapist depending on what patterns of movement are being facilitated or inhibited. Using this technique, the therapist can affect the initiation, speed, range, and end point of the movement as well as the various components involved. Key points of control are changed frequently to avoid dependency on the therapist and promote control by the child.

According to the Bobaths [15], the inhibition

of abnormal reflex activity and facilitation of movement may be used together, alternately, or may follow each other. Whatever combination is used, the child must be allowed the opportunity to move actively. Permanent carryover of treatment will be contingent on the degree of normal movement sequences that can be developed.

NEURODEVELOPMENTAL ASSESSMENT

A systematic assessment of the child's abilities and disabilities is fundamental to planning and carrying out treatment. The assessment aims at determining which motor patterns are missing and how abnormal tone and movement are preventing the development of normal functional skills. It leads directly to the development of treatment measures that provide the child with the most essential patterns needed for functional activity at any stage of development [11].

To assess the child's abilities, the therapist needs knowledge of normal motor development in terms of the acquisition and maturation of postural reflex mechanisms (righting and equilibrium responses that provide the background for normal skilled activity). Knowledge of abnormal motor patterns used by children with CP enables the therapist to identify early signs of abnormal patterns, and thus intervene in their development [12].

Depending on the form used, the actual format for assessment varies. Table 2-8 is an example of an assessment used for a motor evaluation of a child with CP. The assessment must provide the information from which the problems are analyzed. This information includes what the child can do and how it is done, what the child cannot do, whether the child is symmetric or asymmetric, whether the developmental age is equal to the chronological age, what mobility the child has (in terms of joint motion), what the postural tone is, and how adaptable the child is to handling. With this information, the therapist can analyze why the child moves in a certain way, what normal movements are

present, which abnormal movement patterns have developed, what components of movement patterns have developed, what components of movement are missing, why the child cannot move, and the causes of the abnormal mobility and abnormal postural tone [6].

In addition, at the Bobath Centre, observations are an important part of the assessment. They are carried out in an organized manner and include the following:

Behavioral responses to assessment and handling
Respiratory patterns at rest and during movement
Communication and play skills
Feeding and self-care skills
Sensory deficits and associated perceptual problems
Medications and medical history
Equipment used by the child
Home history, including parents' perception of the child and functional level

Reassessment should occur frequently, so that the treatment can be modified or changed according to the child's progress or lack of progress [11]. Assessment, then, becomes an integral part of ongoing treatment.

Spontaneous motor behavior should be assessed in different positions. Change of posture (transitional movements) as well as maintenance of posture should be observed and recorded before the therapist handles the child. The different positions that should be observed include supine, prone, quadruped, progression, sitting, and standing. The assessment should also include upper extremity function (reaching, grasping, and releasing), pattern of walking, and elicited primitive and postural reflexes [54].

PRACTICAL APPLICATION OF
NEURODEVELOPMENTAL TREATMENT

The primary goal of NDT is to provide the child who displays signs of CNS impairment with the sensory experience of normal patterns of posture and movement. The quality of movement patterns is of major concern to the therapist. The NDT approach emphasizes the proper postural alignment and integrated movement patterns of the head and shoulder girdle necessary for the development of coordinated movements throughout the body [54].

The most important motor achievements in treatment include head control, trunk control, weight shifting, weight bearing, and progression. Head control is dependent on balance of neck flexion and extension. Neck flexion provides midline control, and integration of neck flexion and extension allows neck lateral flexion against gravity. The therapist can work to achieve midline orientation of the head and righting into flexion against gravity in supine and supported sit postures. With slow movement, the child's center of gravity can be shifted behind the base of support, and the child responds to correct the alignment of head and trunk. The therapist can guide the proper response and inhibit abnormal patterns through careful placement and degree of support through handling. Neck lateral flexion can be achieved in side-lying, rolling, and supported upright sitting. As the pelvis is rolled to the side, body-righting reaction on the head is facilitated. Neck elongation and chin tucking are important aspects in treatment to provide neck mobility and refined head control.

Trunk control is focused on as head control is beginning to be observed because their development overlaps. Full head mobility is only possible with some degree of shoulder and trunk stability. Integration between flexion and extension of the head and trunk is facilitated in both prone and supine postures. In sitting, righting reactions of the head and trunk can be facilitated by displacing the center of gravity in every direction. Handling should occur at the pelvis, provided sufficient head and trunk control is present.

Rotation of the body can also be facilitated by handling from the pelvis and legs, and shifting weight from one side of the body to the other. Extremity weight bearing is frequently achieved first in prone but should be facilitated in side-lying, reclined sitting, upright sitting, and quadruped. This develops stability of the shoulder girdle and pelvis, protective extension of the arms, and dissociation of arm from shoulder girdle and trunk, and leg from pelvis.

Weight bearing and controlled weight shifting lead to the development of equilibrium reactions that occur first in prone, then supine, sitting, quadruped, and standing postures. As equilibrium reactions develop, the child learns to progress forward, as progression can be viewed as the constant loss and attainment of body balance [6, 54].

Treatment must always be dynamic. Movement into and out of positions or small controlled movements in positions allow the child to actively react to the situation. These active reactions give more normal sensorimotor experiences. Treatment is also preparation for what the child will be doing in the future, as well as working to fill in the gaps in previous development. Treatment techniques are tools with which both the therapist and the child must adapt [6].

To be most effective, treatment must be carried over into all aspects of the child's life: learning, play, daily care, and sleep. Parent training is a vital part of the successful treatment program, since the child spends the majority of time with the parents at home. Parents should be provided with clear explanations of what problems the child has, what the treatment goals are, what is done in treatment, and why it is done. By participating in the treatment sessions, parents can be instructed in proper positioning, handling, and movement of their child in keeping with the therapeutic program [17]. In addition, others involved in the care and management of the child (sitters, extended family members, teachers, doctors) should have knowledge of the specifics needed for carryover of treatment principles [11].

The therapist may find it beneficial to use adaptive devices as part of the therapy pro-

TABLE 2-8. Motor evaluation

Name: Chart no.:   Birth date: Date: Therapist:

I. General impressions (alterness, interaction with parent/environment, communication, reaction to stimuli):

II. Sensory deficits and other pertinent medical information:

III. Motor Functions	Motor patterns: Normal postural adaptations	Abnormal postural responses	Postural tonus
1. Observation of spontaneous behavior 2. Elicit specific reactions if not displayed spontaneously: righting rolling transitions Landau reaction equilibrium protective extension 3. Test for mobility and postural tonus	1. Righting against gravity extension flexion lateral flexion axial rotation 2. Head control face vertical mouth horizontal neck elongated (after 4 mo) 3. Symmetry, midline control (after 4 mo) 4. Shoulder girdle (scapular), stability (after 4 mo) 5. Differentiation and variation of movements 6. Postural stability and mobility equilibrium reactions protective extension of arms (starting at 6 mo)	1. Exaggerated tonic reflexes progravity pull into flexion/extension obligatory asymmetry pronounced abduction at hips pronounced plantarflexion of ankle fisting of hands 2. Hyperextension of head and neck; lack of flexion against gravity (after 3 mo) 3. Persistent scapular protraction/retraction 4. Total extension, pronounced/compensatory flexion 5. Pronounced anterior/posterior pelvic tilt 6. Stereotyped patterns (frog position) 7. Paucity/excess of movement 8. Lack of mobility	Normal Hypotonic Hypertonic Rigid Fluctuating Associated reactions at rest change of tonus in response to stimulation, handling, movement

A. Prone
   Horizontal
   Suspension
B. Supine, pull to sit
C. Sitting
D. All fours
E. Standing, vertical
      suspension
F. Locomotion, gait
G. Manipulation, eye-
      hand coordina-
      tion, protective
      extension of arms

46

TABLE 2-8 (CONTINUED)

IV. Overall quality of motor behavior (variability, grading, sequencing):

V. Predominant motor patterns:

VI. Restricted mobility, (risk for) contractures, deformities:

VII. Reaction to sensory stimulation (kinesthetic, tactile, auditory, visual):

VIII. Additional comments:

IX. Summary:
Displayed behaviors seem to be typical—, if not give apparent reason:

X. Program goals:

IX. Recommended procedures:

Source: A. L. Scherzer and I. Tscharnuter. *Early Diagnosis and Therapy in Cerebral Palsy*. New York: Dekker, 1982. Pp. 160–162. Reprinted by courtesy of Marcel Dekker, Inc.

gram. They may be simply incorporating another person as "an extra set of hands," or using a foam wedge as a stable base on which the child can move to provide proper body alignment. These devices should not be used before the child has experienced movement because they are static [6]. Adaptive equipment such as prone or supine standers, side-lyers, adaptive chairs, rolls, bolsters, wedges, and mobility aids are some examples that are commonly used. More recently, therapists have begun to fabricate inhibitive casts for the ankle/foot or hand/wrist to reduce distal muscle tone. It is important to note that all of these devices are adjuncts to the overall therapeutic program, which is closely monitored by the therapist, and not substitutes for the treatment session.

There are advantages to beginning treatment of the child with CP in early infancy. The young baby with CP frequently displays a paucity of movement rather than abnormal movements. Tone may be fairly normal and contractures and deformities not yet developed. Intervention at this point would have the best effect on the baby's further development. Therapeutic handling to facilitate normal postural tone and normal movement patterns could be incorporated into all aspects of the baby's daily routine [8, 10].

Treatment at this early stage also poses several problems. Diagnosis before 6 weeks of age is difficult except in severe cases. Postural tone may be fairly normal in children who, with time, develop spasticity. Other children may be hypotonic, yet go on to develop athetosis and ataxia. Abnormal movements and postures are usually not present early in life. Babies at this point may just display delayed development with little spontaneous movement. Only as development progresses cephalocaudal, proximal-distal, and gross-fine does the scope of involvement become more evident. However, if treatment was delayed until an accurate diagnosis could be made, the child may have established the abnormal patterns of posture and movement, and treatment may be less effective. The therapist must carefully explore with all team members what to tell the parents of the young baby suspected or at risk for CP. Careful monitoring, frequent reassessment, and treatment (through direct service or parent training) should be available as long as suspicions exist [6, 10].

Oral Motor Skills
Patricia A. R. Laverdure

Children with CNS dysfunction often develop abnormal oral motor patterns. These patterns are occasionally seen at birth but become more pronounced by 4 to 5 months of age. They can include extension of the mandible, known as jaw thrust. The jaw thrust is characterized by a strong, uncontrolled full jaw opening in the absence of a stimulus, while food is being presented, during bolus manipulation, or during swallowing. The child typically demonstrates difficulty closing the mouth to handle the food. This abnormal pattern prevents jaw stabilization and gradation necessary to pull food from a spoon and develop functional chewing patterns.

Tonic-bite reflex is mandible flexion in response to stimulation of the face, lips, teeth, or gums. When food is presented, the jaw closes strongly and uncontrollably. Reopening the mouth is difficult, and the chewing pattern is often poorly coordinated. The child with fluctuating tone will bite down on a spoon as a means of increasing jaw stability but does not demonstrate the reflexive quality seen in the tonic bite reflex [42].

An extensor response of the lip and cheek musculature, which draws the lips back into a straight line across the mouth, is known as lip retraction. At the same time, a flexor response of the orbicularis oris muscle may develop. This "purse-string action" interferes with functional lip abilities.

The infant experiences normal tongue protraction during suckling, with the tongue protruding between the gums or lips during swallowing [18, 43]. Abnormal tongue thrust occurs when the tongue protracts to a greater extent and force than normal during swallowing. This child demonstrates an exaggerated contraction of the intrinsic extensor musculature of the tongue, resulting in a thicker appearance. Placing the nipple, spoon, or cup to the oral cavity during tongue thrusting is difficult, and food may be pushed from the mouth during the chewing or swallowing process.

Tongue retraction occurs when the tongue is elevated to the roof of the pharyngeal space with the tip pressing against the anterior aspect of the soft palate or the posterior aspect of the hard palate. It can be the result of abnormal extensor tone of the body or as a result of a protective response to poor swallowing. It interferes with respiration and feeding, making food insertion inefficient.

Nasal regurgitation occurs when soft palate musculature is not synchronized with other oral motor patterns and if a cleft palate exists [42]. It too compromises the efficiency of feeding behavior.

Hypertonicity severely decreases the amount of spontaneous gross motor activity a child may experience, limiting the necessary movement for respiration. Poor neck and trunk control coupled with spasticity of the abdominal musculature often leave respiration shallow and vocalizations breathy. Oral motor control is compromised due to tongue retraction or protrusion, lip retraction, jaw thrust, and poor stability. The child often exhibits difficulty in maintaining velopharyngeal closure. Finger feeding is difficult due to the inability to control the body and establish a hand-to-mouth pattern.

Hypotonicity results in an inability to maintain neck and trunk control against gravity necessary for adequate oral motor functioning. An inability to provide proximal stability of the abdominal, thoracic, and laryngeal areas interferes with sucking, swallowing, biting, and chewing.

Children with fluctuating or athetoidlike tone exhibit poorly coordinated movement patterns. Smooth oral movement is inadequate, which results in jaw thrusting and deviation, poor lip closure, tongue thrusting, and poorly coordinated swallowing. Facial grimacing may also be evident.

If flexion and neck elongation fail to develop, shoulder elevation is seen in an attempt to

48

provide stability to a poor head control [1]. During feeding, shoulder elevation provides stability to the jaw, which encourages thrusting or tonic biting. Lips and cheeks retract in an attempt to increase stability, and the tongue retracts and elevates to the hard palate. Lips may purse to approximate lip closure.

Children with abnormal muscle tone often develop scapular retraction and scapulohumeral tightness in an effort to achieve shoulder girdle control [1]. Upper-trunk flexor control does not develop efficiently, resulting in decreased forward movement of the upper extremities. Decreased active horizontal adduction reduces the elasticity of the musculature of the scapula and humerus, limiting scapulohumeral disassociation and fine motor abilities. In an attempt to stabilize the shoulder girdle, shoulder elevation, capital and cervical hyperextension, and compensatory oral motor functioning are increased.

An exaggerated response to oral tactile stimulation is often observed in children with CNS damage. Such a response interferes with the development and control of oral motor structures and can result in a failure to develop normal feeding behavior. When the oral or facial areas are touched, abnormal postural tone may be seen, making feeding difficult. The child may avoid hand-to-mouth experiences, which can affect the development of finger-feeding skills and perceptual awareness of body parts. On tactile stimulation of oral structures, the jaw may thrust or bite, the lips and tongue may retract, and an abnormal gag reflex may be elicited [20]. Facial grimacing may be evident on oral or facial stimulation, and the child may reject changes in temperatures or textures of food.

FEEDING EVALUATION

The feeding evaluation includes the child's history of feeding difficulties and therapeutic interventions used, changes in feeding abilities, types of food eaten and equipment used, and current feeding problems. It is beneficial to assess the child while being fed in the typical routine position using familiar foods and the child's own utensils.

General postural tone is established during rest, activity, and prior to and during the feeding assessment [44]. Upper-extremity function is noted during play and feeding. Voluntary motor control of the facial musculature, jaw, lips, and tongue is assessed during feeding. Oral structures are observed in their response to flexion and extension movements and during rest. Asymmetry of oral structures is noted.

Reflexive behavior is assessed during the oral motor evaluation [48] by methods previously discussed. The first pattern of controlled feeding is suckling. It is generally associated with emerging extensor tone and involves protraction and retraction of the tongue combined with vertical jaw excursion and lip approximation to the nipple. The lateral aspects of the lips are open, often resulting in lateral liquid spillage. At the age of 6 months when spoon feeding is generally initiated, it is the suckling pattern that draws the food back into the oral cavity [40]. Because lip activation is limited, food is typically scraped off of the spoon by the upper-gum ridge.

As flexor control of the body develops, intrinsic tongue, cheek, and lip musculature is activated, and suckling gives way to sucking. In sucking, jaw movement is minimal, and the tongue gradually begins to move in an up and down pattern independently of the jaw [40]. The lips form a firm seal on the nipple, and the cheeks assist in developing negative pressure in the oral cavity. A sucking pattern in a young infant should be assessed as a possible indicator of abnormally high flexor tone.

As lip activity is increased, coughing, spitting, and liquid loss during cup drinking are reduced. Up until approximately 1 year of life, a combination of suckling and sucking tongue motion is used [40]. The jaw does not have the necessary stability to allow independent tongue and lip mobility; therefore, the oral mechanism tends to act as one unit in a vertical excursion pattern.

Suckling and sucking initiation and rhythmicity should be noted with respect to their interference with the feeding process. Suckling and suck patterns, typically initiated before the nipple is inserted into the oral cavity, normally demonstrate a very precise and consistent rhythm [41]. The coordination of the sucking with other oral motor function such as swallowing and breathing should be addressed during the feeding evaluation.

Suckling and sucking provide the stimulus for the automatic response of swallowing. Swallowing, although difficult at times to discern from its counterpart stimulus, is considered the passage of the bolus of food down the esophagus, producing elevation of the hyoid and larynx. An ineffective or poorly coordinated swallow can produce recurrent aspiration pneumonia and other medically threatening conditions. It is best evaluated during barium swallow or other radiographic procedures.

As jaw stabilization improves through the active contraction of muscles about the temporomandibular joint, the control of liquid and semisolid intake occurs through the lips in cup drinking and spoon feeding [40]. The tongue remains in the oral cavity and approximates to the hard palate, and a sucking pattern no longer provides the stimulus to swallow. Independent tongue and lip elevation occurs in mature swallowing.

The development of jaw, lip, and tongue control are necessary prerequisites to the production of biting and chewing. Biting is present at birth in the form of an automatic phasic bite release pattern. This reflexive action continues normally until the age of 4 to 5 months when it gradually evolves to a munching, chewing pattern with the emergence of a jaw stability. The therapist should note a bite reflex with a tonic quality, along with poorly graded jaw movement. In addition, the ease in which a bite and holding pattern releases on a cup or spoon should be identified as a function of increased jaw stability [26, 40, 48].

Munching is characterized by a vertical excursion of the jaw with flattening of the tongue. The chewing surface is between the tongue and the hard palate during this early period. Munching emerges as the combination and coordination of two primitive patterns: the automatic phasic-bite release pattern and sucking. As tongue disassociation and lateralization develop, lateral and rotary components emerge, which allow the development of mature chewing [40].

The child's response to vestibular, gustatory, olfactory, auditory, and visual stimuli is assessed to determine its effect on total body functioning during play and feeding. The child's tolerance to varying intensities and quick changes of stimulation is noted. Foods such as soft and hard cookies, raisins, and juice are useful evaluation tools because the child will voluntarily select the movement pattern that most efficiently fulfills the objective of successful feeding. Hypersensitivity and abnormal oral motor patterns in response to tactile stimulation provided through food textures, temperatures, and utensils should be noted.

Deformities and deviations of oral mechanism are assessed, and consultation with an orthodontist or otorhinolaryngologist may be necessary. Structural deformities of the mandible and maxilla are noted as well as asymmetries of the face and head. The presence and condition of erupted teeth and their placement during jaw closure are essential to the masticatory function of the oral mechanism. The tongue is assessed as it relates in size to its masticatory space and its mobility within the mouth. The lingual frenulum should allow lateral tongue mobility. The presence of a cleft lip/palate or surgical repair is noted as is the height of the hard palate.

At birth, a child lacks full extensor control against gravity. As a result, respiration is shallow and rapid, involving a lowering of the diaphragm to expand the lungs. As the child matures and extension components of movement develop, the intercostals and the diaphragm play a more integrated role in respiration. As a child gains control in an upright position and flexion and extension components become balanced, the thoracic cavity is elongated. Respiration becomes diaphragmatic-thoracic in nature, characterized by increased thoracic excursion during inspiration [1].

Thus, evaluation of respiratory function includes the tone of breathing musculature. If hypotonicity is present, the chest may present in a barrel shape with abdominal breathing predominating. If tone is increased, the rib cage is typically flared and flattened, and clavicular breathing may be present [50].

The coordination of the child's suck, swallow, and breathing pattern should allow adequate nutritional intake without the danger of aspiration. The rate and rhythm of the pattern are determined during bottle, breast, or cup drinking. A history of aspiration pneumonia, excessive coughing, or choking should be noted.

TREATMENT OF ORAL MOTOR PROBLEMS

Proper positioning of the child is critical for effective feeding. It assists in normalizing tone and prevents aspiration and back flow of food and liquid into the nasal passages [60]. The child is positioned so that the neck is slightly flexed and the chin is forward. Swallowing is more difficult, and aspiration is more probable when the neck is hyperextended. The trunk is positioned in a vertical position to facilitate breathing. In bringing the shoulder and arms forward and flexing the hips and knees to 90 degrees, hyperextension is inhibited. The ankles should be flexed to 90 degrees and the feet supported on a stable surface.

Adaptive seating may become necessary for the handicapped child, which should be appropriate to a child's age. Although not ideal, the child can be fed while positioned in the lap. This position does avoid aspiration and extensor thrust [59]. When the child is fed in a semireclining position, the child's arms and legs are crossed. Head support is placed behind the neck to achieve neck flexion and midline orientation. The trunk should not be curved. To reduce hyperextension the hip flexion can be increased by lowering the leg on which the buttocks are resting.

The child with severe suckling and swallowing problems may demonstrate increased coordination when fed in a prone position at a 45-degree angle [60]. A child with increased extensor tone may require a bolster placed at the base of the neck to enhance flexion. A hypotonic child may need to be held in place with shoulder and chest straps. These straps are fastened to the back of the chair to maintain an upright position. A child with increased trunk and lower extremity tone may require positioning over a roll [24] to achieve hip abduction and knee and ankle flexion.

Frequently jaw control is compromised even when proper positioning is achieved. The child may lack the necessary tone in the jaw, neck, and shoulder girdle to develop smooth gradation of jaw movement. Normal jaw control can be provided by the side or front of the face to enhance the stability of the oral mechanism. As in Figure 2-4, when provided from the front, place the middle finger of the nonfeeding hand posterior to the bony portion of the chin. Place the thumb below the bottom lip, and place the index finger parallel to the child's mandible to provide added stability. Manual jaw control provided from the side assists with poor head control, neck and trunk hyperextension, and jaw stabilization. As in Figure 2-5, place the middle

FIG. 2-4. Manual jaw control provided anteriorly.

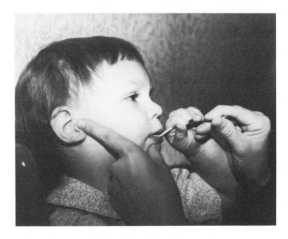

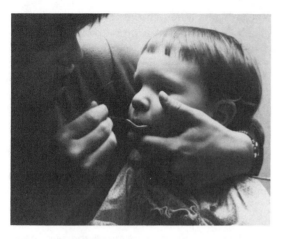

FIG. 2-5. Manual jaw control provided posteriorly.

finger of the nonfeeding hand posterior to the bony portion of the chin. Place the index finger on the chin below the lower lip. The thumb is placed obliquely across the cheek to provide lateral jaw stability. If a strong tongue protrusion pattern is present, a firm upward and backward motion of the middle finger will stimulate the proprioceptors of the tongue, facilitating retraction.

Jaw control technique can be used during spoon feeding and cup drinking. On presentation of the spoon, open the mouth slightly as the spoon touches the lips to allow its entrance. Slowly pull the spoon from the mouth without tipping it to facilitate activation of the upper lip to pull food from the spoon. Close the jaw as soon as the spoon is removed.

Using either jaw control technique, place the cup on the bottom lip, and tip the cup up while keeping the mouth closed. By facilitation of the upper lip and swallowing with the tongue in the mouth, a more mature drinking pattern emerges, which leads to controlled consecutive swallowing.

Jaw control techniques may, in addition, be adjuncts to a therapeutic program to enhance appropriate chewing skills. While providing jaw control, place a strip of meat, dried fruit, or fruit wrapped in cheese cloth on the biting surface of the premolar or molar teeth. Munching or rotational chewing pattern can be enhanced in this manner.

If chewing is developmentally appropriate, manual jaw control may not be necessary. If adequate jaw control is present to open and close the mouth voluntarily, alternative means to enhance chewing may be indicated. A gradual presentation of successively more difficult chewing foods is designed to include lumpy foods, soft chewy foods, and finally gummy-type foods. As the child learns to tolerate each level of food, biting and chewing on each side of the mouth as well as tongue lateralization should be encouraged.

With the development of fine jaw control, the tongue has a point of stability that encourages the mobility necessary for eating, swallowing, and phonation. A small amount of food presented on the spoon results in a more mature sucking or chewing motion of the tongue. A slight downward pressure of the spoon on the center of the tongue stimulates the proprioceptors, which facilitate a backward and upward motion of the tongue. Keeping the jaw closed inhibits protrusion of the tongue through the lips when swallowing.

When the jaw is maximally controlled either externally by the feeder or internally by adequate jaw tonus and stability, the lips are facilitated for activation. Using a spoon with a flat bowl, place the spoon in the mouth. Allow a few moments for the upper lip to assist in the removal of the food. Direct facilitatory stimulation to the lips enhances lip closure. Vibrating, tapping, and rubbing the orbicularis oris muscle facilitates contraction, resulting in closed lips. A quick stretch in a lateral motion from both corners of the mouth biases the muscle spindles toward lip closure. Strict stimulation should be done at least 30 minutes before feeding [45].

Learning to suck and swallow combines the voluntary action of the jaw, tongue, and lips in one controlled pattern. Proper positioning is essential for adequate sucking in the young child. Sucking can be enhanced by many forms of sensory stimuli. The tactile stimuli of the nipple touching the lips or moving inside the mouth, cold temperature, and sweet gustatory stimuli can enhance sucking.

Complete lip closure is a necessary prerequisite to adequate sucking. Assistance may be required from the feeder or obtained with the use of an adapted nipple. The feeder places a finger on each cheek and pushes anteriorly, which assists with lip pursing and gaining lateral lip closure. In addition a downward bilateral stroke on the cheeks stimulates a sucking reflex.

As tongue control and sucking improve, swallowing becomes more coordinated and consecutive. Techniques that increase the production of saliva subsequently enhance swallowing. Rubbing the outer gums and icing the orbicularis oris may increase saliva production [60]. It is cautioned, however, that some children may demonstrate increased seizure activity if icing crosses the midline of the body. Swallowing is also elicited by a firm stroke with the fingers in an upward direction on either side of the throat.

Profuse drooling frequently accompanies oral motor problems. Therapeutic intervention should be aimed at reducing the oral motor difficulties rather than the drooling itself. Therapy may take the form of increasing jaw and lip control, improving tongue mobility, and coordinating the suck-swallow pattern.

Mature oral motor abilities often fail to develop in the presence of abnormal tactile sensitivity about the facial and oral area [45]. If tactile hypersensitivity or defensiveness is present, an oral tactile stimulation program should be initiated. During activities that are familiar and comfortable, begin providing tactile stimulation in the areas that are most tolerable. For example, deep pressure is provided in a gradual manner in the direction of the face and mouth. As the child becomes less acceptant of the stimuli, the approach should be withdrawn to areas of less defensive reactions.

As facial sensitivity becomes normalized, stimulation to the mouth is provided. Often games and riddles can be devised to facilitate stimulation to the lips, gums, palate, and tongue. Many techniques that parallel normal developmental activities can be used to desensitize the mouth, such as tooth brushing, licking a lollypop and Popsicle, and eating foods of varying textures.

Self-initiated hand-to-mouth behavior is often considered the most effective means of normalizing oral motor sensitivity. During self-modulated tactile exploration, the child can control the intensity and duration of the stimulation being experienced. The development of hand-to-mouth activities such as toy mouthing and finger feeding may also assist in reducing tactile hypersensitivity.

SELECTION OF FOODS

The texture, temperature, taste, and smell of the foods can enhance the development of more normal oral motor patterns during a feeding program. It is essential that proper nutrition is kept in mind when choosing foods, so that general good health is not compromised for oral motor development [46].

Thickening the consistency of food increases its tactile and proprioceptive qualities, making swallowing more efficient. Food can be thickened by the addition of rice cereals for the young child, and as digestive abilities mature, untoasted wheat germ may be used. When blending table food to a puréed form, less liquid can be added. Liquids can be thickened by adding fruit pulp and sauce to juice and yogurt, and ice milk and cream to milk. The processed sugar content of the additives should be monitored closely and eliminated where possible. Calcium products, including cheese, yogurt, and powdered milk, should be limited in the diet of a child with severe swallowing and drooling problems. Milk and sweetened foods and liquids generally increase salivatory action, making it difficult to effect adequate feeding [46].

By altering the consistency of the food product from a puréed or soft food to a lumpy or hard food, the emphasis of the therapeutic program can be focused on increasing jaw stability and function. Munching and rotary chewing can be enhanced by the introduction of gummy or crunchy foods. Strips of rate beef, cheeses, and dried fruit provide excellent media to stimulate chewing [46]. To reduce the threat of aspiration in children with swallowing difficulty, food items can be wrapped in a small piece of cheese cloth and stabilized by the caregiver as they are held between the chewing surfaces.

As chewing develops, tongue lateralization and cheek activation can be enhanced by introducing foods that may break into many fine pieces as the child chews. Rough cereals, granolas, rice cakes, and crackers provide nutritional alternatives to cookies. If a child has not developed the necessary skill to handle this type of food, a sucking pattern may be elicited, resulting in coughing or choking on larger pieces [46].

Food of varying consistency provides the stimulus for the development of coordinated and integrated oral motor functioning [46]. For example, as the child chews one portion of the item, he or she must swallow another portion, which demands considerable control of the oral pharyngeal system. Coughing and choking can result if the child is not yet demonstrating such oral motor control.

Selection of proper foods can play a large role in normalizing sensitivity to the oral region. The introduction of larger pieces of food reduces the risk of stimulation of a gag reflex [46]. Small pieces of food tend to stimulate various tactile receptors in the mouth, creating an aversive reaction.

ADAPTIVE FEEDING EQUIPMENT

A wide variety of adaptive feeding supplies are available commercially through therapeutic and educational equipment vendors as well as local stores that sell infant and toddler products.

Poor lip closure and sucking difficulties may necessitate the use of a specialized nipple during bottle drinking. A "premie" nipple is soft, there is less resistance to the "milking," suckling motion of the tongue, allowing the child to draw the necessary liquid into the oral cavity before tiring, and thus allowing the development of suck-swallow patterns. Enlarging the hole of a nipple is generally not an accepted practice because it allows more sucking, swallowing, and breathing and increases the risk of aspiration. Ribbed nipples facilitate lip closure and prevent liquid loss from the lateral aspects. The Nuk orthodontic nipple also facilitates lip closure by providing continual tactile stimulation to both lip surfaces. In addition, it has also been found useful in reducing tongue thrust and a bite reflex [46].

Lip closure can also be enhanced with a Tupperware 2-oz cup. The flared lip on the cup provides direct stimulation to the lips, enhancing lateral closure on the cup. In addition, the Tommy-tippy cup with spout cover enhances lip closure and provides an efficient transition from bottle to cup drinking. When tongue thrusting is being inhibited, the Tommy-tippy cup with inserted cover allows the mouth to maintain closure, encouraging tongue-tip elevation with swallowing. When a strong extensor thrust is present, a cut-out cup, available commercially and easily constructed from a soft plastic cup, will enhance the maintenance of a flexed posture (Figure 2-6).

Spoons vary in their size and shape, and the qualities of the spoon should be considered carefully before its use in a therapeutic program. The width should be appropriate in size to the child's mouth to avoid excessive mouth opening for spoon entrance. A spoon with a flat bowl reduces the tendency of a bite reflex and may reduce tongue thrusting and increase lip closure by depressing the spoon bowl on the back and center of the tongue. A bite reflex and temperature hypersensitivity are reduced when a latex-covered spoon is introduced [46]. As the child begins to self-feed, a number of spoons are available, which include a bent spoon, a swivel spoon, a weighted spoon, and a spoon with a built-up handle.

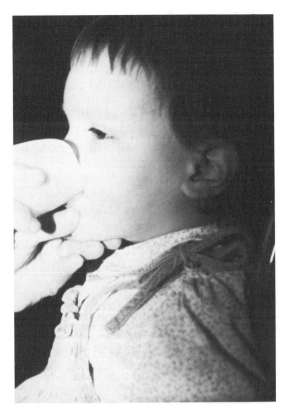

FIG. 2-6. Manual jaw control while drinking from a cut-out cup.

FUNCTIONAL SKILLS

Due to the variety of motor problems a child with CP can exhibit, a functional program must be designed with individual problems and limitations in mind. Additionally, associated problems of vision, hearing, seizures, or intellectual deficits can also influence the program. Some children can control the position of the head and use of their hands, yet others find it impossible. Some may manipulate an object yet not understand its use. The child may be limited to a few inadequate, stereotyped movements that form the basis of new motor learning. Unlike the normal child who can adapt movements, repetition of faulty movements can lead to contractures and deformities in the child with CP.

Finnie [24] describes some general principles of handling the child that apply whether the child is carried, bathed, dressed, or moved in the environment. These principles reinforce an NDT approach to the child's therapy program.

1. Handling the child at key points will make certain movements easier. These key points include the head, neck and spine, shoulder and shoulder girdle, hips and pelvis.
2. Techniques of handling may vary. For example, the spastic child may need to be inhibited, whereas the athetoid or floppy child needs pressure and stability.
3. Emphasis is on symmetry.
4. The therapist must become sensitive to changes in the child's muscle tone.

POSITIONING

Positioning the child to prevent contractures and deformities while facilitating normal movement patterns may require the use of special equipment such as wedges, bolsters, and Tumble Forms. These devices are particularly useful when the child is on the floor, a low mat, or in bed. They enable the child to lie in various positions that are often impossible to assume without some type of support. An example is the use of a side-lying positioner, which enables the hypotonic child to have more control over movement. In such a device, the child rests on one side of the body. This is usually accomplished in such a manner that the child can use the upper extremities. By placing the shoulders and arms well forward, the child can turn the head to the side. In this position the under leg is straight and the leg on the top is in a flexed, slightly forward position.

The prone stander may be used to provide the child with an opportunity to stand with the body in proper alignment. This device allows the child to stand while supporting the knees, trunk, and upper body. Often this is accomplished with the prone board at a 30-degree angle. Some children with good head, neck, and trunk control participate more successfully in upper-extremity activities while positioned in this manner.

SEATING

A major consideration with seating devices is that proper support is provided. For example, if the child lacks head control, care must be taken that the child does not fall forward or to the side, or push against the head rest causing the body to extend. Moreover, while seated the child should maintain appropriate posture. For example, a too soft seat can lead to abnormal posturing. Thus a firm seat insertion of a triangular shape is suggested.

Among the many seating devices available are the Tumble Forms seat, bean bag chair, corner seat, and Rifton chair. Care must be taken, however, that the seating device does not encourage abnormal postures, and that the child changes positions frequently throughout the day.

Trefler [62] recommends seating devices that enable the child's head, neck, trunk, and pelvis to be in midline. Additional recommendations include

1. *Head and neck:* Head rests are useful for hypotonic children who do not demonstrate extensor hypertonicity. Neck collars can be helpful in holding the head in midline with minimal support. They do not facilitate the occipital area, which is a trigger point for extensor tone.

2. *Trunk:* Lateral thoracic supports placed symmetrically can help support floppy children in midline. If the child has a scoliosis, pads can be placed under the apex on the convex side of the curve and high under the axilla on the opposite side. Chest straps can be useful if the child has poor trunk stability.

3. *Pelvis:* Lateral edges on the chair or blocks built into the insert cab help maintain the pelvis in midline. The goal is to stabilize the pelvis in midline, not immobilize. Usually, the hips are flexed 90 degrees to assist in decreasing extensor tone. If an angle less than 90 de-

grees is necessary, the therapist must be careful not to tip the pelvis posteriorly, thus reducing the lumbar curve. A wedge or anterior roll will help maintain the desired hip angle, keep the child well back in the chair, and encourage lower extremity abduction. A lap belt is suggested at a 45-degree angle to the seat base. A lapboard should also be considered for support as well as to allow increased use of the upper extremities.

4. *Low extremities:* Hips, knees, and ankles are usually at 90 degrees. If severe extensor tone is evident, the angle at the hips can be reduced and the ankles placed in slight dorsiflexion. Feet should always be supported.

MOBILITY

Early on the child typically requires a mobility device. Depending on the physical involvement, this may be a pediatric wheelchair, although for the infant an umbrella stroller and for the young child a travel chair are adequate. In more severe cases a Mulholland or similar support chair may be necessary.

A wedged scooter board with abduction triangle can offer mobility and proper positioning for the child with spasticity. In addition, the child can self-propel the device using hands to the floor. Other devices of this type include the Tumble Forms Jettmobile.

The recommendation of a mobility device can be difficult for the parents to accept, as denial can be a coping strategy used to deal with the child's physical handicap. The wheelchair becomes an obvious reminder of the significance of the disability. As the child grows and develops, a standard rehabilitation program continually assesses at timely intervals the child's need of adaptive equipment.

If ambulation is a goal, an assistive device may be recommended by the physical therapist. Often orthopedic surgery is suggested relative to ambulation potential (see Table 2-7), which may result in a recommendation for bracing. When there is increased tone in the lower extremity, a short leg brace may be recommended. This brace consists of a metal bar attached to the shoe, which maintains the foot in dorsiflexion. A strap around the calf is used to hold the brace in place. The popular alternative is the ankle-foot orthosis (AFO), which is a lightweight plastic brace. It is molded to the foot and lower leg and worn inside the shoe. The child is often fitted with AFOs at an early age in the belief that their use will prevent heel cord shortening. Each type of brace requires replacement or adjustment, or both, as the child grows.

SELF CARE

Self-care activities should be encouraged even if the child has limited motor control. Toileting, bathing, and dressing are activities that follow a normal developmental sequence.

Sitting balance and relaxation are often the most significant problems encountered in toilet training a CP child. There are several suggestions to address these problems. The correct type of toilet device, its position, and the child's position help to address the problem with sitting balance. Finnie [24] recommends that a trainer commode be placed on the chair between the parent's knees. The child's back is supported by the parent while the legs are held apart with hips flexed and upper extremities forward. A relaxed position is encouraged with a trainer commode that has good back support and a wide firm base. Commercially made devices, such as the Posture Commode Chair or a commode in a triangle chair, can be used once the child's trunk control and balance improve. A wooden block or stool placed under the feet can help the older child use an ordinary toilet seat and relax the abdominal muscles. A nonskid mat in front of the toilet, toilet paper at the child's height, toilet grab bars, and adapted flush handle are all means to improve the child's independence in toileting.

BATHING

A baby bath that has a slope for back support and a nonskid bath mat are recommended for bathing the baby. Support is required when placing the child in the bath water and when lifting out of the bath to avoid hyperextension of the body. As the child grows, the normal size tub is used with a special tub seat that provides adequate support. Typically, the occupational therapist will try different seats with the child and parents to find the one that meets their particular requirements. Play can be incorporated into bath time by adding floating toys to the water. These toys are often easier for the child to move about and manipulate. To encourage independent bathing as the child grows, the following devices can be helpful: bath mitt, long-handled bath sponge, soap holder, nail brush with suction cups, plastic liquid-soap container, adapted faucet handles, large terry robe, and tub grab rails.

DRESSING

Positioning the child with hips and knees flexed, shoulders raised, and arms forward facilitates the dressing process. When the child is very young, this position is easily adopted by the child lying supine across the parent's lap. As the child grows, it may be easier to dress sitting in a parent's lap or on a table, stool, or floor. This allows the parent to control the child's balance from the back, maintaining the posture mentioned above. This is a good position to see the child and clothing as well as to encourage the child to take part in the activity. The child can also see the clothes in easy reach, which is an important step in developing independence in dressing. Other suggestions for easier dressing include positioning the child symmetrically with hips and knees flexed, shoulders and arms forward, and trunk slightly flexed. This position is quite useful when donning and doffing socks and shoes. Clothes can be put on the more involved arm, leg first. A pillow placed under the head of the child facilitates diaper changing, and side-lying may be a useful position for more mobility and participation.

Children with CP want to wear the same clothing that peers wear. Contemporary designs of children's clothes are suitable for many handicapped children, requiring a minimum of adaptations. In general, shirts, pants, and dresses should be loose fitting with simple or no fastenings. Elastic waist bands are helpful as are Velcro closures. Socks and shoes should fit well, and boots should have a side opening for easy manipulation. The Appendix includes resources for equipment, accessories, clothing, and toys especially designed for children with disabilities.

HAND FUNCTION

Hand function can play a critical role in the child's ability to succeed with activities of daily living. The therapist should pay particular attention to the normal development of hand use. Some therapists find that splints are helpful in preventing deformity and enable increased hand function. A resting pan splint is often recommended, which allows thumb abduction, wrist extension, and functional positioning of the digits.

A wide variety of adaptive devices are available for the disabled child including self-care and writing devices. These are designed to optimize existing function in the hands. The Appendix provides information on the types of devices commercially available and names and addresses of vendors.

EDUCATION

With the institution of Public Law 94-142, all handicapped children are entitled to an education in the least restrictive environment. As Hallahan and Kauffman [28] point out, the educational problems of children with CP are as multifaceted as their handicaps. Some may require special equipment and facilities due to physical limitations, whereas others may need special educational procedures and programs.

Physical handicaps can also affect the cognitive, emotional, and social development of the child. Thus, the educational program must be sensitive to these issues and seek ways to handle the problems posed by physical limitations. This child may require special classes or devices. For example, the use of a nonvocal communication device may be essential to the academic and social success of a child with athetoid CP.

Continuous educational assessment is essential to prevent an underestimation of the child's performance capacity [28]. Additionally, as the child grows, vocational interests should be considered and plans for independent living kept in mind by parents, teachers, and therapists. All must recognize the continually changing needs of the child, who despite physical limitations or slowed development, is growing and developing.

REFERENCES

1. Anderson, R. Early Feeding, Sound Production and Prelinguistic/Cognitive Development. Comprehensive Training Program for Infant and Young Cerebral Palsied Children. Curative Rehabilitation Center, 9001 West Watertown Plank Road, Wauwatosa, WI 53226, 1980.
2. Thomas, A. Chesni, Y., and Saint-Anne Dargassies, S. *The Neurological Examination of the Infant*. Little Club Clinics in Developmental Medicine, No. 1. London: Heinemann, 1960.
3. Batshaw, M. L., and Perrett, Y. M. *Children with Handicaps: A Medical Primer* (2nd ed.). Baltimore: Brookes, 1986.
4. Black, P. D. Ocular defects in children with cerebral palsy. *Br. Med. J.* 281:487, 1980.
5. Bleck, E. E. *Cerebral Palsy: Orthopedic Aspects*. Boston: Pediatric Rehabilitation, Tufts Research and Training Center, 1982.
6. Bly, L. Notes from NDT baby course. New York Hospital, 1980.
7. Bobath, B. *Abnormal Postural Reflex Activity Caused by Brain Lesions*. London: Heinemann, 1965.
8. Bobath, B. The very early treatment of cerebral palsy. *Dev. Med. Child Neurol.* 9(4):373, 1967.
9. Bobath, B. The Neurodevelopmental Approach to Treatment. In P. Pearson and C. Williams (eds.), *Physical Therapy Services in the Developmental Disabilities* (5th ed.). Springfield, IL: Thomas, 1977.
10. Bobath, B. Motor Development and its Application to Treatment and Management of Cerebral Palsy. Lecture, Boston, 1982.
11. Bobath, B. The Concept of Neuro-developmental Treatment. Lecture, Boston, 1982.
12. Bobath, B., and Bobath, K. *Motor Development in the Different Types of Cerebral Palsy* (2nd ed.). London: Heinemann, 1978.

13. Bobath, K. The motor deficit in patients with cerebral palsy. *Clin. Dev. Med.* No. 23, 1966.
14. Bobath, K. The normal postural mechanism and its deviation in children with cerebral palsy. *Physiotherapy* 57:85, 1971.
15. Bobath, K. *A Neurophysiological Basis for the Treatment of Cerebral Palsy* (2nd ed.). Philadelphia: Lippincott, 1980.
16. Bobath, K., and Bobath, B. The facilitation of normal postural reactions and movements in the treatment of cerebral palsy. *Physiotherapy* 50:3, 1964.
17. Bobath, K., and Bobath, B. Student papers (unpublished). London: The Bobath Centre, 1981.
18. Bosma, J. Structure and Function of Infant Oral and Pharyngeal Mechanisms. In J. M. Wilson (ed.), *Oral-Motor Function and Dysfunction in Children*. University of North Carolina at Chapel Hill, Division of Physical Therapy, 1977.
19. Bryce, J. The management of spasticity in children. *Physiotherapy* 62:11, 1976.
20. Cambell, S. Oral Sensorimotor Physiology. In J. M. Wilson (ed.), *Oral-Motor Function and Dysfunction in Children*. University of North Carolina at Chapel Hill, Division of Physical Therapy, 1977.
21. Connor, F. P., Williamson, G. G. and Siepp, T. M. (eds.). *Program Guide for Infants and Toddlers with Neuromotor and Other Developmental Disabilities*. New York: Teachers College, 1978.
22. Denhoff, E. Current status of infant stimulation or enrichment programs for children with developmental disabilities. *Pediatrics* 67:32, 1981.
23. Dichter, M. A. *Seizure Disorders and Epilepsy. Fundamentals of Neurology.* Boston: Massachusetts General Hospital, 1982.
24. Finnie, N. R. *Handling the Young Cerebral Palsied Child at Home* (2nd ed.). New York: Dutton, 1974.
25. Gans, B. *Rehabilitation Management of Cerebral Palsy.* Boston: Pediatric Rehabilitation, Tufts Research and Training Center, 1982.
26. Gesell, A. *The First Five Years of Life.* New York: Harper, 1940.
27. Gesell, A., and Amatruda, G. *Developmental Diagnosis* (2nd ed.). London: Harper, 1981.
28. Hallahan, D. P., and Kauffman, J. M. *Exceptional Children*. Englewood Cliffs, N.J.: Prentice-Hall, 1978.
29. Haynes, U. B. The National Collaborative Infant Project. In T. D. Tjossem (ed.), *Intervention Strategies for High Risk Infants and Young Children*. Baltimore: University Park, 1978.
30. Holt, K. S. Neurological and Neuromuscular Disorders. In S. Gabel and M. T. Erickson (eds.), *Child Development and Developmental Disabilities*. Boston: Little, Brown, 1980.
31. Hoth, A. *The Role of Occupational Therapy in Early Childhood Intervention*. Rockville, MD: American Occupational Therapy Association, 1981.
32. Illingworth, R. *The Development of the Infant and Young Child, Normal and Abnormal*. London: Livingstone, 1960.
33. Keats, S. *Cerebral Palsy*. Springfield, IL: Thomas, 1965.
34. Levine, M.S. Cerebral palsy diagnosis in children over age 1 year: Standard criteria. *Arch. Phys. Med. Rehabil.* 61:9, 1980.
35. Little, W. On the influence of abnormal parturition, difficult labours, premature birth, and asphyxia neonatorum on the mental and physical condition of the child, especially in relation to deformities. *Trans. Obstet. Soc. London.* 3:293, 1861.
36. Low, N. L. Cerebral palsy. *Med. Clin.* 56, (6):1972.
37. Magnus, R. some results of studies in the physiology of posture. *Lancet* 2:531, 1926.
38. McGraw, M. *The Neuromuscular Maturation of the Human Infant.* New York: Columbia University Press, 1943.
39. Menkes, J. H. *Textbook of Child Neurology* (2nd ed.). Philadelphia: Lea & Febiger, 1980.
40. Morris, S. E. Differential Diagnosis of Sucking, Swallowing, Biting and Chewing. In M. M. Palmer (ed.), *The Normal Acquisition of Oral Feeding Skills*. New York: Therapeutic Media, 1982.
41. Morris, S. E. Feeding Patterns of the Normal Infant. In M. M. Palmer (ed.), *The Normal Acquisition of Oral Feeding Skills*. New York: Therapeutic Media, 1982.
42. Morris, S. E. Oral-Motor Development: Normal and Abnormal. In J. M. Wilson (ed.), *Oral-Motor Function and Dysfunction in Children*. University of North Carolina at Chapel Hill, Division of Physical Therapy, 1977.
43. Morris, S. E. Overview of the Anatomy and Physiology of the Oral Pharyngeal Mechanism. In M. M. Palmer (ed.), *The Normal Acquisition of Oral Feeding Skills*. New York: Therapeutic Media, 1982.
44. Morris, S. E. Principals of Oral-Motor Assessment. In J. M. Wilson (ed.), *Oral-Motor Function and Dysfunction in Children*. University of North Carolina at Chapel Hill, Division of Physical Therapy, 1977.
45. Morris, S. E. *Program Guidelines for Children*

with Feeding Problems. Edison, NJ: Child Craft Education, 1977.

46. Morris, S. E. Selection of Food and Equipment for Effective Feeding Therapy. In J. M. Wilson (ed.), *Oral-Motor Function and Dysfunction in Children.* University of North Carolina at Chapel Hill, Division of Physical Therapy, 1977.

47. Rademaker, G. *Reactions Labyrinthiques et Equilibre.* Paris: Masson et Cie, 1935.

48. Radtka, S. Feeding Reflexes and Neural Control. In J. M. Wilson (ed.), *Oral-Motor Function and Dysfunction in Children.* University of North Carolina at Chapel Hill, Division of Physical Therapy, 1977.

49. Robinson, R. O. The frequency of other handicaps in children with cerebral palsy. *Dev. Med. Child Neurol.* 15:305, 1973.

50. Salek, B. *Normal Motor Development as a Base for Normal Respiration and Prespeech Function. Physiological Aspects of Prespeech and Language Development.* Baltimore: University of Maryland Medical School. Department of Physical Therapy, 1975.

51. Sandow, S., and Clark, A. *Home Intervention with Parents of Severely Subnormal Preschool Children: An Interim Report.* Boston: Blackwell, Child and Health Care Development 4, 1978.

52. Schain, R. J. *Neurology of Childhood Learning Disorders* (2nd ed.), Baltimore: Williams & Wilkins, 1977.

53. Schaltenbrand, G. The development of human motility and motor disturbances. *Arch. Neurol. Psych.* 18:944, 1927.

54. Scherzer, A. L., and Tscharnuter, I. *Early Diagnosis and Therapy in Cerebral Palsy.* New York: Dekker, 1982.

55. Schilling, M., Siepp, J., and Patterson, E. *The First Three Years: Programming for Atypical Infants and Their Families.* New York: United Cerebral Palsy Associates, 1974.

56. Simeonsson, R. J., Cooper, D. H., and Scheiner, A. P. A review and analysis of the effectiveness of early intervention programs. *Pediatrics* 69:5, 1982.

57. Simeonsson, R. J., and Wiegerink, R. Accountability: a dilemma in infant intervention. *Except. Child.* 41:474, 1975.

58. Singer, W. *Cerebral Palsy: Neurological Aspects.* Boston: Pediatric Rehabilitation, Tufts Research and Training Center, 1983.

59. Smith, M. H., Connelly, B. Mcfadden, S., et al. *Feeding Management of a Child with a Handicap: A Guide for Professionals.* University of Tennessee Center for the Health Sciences, Child Development Center, Memphis, Tennessee, 38105, 1982.

60. Stainback, S. B., and Healy, H. A. *Teaching Eating Skills.* Springfield, IL: Thomas, 1982.

61. Tjossem, T. D. Early intervention: Issues and Approaches. In T. D. Tjossem (ed.), *Intervention Strategies for High Risk Infants and Young Children.* Baltimore: University Park, 1978.

62. Trefler, E. Seating systems for children with cerebral palsy. *Rx Home Care* 41, 1984.

63. Walshe, F. On certain tonic or postural reflexes in hemiplegia with special references to so-called associated movements. *Brain* 46:1, 1923.

64. Weisz, S. Studies in equilibrium reactions. *J. Nerv. Ment. Dis.* 88:153, 1938.

SUGGESTED READING

GENERAL

Amiel-Tison, C., and Gremer, A. *Neurologic Evaluation of the Newborn and the Infant.* New York: Masson, 1983.

Berk, R. A., and DeGangi, G. A. Technical consideration in the evaluation of pediatric motor scales. *Am. J. Occup. Ther.* 33(4):240, 1979.

Cattell, P. *Cattell Infant Intelligence Scale.* New York: Psychological Corp., 1960.

Dubowitz, I. M. S., Dubowitz, V., and Goldberg, C. Clinical assessment of gestational age in the newborn infant. *J. Pediatr.* 77:1, 1970.

Egan, D. F., Illingworth, R. S., and Mackeith, R. C. *Development screening 0–5 years. Clin. Dev. Med.* No. 30. London: Spastics International Medical in association with Heinemann, 1979.

Fiorentino, M. *Reflex Testing Methods for Evaluating CNS Development.* Springfield, IL: Thomas 1973.

Hiskey, M. S. *Manual: Hiskey-Nebraska Test of Learning Aptitude.* Lincoln: University of Nebraska Press, 1966.

Kearsley, R. Cognitive assessment of the handicapped infant: the need for an alternative approach. *Am. J. Orthopsychiatry* 52:43, 1981.

Kearsley, R., and Sigel, I. (eds.). *Infants at Risk: Assessment of Cognitive Functioning.* Hillsdale: N. J. Erlbaum, 1979.

Koontz, C. *Koontz Child Development Program.* Los Angeles: Western Psychological, 1974.

Pless, I. B. Clinical assessment: physical and psychological functioning. *Pediatr. Clin. North Am.* 31(1):33, 1984.

Simeonsson, R. J., and Huntington, G. S. *A Multivariate Approach to Plan and Evaluate Child Progress.* Chapel Hill: University of North Carolina, 1980.

EARLY INTERVENTION

Bagnato, S. J., and Neisworth, J. T. The intervention efficiency index: an approach to preschool program accountability. *Except. Child.* 46:4, 1980.

Bricker, D. Dow, M. Early intervention with the young, severely handicapped child. *JASH* 5(2):130, 1980. *Sci.* 1:4,

Browder, J. A. The pediatrician's orientation to infant stimulation programs. *Pediatrics* 67:1, 1981.

Brown, C. C. (ed.). *Infants at Risk: Assessment and Intervention—An Update for Health Care Professionals and Parents.* Boston: Summar, Johnson & Johnson, 1981.

Field, T. M. (ed.). *Infants Born at Risk: Behavior and Development.* New York: SP Medical and Scientific, Spectrum, 1979.

NEURODEVELOPMENTAL TREATMENT

Bly, L. *The Components of Normal and Abnormal Movement During the First Year of Life.* Proceedings from Development of Movement in Infants, May 1980. Division of Physical Therapy, University of North Carolina, Chapel Hill, N.C., 1981.

ORAL MOTOR SKILLS

Bosma, J. F. *Fourth Symposium on Oral Sensation and Perception.* Bethesda: National Institutes of Health, 1973.

Bosma, J. F. *Second Symposium on Oral Sensation and Perception.* Springfield, IL: Thomas, 1970.

Bosma, J. F. *Symposium on Oral Sensation and Perception.* Springfield, IL: Thomas, 1967.

Bosma, J. F. *Third Symposium on Oral Sensation and Perception.* Springfield, IL: Thomas, 1972.

Fisher, S. E., Painter, M., and Milmoe, G. Swallowing disorders in infancy. *Pediatr. Clin. North Am.* 28:4, 1981.

Hanson, M. L. Toward more effective therapy for tongue thrust. *Int. J. Orthod.* 19:3, 1981.

Lebowitz, J. M., and Holcer, P. Building and maintaining self feeding skills in a retarded child. *Am. J. Occup. Ther.* 28:9, 1974.

McClannahan, C. *Feeding and Caring for Infants and Children with Special Needs.* Rockville, MD: American Occupational Therapy Association, 1987.

McCracken, A. Drool control and tongue thrust therapy for the mentally retarded. *Am. J. Occup. Ther.* 32:2, 1978.

Moore, J. *Oral-Facial Development and Function.* Vermillion, SD: Department of Anatomy, University of South Dakota, School of Medicine, 1981.

Stratton, M. Behavioral assessment scale of oral functions in feeding. *Am. J. Occup. Ther.* 35:11, 1981.

CHAPTER 3

Mental Retardation

Judith D. Ward

Mental retardation is a condition associated with a variety of social, psychological, and physical factors, which may be the cause or the result of the retardation.

The most widely used definition of mental retardation is that of the American Association on Mental Deficiency (AAMD): "Mental retardation refers to significantly subaverage general intellectual functioning existing concurrently with deficits in adaptive behavior, and manifested during the developmental period" [17].

An individual is not considered to have *significantly subaverage general intellectual functioning* unless his or her IQ score is more than two standard deviations below the mean for the test. The AAMD describes *adaptive behavior* as "the effectiveness or degree with which an individual meets the standards of personal independence and social responsibility expected for age and cultural group" [17].

Mental retardation is found in 1 [1] to 3 percent [11] of the population and is twice as common in males as in females [1]. There are many causes of retardation (Table 3-1). At least 80 percent of retarded individuals are only mildly retarded, and for most of these the cause is unknown; the more severe cases are less prevalent, and their causes usually are known [25].

TABLE 3-1. American Association of Mental Deficiency (AAMD) Medical Classification

Major categories of etiology*
  Infections and intoxications
  Trauma and physical agent
  Metabolism or nutrition
  Gross brain disease (postnatal)
  Unknown prenatal influence
  Chromosomal abnormality
  Gestational disorders
  Following psychiatric disorder
  Environmental influences
  Other conditions
Additional medical information*
  Genetic component
  Secondary cranial anomaly
  Impairment of special senses
  Disorders of perception and expression
  Convulsive disorders
  Psychiatric impairment
  Motor dysfunction

* More specific subdivisions are listed under each category. Source: Adapted from H. J. Grossman (ed.). *Manual on Terminology and Classification in Mental Retardation (1977 revision)*. Washington, DC: AAMD, 1977.

EARLY IDENTIFICATION AND RISK FACTORS

Some children can be identified as mentally retarded at birth. Those with cerebral malformations, craniofacial anomalies, and meningoencephalocele have obvious indications. Certain chromosomal abnormalities, such as Down's syndrome, are associated with varying degrees of mental retardation and present characteristic physical symptoms: epicanthal folds, protruding tongue, broad bridged nose, muscular hypotonia, and, often, congenital heart disease [17].

Some children are considered at risk for retardation because of *biomedical factors:*

Maternal infectious diseases, particularly during the first trimester of pregnancy
Pregnant mother's intoxication due to drugs, alcohol, or exposure to other chemicals
Premature birth or low birth weight (less than 5 lb, 8 oz)
Difficult birth
Low APGAR score

Infants may also be considered at risk for retardation because of *environmental factors*. The AAMD attributes mental retardation to environmental factors if the child shows retardation in the absence of organic disease coupled with adverse environmental conditions [17].

A common form of environmental deprivation is due to psychosocial disadvantage, which is associated with poverty and all its ills—inadequate diet and medical care, poor housing [17], neglect. The AAMD specifies that there must be "evidence of subnormal intellectual functioning in at least one of the parents and in one or more siblings" to identify retardation due to psychosocial disadvantage [17]. Although this criterion would seem to restrict candidates for this classification, about 75 percent of retarded individuals in the United States come from socioeconomically deprived homes [9], most are mildly retarded, and most are being raised by at least one parent who is intellectually subnormal [30]. In the preliminary study for the Milwaukee Project, a program from the 1960s often used as a model of intervention in cases of retardation due to psychosocial deprivation, it was found that in one sample, 45 percent of the mothers were responsible for nearly 80 percent of the children with IQs below 80, that the mothers themselves had IQs of 80 or below, and that their children showed a decline in IQ from normal to retarded between infancy and maturity. Children of mothers with the same sociocultural background but higher IQs did not show the same decline [14].

See Early Intervention in Chapter 2 for a full discussion of early intervention and the team members involved.

CLASSIFICATION

The most common system of classifying mental retardation is by IQ scores. Educators use a classification system based on the educational level the child can be expected to achieve. The AAMD suggests a dual approach for classification using a biomedical system, which classifies retardation according to etiology and other medical information (see Table 3-1), and a behavioral system, which classifies individuals according to their measured intelligence and adaptive behavior.

Intelligence tests and *adaptive behavior scales* are tests and scales that measure different kinds of skills: IQ tests measure the individual's *potential for academic achievement,* while adaptive behavior scales measure *current everyday coping skills.*

The IQ test is given in a controlled environment; it should be administered individually, not in a group situation, by a person who has been specifically trained to use that test and who has been supervised in its use with the retarded [17]. The test should be standardized for the age of the child. Intelligence testing is a controversial issue. Some argue that intelligence tests are culturally biased against ethnic minorities [30]; others claim that a single IQ score is viewed as a "sacred permanent quantity" used to label people [11, p. 54]. However, when properly administered and when all behavioral correlates are considered, standard intelligence tests are the most efficient and reliable means of predicting academic success [30].

Adaptive behavior is usually obtained by interviewing a third party who knows the child's typical behavior. Deficits in adaptive behavior are reflected in different areas for different age groups [17]:

During infancy and early childhood in:
Sensory motor skills dvelopment
Communication skills (including speech and language)
Self-help skills
Socialization (development of ability to interact with others)
During childhood and early adolescence in:
Application of basic academic skills in daily life activities
Application of appropriate reasoning and judgment in mastery of the environment
Social skills (participation in group activities and interpersonal relationships)

During late adolescence and adult life in:
Vocational and social responsibilities and performances [17]

Since 1961, when the AAMD included adaptive behavior in its definition of mental retardation, there has been a push to develop instruments to measure it. There are now over 100 adaptive behavior scales in use. (For information on the AAMD Adaptive Behavior Scale, see the Test Appendix in Chapter 5.) Some scales include norms, some cover a wide variety of behaviors, and others concentrate on specifics such as school-related behavior. Many scales include maladaptive behavior because such behavior interferes with the child's integration into community life [32] and because it is important to know what the child is doing when not engaged in activities that show positive adaptation [28]. The populations for which the scales are intended are diverse, ranging from the severely or profoundly retarded, to the moderately (trainable) or mildly (educable) retarded, to even the learning disabled [32].

Most adaptive behavior scales obtain information from a third party, but a few require direct observations of the child [32]. Most include the following domains:

1. Self-help skills
2. Physical development
3. Communication skills
4. Cognitive functioning
5. Domestic and occupational activities
6. Self-direction and responsibility
7. Socialization

The measurement of adaptive behavior is less refined than that of intelligence, but the value of adaptive behavior scales is that they provide a description of current, typical functioning, which can be used in developing programs for the individual. They also provide a baseline against which progress can be measured and programming can be evaluated [32].

Generally, retardation is divided into four levels of severity [1, 9]:

LEVELS	INTELLIGENCE QUOTIENT	EDUCATIONAL CATEGORY
Mild	50–70	Educable
Moderate	35–49	Trainable
Severe	20–34	Dependent
Profound	<20	Life support

Mild retardation is the most common form. These children can be expected to acquire some academic skills and the life skills necessary to live independently [38]. As adults, they will be able to assume responsibility for routine personal care, carrying on everyday conversation, using the telephone, and writing simple letters. Socially, they are able to cooperate with others and compete in recreational games, and they will be able to belong to social groups and undertake hobbies that do not require complex planning. They can engage in simple or semi-skilled jobs, perform everyday household activities, and assume routine responsibilities. They need guidance in money management although they can be expected to learn to make change. And they will need help in health care and care of others [17].

Moderately retarded individuals are considered trainable. They can develop skills in hygiene, feeding, toileting, and communication. They can learn homemaking and home maintenance skills, although they cannot be expected to achieve social or economic independence [38]. Academic skills are minimal, and instruction is concerned with recognizing words. They can converse and cooperate with others and they may show initiative in their own activities [17].

Severe mental retardation may be associated with physical handicaps. With training, these children can learn simple self-care tasks and some communication skills [38]. They can participate in simple group activities and may carry out short-term household responsibilities [17].

Profound mental retardation is frequently associated with physical handicaps, and these children are often nonambulatory. Their self-help skills are poor, but they may try to help

feed, dress, and bathe themselves. Toilet training is a problem. They may understand simple commands and have some verbal or nonverbal communication skills. Some can participate in simple expressive activities and games [17].

EDUCATION

Public schools have become central in the education, treatment, and training of mentally retarded children since the institution of Public Law 94-142. This law provides handicapped children with access to appropriate, free public education from the ages of 3 to 21 years [24]; it gives the schools these reponsibilities: (1) locating and identifying mentally retarded children, (2) evaluating them for appropriate educational placement and program planning, and (3) developing an individualized educational plan to meet the child's needs. All planning must include the parents, and the services of a variety of professionals must be available through the schools.

Most parents of mentally retarded children and the professionals who work with them consider the legislation regarding "mainstreaming" a positive step in integrating retarded people of all ages into community life. However, the implications are enormous. First, the label of mental retardation says nothing about the degree of intellectual impairment of a specific chid. The difference between a mildly retarded child and his or her "normal" peers may be much less than the difference between the mildly retarded and the severely retarded child. The appropriate educational placement of the child depends more on the severity of retardation than on the general label of mental retardation.

A second consideration in educational placement of retarded children is their physical, medical, and communication problems. Some children require environmental modifications to account for their visual or hearing deficits, their mobility problems or special medical needs. Public Law 94-142 calls for handicapped children to be educated with nonhandicapped children to the "maximum extent appropriate" in the "regular eductional environment" unless their handicap is so severe that "education in regular classes with the use of supplementary aids and services cannot be achieved satisfactorily" [24]. Although the more severely retarded children tend to have the most physically handicapping conditions, it is quite possible for a mildly retarded child to have major physical problems. Is the mildly retarded, physically handicapped child to be placed in an educational setting based on intellectual potential, or will the need for an adapted physical environment become the most critical factor in placement?

A third consideration in educational placement is the child's social adaptation to school. Some believe that even mildly retarded children should be trained in classroom behavior before they are integrated into regular classes, to prevent rejection by their nonhandicapped peers and teachers [15].

Mentally retarded children benefit from *early education;* the goal is to provide the developmental stimulation that serves as a precursor for learning, and to provide remedial educational programs to prevent the pattern of failure that occurs in children whose needs are not met [22].

PRESCHOOL SCREENING

The first task of the schools is locating and identifying children who need special education services. Some children are referred by community agencies or medical professionals, but the majority of educationally handicapped children must be detected by the schools. Most school systems use developmental screening procedures to screen all children of kindergarten age [22], since delays in language, social, and motor development provide the first clues to educational problems (see Test Appendix in Chapter 5). For children who show developmental lags there must be sufficient time available to do further diagnostic testing and program planning before the child is placed in an education program.

ASSESSMENT FOR INDIVIDUALIZED EDUCATION PLAN

Publically funded schools are required by law to develop an *individualized education plan* (IEP), which must be in place before the child can receive special education or other services [3]. The IEP must include the following [3]:

The present level of educational performance

Specific educational services to be provided

Projected date for initiation and anticipated direction of services

Statement of appropriate objective criteria and evaluation procedures

Method of determining, at least annually, whether instructional objectives are being met

The *initial educational assessment* addresses the child's present educational level and a behavioral or psychoeducational profile. It also includes physical and social factors as well as academic skills [21] and is done by an interdisciplinary team, which may include a psychologist; nurse; audiologist; and speech, occupational, and physical therapists; in addition to the teacher. Information is gained through several sources: tests and observations, school records and other records, and interviews with parents [40]. The following are the specific areas to be assessed [29, 40]:

I. Sensory motor domain
  A. Sensory reception and acuity
    1. Vision
    2. Hearing
  B. Perception
    1. Visual
    2. Auditory
    3. Other
  C. Motor ability
    1. Gross and fine motor skills
    2. Locomotion
    3. Manipulation
    4. Activity level

II. Speech and language skills
   A. Reception
   B. Expression
   C. Nonverbal
III. Psychological domain
   A. Adaptive behavior
   B. Motivation
   C. Attention
   D. Organization
   E. Interpersonal skills
   F. Cultural factors
IV. Cognition
   A. Intelligence
   B. Cognitive processes
 V. Educational skills
   A. Achievement in subject areas
   B. Learning style

The child's *current level of functioning* and the child's *learning style* are two general areas that must be assessed for program planning. Current functioning is assessed through IQ tests and adaptive behavior scales (discussed earlier in the chapter); educational achievement tests, which identify strengths and deficits in academic content; and sensory, motor, and cognitive development tests, which assess current skills in those areas (see Test Appendix in Chapter 5).

Identifying the child's learning style is more complex than identifying what to teach. Although IQ tests suggest certain levels of potential achievement, the identification of deficits does not identify learning potential, and success depends on the use of teaching strategies that are meaningful to the child. Things that should be considered include environmental factors, motivation, responses to instruction, behavior, and communication [19, 23]

EDUCATIONAL SETTINGS AND GOALS

By law, handicapped children are to be educated with nonhandicapped children to the maximum extent appropriate [24]. The options for educating retarded children in public school range from full-time attendance in regular class-

rooms to full-time attendance in self-contained special education classrooms. Between these extremes are various combinations of settings geared to the needs of the individual child: the child can spend most of their time in regular classrooms with the help of a resource teacher for special needs [25], or he or she may attend special classrooms for academic subjects and be integrated with other children for art, music, or physical education.

MILDLY RETARDED (EDUCABLE) CHILDREN

The controversy of regular classrooms versus self-contained classrooms is most heated with regard to the mildly retarded child. The issues involved are not merely academic. Proponents of self-contained classrooms argue that the teacher is specially trained to work with handicapped students, and the material and methods can be geared to special needs. The children can receive more individual attention, they will not suffer from being compared with nonretarded children, and they will not interfere with the learning of nonretarded children [20]. The arguments against self-contained classrooms are that mildly retarded children have not been proven to do better in self-contained classes. Teachers in special classes may have lower expectations of their students, and self-contained classes may become dumping grounds for difficult children. Self-contained classes reinforce stereotypes held by nonretarded children and perpetuate social isolation. They also tend to separate children racially and ethnically [20]. Instruction for all children in regular classes is currently more individualized and can accommodate slow learners.

In elementary school, the educational goals of mildly retarded children are similar to those for nonretarded children [20], and probably the best setting is attendance in regular classrooms with supplemental help from special education teachers and other professionals. Ingalls [20] claims that this gives the child the benefit of being with nonretarded peers while still receiving the needed special instruction. Because other children with special needs (learning disabled, physically handicapped) would be receiving help from specialists, the retarded child would not be stigmatized.

In higher elementary school grades and in junior high school, the educational goals for the mildly retarded diverge more from those of the nonretarded, becoming more technical with a vocational orientation. The children can be integrated for music, physical education, industrial arts, and home economics [25]. In any setting, retarded children learn best in small classes with individualized instruction [30].

The educational goals for the educable retarded child are to enhance social competence, develop personal adequacy, and teach occupational skills [30]. Academically, the mildly retarded child can be expected to gain basic, practical reading skills [38]; the emphasis in math is on calculation for money management and telling time [20]. The development of communication skills includes simple writing, conversing, and using the telephone. The mildly retarded person can be expected to learn personal care, the preparation of simple meals, household tasks, and independent travel in a familiar environment [25]. Vocational training for semiskilled jobs is an important goal of education. This includes the social skills necessary to work with others. Finally, the ability to use leisure time in a way that is satisfying is important for the quality of life of the retarded individual.

The educable retarded child may have physical, speech, language, and behavioral problems. Although mildly retarded children are less likely to have associated physical problems, they can have perceptual motor immaturity or dysfunction. These children benefit from a physical education program greared to their needs. Occupational or physical therapists can provide developmental programs of gross motor or sensory integrative activities, and speech therapists work with tongue control and articulation problems.

Disadvantaged children may not have been encouraged to develop verbal communication skills: Their vocabularies may be limited, and they may have learned poor articulation and grammar [20]. These children need stimulation of expressive and receptive language and encouragement in expressing ideas [20]. Children from families that devote most of their energies to basic survival may not have learned to value education. Their parents may seem apathetic about school performance, distrust school personnel, or feel incompetent to deal with their child's problems. Some children exhibit behavior problems, are indifferent to learning, and are likely to become school dropouts before they have acquired adequate academic or vocational skills [35].

The social skills of mentally retarded children are important to their adjustment in school. It was believed that mentally retarded children would be less stigmatized in regular classes than in self-contained classes. Gottlieb [15] says that educable retarded children are not more accepted by their peers in regular classrooms, perhaps because of "behavior that violates group norms." Budoff [8] observed the behavior of handicapped (including retarded) and nonhandicapped children in regular classrooms and found that the behavior of handicapped children was different from that of their nonhandicapped peers. The handicapped children were more frequently at the periphery of group activities, and they had fewer conversations. When working alone, they emitted more noises and made more "strange movements and gestures" than nonhandicapped children. Older children made fewer noises than younger children, but they maintained a high level of irrelevant movements and gestures [8]. Gottlieb [15] suggests that retarded children need training in classroom behavior prior to attending regular class. "It may be too late to train EMR children's behavior once they are integrated into regular classes because considerable research data suggests that first impression form easily and are durable" [15].

Moderately Retarded (Trainable) Children

Although the trainable child can learn at home, school experiences are desirable because teachers have more continuity of observation and can do a better assessment than a professional who sees the child briefly to develop a home program. School gives the child new social experiences, and it takes some of the burden off the parents, who might otherwise have to institutionalize the child [34].

The educational goals for the trainable mentally retarded child are to achieve maximum independence in self care and to promote social adjustment in a supervised environment [38]. Most feel, however, that the moderately retarded child who has physical handicaps and deficits in toileting and self-care skills, does not benefit from placement in the regular classroom [24, 28, 43]. Self-contained classes are more appropriate. Other training settings are special day school, 5-day boarding schools, home-based programs [38], or residential facilities.

Early educational programs for moderately retarded children involve helping them learn things that their normal peers learn easily at home [38]. The three-year-old moderately retarded children will probably not be toilet trained but will be ready to begin [25]. They feed themselves, messily, and their vocabulary may be quite limited, although they can communicate with gestures [25]. The child who is not physically handicapped can walk at this age, but may have trouble with stairs [25]. Many of the children have physical, sensory, and perceptual handicaps.

The education and training of the trainable child require the services of many child development specialists. The child's developmental delays may be due to intelligence, maturational lag, perceptual deficits, lack of experience, or lack of language stimulation, and all these areas need attention. Occupational, physical, and speech therapists address the delays in perceptual motor and language development. The specialist in early childhood education provides an environment that will stimulate social and cognitive development [11]. Physical activities that provide the opportunity to explore the environment are important at this stage. Toilet training and training in feeding and dressing are part of the preschool curriculum [25], but equally important, is learning to get along with others.

During elementary school years, the focus continues on the development of language, sensorimotor training, practical self-care skills [20], and social skills. Later, skills in practical reading and some use of money may be developed. These children cannot be expected to live independently in the community. However, with proper training, they can perform unskilled jobs with supervision and be useful members of a family.

Severely and Profoundly Retarded Children

Severely and profoundly retarded children have the right to public education, although the severity of their problems, both physical and intellectual, may preclude them from the regular classroom. Educational programs are usually in either a special school or a special program within the regular school. The student-teacher ratio should be lower, and there is greater need for ancillary personnel within the school. Teachers who have been trained to work with non-handicapped children cannot be expected to shoulder full responsiblity for teaching handicapped children. Special education teachers; speech, occupational, and physical therapists; and nurses are very important. These children have more medical problems than the mildly or moderately retarded children, and they need intensive training in language, motor skills, and activities of daily living (45). Teachers and other staff must be able to deal with behavior problems, seizures, and dependency. The environment must be free of architectural barriers because just transporting these children to school is a major undertaking.

Programs for severe and profoundly retarded students are not as specific as those for educable and trainable students [30]. In addition to sensorimotor development, developing skills to increase independence is more important. Basic self-care skills such as toileting and feeding are necessary. Helping the children become as mobile as possible increases independence and provides wider horizons for them to explore. The goal for some children may be to prepare them for classes for the trainable retarded [30].

TEACHING/LEARNING

Whether one is an occupational therapists working in a child development center, a speech therapist in a speech and hearing clinic, or a teacher in the public schools, a knowledge of how mentally retarded children learn is critical. There are certain learning characteristics that mentally retarded people share, to varying degrees, depending on the extent of retardation. They are slow to learn and have memory impairments. They have trouble with abstract concepts, and they often will not use skills learned in one setting in other situations.

MEMORY AND REHEARSAL STRATEGIES

Memory involves the ability to attend to stimuli, process and store information, and recall that information for use. Rehearsal strategies are employed in processing information. A simple repetition of information will hold it in short-term memory, but to hold information in long-term memory, a more elaborate rehearsal strategy is needed. Information is organized, classified, grouped into categories, and associated with past experiences in order to be stored in long-term memory [27].

Mentally retarded individuals lack rehearsal strategies. Lawson [27] calls the mentally retarded "passive processors of information." They "do not group items for rehearsal, rehearse less frequently than normals, and they are less flexible in apportioning the time which is available to them for rehearsal" [27].

Mildly retarded individuals can be trained to use rehearsal strategies [27, 26], and they can

retain mnemonic strategies for performing a task if it is the same as the training task. However, they have problems generalizing these strategies to new tasks [26]. To help retarded learners remember, teaching materials and tasks should be meaningful and interesting to them. The materials can be organized into small chunks of information that can be repeated over time. The learner can also be helped to make verbal associations and learn rehearsal strategies.

GENERALIZATION OF LEARNING

Generalization of learning is evident when skills acquired in one setting are used in other situations [7]. Teachers and therapists want retarded children to use the skills they learn in a variety of settings. Math is taught so they can handle money. Children learn social behaviors that will help them get along with their peers or enable them to be accepted by employers. If children do not use the skills they are taught, or if their behavior depends on very specific cues (stimuli), then generalization of learning has not occurred.

There are teaching strategies that help foster generalization. One must consider the stimuli involved in learning a specific skill: the setting, the teaching methods, and the teacher. Teaching a skill in a variety of settings encourages less dependence on a specific environment. More than one teacher, using a variety of teaching methods, encourages the use of newly learned behavior in response to varied stimuli.

Behavior that is reinforced will be repeated. Transfer of learning is more likely if reinforcements are used that occur naturally in the child's environment. If reinforcement of a behavior is unlikely to occur in the child's natural environment, the use of intermittent or delayed reinforcement encourages the use of desired behavior in settings where it is not automatically reinforced. Baer and Stokes [4] describe teaching institutionalized individuals to ask for approval from the staff, an example of teaching the learner to seek out reinforcement.

Sometimes the natural environment needs to

be modified to provide reinforcement of newly learned behavior. Children who have learned to button their coats at school should be allowed to do this at home, too.

VARIABLES IN LEARNING

A number of variables affect learning: maturation, attention, motivation, language, and reinforcement.

Maturation is the individual's developmental level. Mentally retarded individuals experience delays in development in one or more domains: sensorimotor, cognitive, social, and language. Those who work with retarded children need a strong background knowledge in child development. This is not just to identify the retarded child's developmental level. Teachers and therpists must know when the child is ready to learn a particular skill. For instance, neuromotor development provides the foundation on which all other skills are built. Trying to teach cognitive, social, or langugage skills without consideration of sensorimotor skills is futile.

Attention is "the process by which an individual receives and processes information about the environment" [39]. It involves scanning stimuli, responding to those stimuli that are most important, and inhibiting responses to the irrelevant [7]. Thus, attention involves perception and discrimination of stimuli. Mentally retarded children are easily distracted [7]. One of the reasons it takes them longer to learn is because they attend to irrelevant dimensions of the task. They seem to be unable to discriminate between relevant and irrelevant stimuli. If they are helped to focus on relevant stimuli, their performance improves [41]. Attention also improves when a novel stimulus is introduced. Just like the rest of us, retarded children become more alert and attentive when something new and different occurs.

Attention is also affected by expectation. Retarded people expect to fail, and their lack of attention, in some circumstances, may be avoidance of a task that they believe they will fail to accomplish [25].

Therapists and teachers can help children overcome attention problems by

1. Teaching new skills in an environment free of extraneous stimuli [25]
2. Using relevant, novel stimuli to gain attention and speed up learning [25]
3. Drawing attention to important aspects of the task and giving auditory, tactile, and visual cues [7]
4. Grading tasks for the amount of stimuli, at first, presenting only small bits of information (stimuli), gradually introducing more elements [25]
5. Organizing material (stimuli) into meaningful parts and teaching the child to make associations between similar bits of information [25]
6. Rewarding attention to relevant stimuli [25]

"A motivated person wants something" [44] *Motivation* results from a drive to meet a need. It has been said that retarded people lack motivation. Actually they lack motivation to do certain things under certain conditions.

Mentally retarded people experience many failures, and one of the biggest stumbling blocks in learning new skills is their expectation of failure [25]. They avoid new situations and situations where they have previously failed [25]. It has been found that retarded children in mainstream classes have lower expectations of success than retarded children in special classes, and retarded children are more anxious than their nonretarded peers, which interferes with motivation and learning [5].

When teaching retarded children, the chances of failure are less if the activities are graded so that the first steps are easy, and the difficulty of the task is gradually increased. This gives the child a chance to gain confidence and decreases anxiety in new situations [25].

Trust and confidence in the teacher influences motivation for learning. Children whose retardation is due to social deprivation do not trust adults. Balla and Zigler [5] report that they have both a "a heightened motivation to interact with supportive adults and a wariness to do so." Winning the child's trust is no easy task, but the teacher who is associated with successful experiences is more likely to be trusted.

Retarded children are less intrinsically motivated than children of average intelligence [5, 30]. They are more likely to work for tangible rewards than for their own feeling of accomplishment. Tangible reinforcement heightens motivation because these children are externally oriented, the use of other children as role models of desired behavior enhances motivation and learning [25].

Language is central to learning. It provides a system of symbols to help us learn about things that are not physically present and observable [7]. Even educable children have inadequate language skills. Their vocabularies are limited, and their speech is repetitive and stereotyped [20].

The development of language skills is important for the development of cognitive skills. Since written language skills are not highly developed in retarded people, it is especially important for them to develop good oral language [20]. They need help with articulation, vocabulary, and grammar. All who work with them need to encourage them to express ideas verbally [20].

Because retarded children are extrinsically motivated, tangible rewards are used to *reinforce learning*. Immediate reinforcement is often necessary because if rewards are delayed, irrelevant aspects of the task may inadvertently be reinforced. Behavior modification is extensively used in teaching the mentally retarded person.

BEHAVIOR MODIFICATION

Many retarded children do not acquire incidental learning from being exposed to information. Each skill must be specifically taught. They have trouble with generalization of learning, and one cannot assume that they are motivated to learn [20]. They are less flexible than other children in their approach to tasks and do not adapt easily to changes. Retarded children respond best to concrete teaching materials. For instance, making change with real money is more effective teaching strategy than talking about money management [37].

Because retarded children require a structured learning environment, the principles of behavior modification provide a useful framework for teaching cognitive, social, language, or motor skills. Behavior modification is systematic and individualized. Assessment provides observable, measurable descriptions of behavior and accounts for the environment. Behavioral objectives clearly specify target behaviors so that they are clear to everyone who works with the child. In behavior modification, the skills being taught are analyzed and broken down into sequential subskills. It is easy to chart progress and to identify skill levels. Furthermore, there are published behavioral curricula designed for the retarded [20].

Behavioral techniques are effective with people of all levels of retardation. Whitman and Scibak [49], when studying research reports on behavior modification with severely and profoundly retarded institutionalized individuals, concluded that the introduction of behavioral techniques has changed institutions from custodial to developmental in orientation. The objectives of behavior therapy with this population focus on increasing adaptive behavior and decreasing maladaptive responding [49]. Behavioral techniques are quite effective for teaching toileting and self-feeding. They are good for teaching basic imitative, social, and language skills but are not as well developed for teaching more complex social and language skills [49].

Retarded children, especially the more severely retarded, may demonstrate serious behavior problems. Problems can range from stereotypical, autistic behavior, which causes the child to be ostracized, to self-injurious behavior, which can cause physical harm. When working to diminish these behaviors, an analysis is done of the antecedents and consequences of the behavior to identify what is causing (reinforcing) it. It is thought that several conditions contribute to the development of autistic or self-abusive behaviors. They may occur in response to frustration, tension, and discomfort [6] or when there has been some disruptive occurrence [42]. They can be associated with isolation or sensory deprivation where abusive and autistic behavior serve as vestibular and kinesthetic self-stimulation [6]. Balthazar [6] reports that autistic behavior is associated with periods of inactivity. It is thought that repetitive, stereotypical behavior may also serve to soothe the individual by decreasing arousal [6]. Abnormal behavior may be inadvertently reinforced by caretakers when the child gets more attention for abnormal behavior than when acting appropriately [42].

DIMINISHING SELF-ABUSIVE OR
DISRUPTIVE BEHAVIOR

The strategies used to intervene in maladaptive behavior depend on the cause. If the behavior seems to serve as self-stimulation, then alternative purposeful activity that affords noninjurious stimulation is provided [42]. Systematically reinforcing desirable behavior may be all that is necessary to extinguish undesirable behaviors. The biggest challenge in working with profoundly retarded individuals is selecting appropriate reinforcers, because these children are more restricted in their ability to respond to the environment [49]. Since these children are difficult to reach verbally, nonverbal approaches are commonly used to suppress severely abusive or disruptive behavior [18].

Differential reinforcement of other behaviors (DRO) reinforces actions that are incompatible with maladaptive behavior. If a child picks at her face, the therapist might reinforce play behavior that involves the hands [31]. DRO is most often used in combination with time-out or other strategies. It is effective if the child shows alternative behaviors that can be reinforced [18].

Contingent removal of reinforcement is a form of time-out used when the child is functioning in a rewarding environment [18]. The rewarding stimuli are terminated when the child emits undesirable behavior. For instance, if a child plays around with food at mealtime, the therapist would withdraw the plate of food, for a second or two, every time he or she starts to play with the food. This technique is used for sleeping and eating behavior, tantrums, and inappropriate attention seeking [18].

Overcorrection or *restitution* is a procedure developed by Foxx and Azrin [13] which eliminates disruptive behavior and teaches the individual responsibility for actions. The aggressive or disruptive individual is required to restore any damage he or she has done, leaving the environment in a better condition than before the disruption [13].

An overcorrection program with Ann, a profoundly retarded woman, who frequently and unpredictably threw furniture, is described by Foxx and Azrin. Each time Ann threw furniture, she was required to not only straighten the furniture on the ward, but also to dust it and clean all the ashtrays. She had to apologize to everyone whose possessions she disturbed and everyone present during the disturbance. Ann needed to be taught to make beds and arrange furniture. This *restitution training* was given through instruction, demonstration, and physical guidance through the task [13].

Restitution should relate directly to the maladaptive behavior. It should occur immediately following the act and should be extended in duration. Instruction and interaction with the individual during restitution training should not include praise since this may serve to reinforce the destructive act. Nonverbal individuals apologize by nodding their heads in agreement with the therapist's reassurance of the harmed or annoyed bystanders [13].

Electric shock, most often administered with a battery-operated prod, is effective in immediately suppressing behavior. It has been used with retarded or autistic children who cannot understand instruction, to control severe self-in-

74

jurious behavior [18]. The use of electric shock, like the use of other forms of corporal punishment, is controversial. Harris and Ersner-Hershfield [18] state that "in spite of its initial promise, electric shock has been found to have limitations. Problems of generalization, maintenance, potential side effects, method of delivery, and schedules of punishment, as well as lay and professional resistance to the use of such a painful modality, demanded a careful examination of this approach" [18].

Restraint conjures up the image of a straight-jacket, but brief, partial restraint, such as holding a child's hand to prevent self-injurious behavior may be appropriate in some circumstances [31, 18].

BRINGING ABOUT DESIRABLE BEHAVIOR
The elimination of self-injurious, self-stimulating, and severely disruptive behavior enhances the child's ability to attend to behavioral procedures that are less punitive and that account for limited cognitive and social abilities.

In general, reinforcement should be consistent and immediate. Even a slight delay in reinforcement might serve to accidentally strengthen the wrong response [46]. Initially the children may require primary reinforcers such as food. They can be gradually introduced to social (secondary) reinforcers by pairing primary and secondary reinforcers and gradually fading the primary ones [31]. The child's perceptual and attentional abilities and the intensity of reinforcing stimuli required must be considered [46]. The child must perceive the reinforcement, and yet the reinforcing stimuli should not detract from the child's attention to the task [31]. Simple tasks are easier to reinforce than complex ones. Tasks can be graded in a series of steps, and appropriate behavior can be rewarded at the completion of each small step [46].

A behavior must occur for operant conditioning to take place. If the behavior does not occur, then the individual never has the opportu-
nity to experience its consequences. Obviously, with most people, one can give information about how and when to perform the desired action. The action can be modeled and the performance guided. One can give auditory and visual feedback about the quality of performance and reinforce the individual when the behavior is demonstrated. With children who cannot understand directions or who have disabilities that interfere with communication, the more intricate processes of response shaping and fading may be required to get the desired behavior to occur.

Shaping is the reinforcement of successive approximations of the desired response. A therapist might use shaping to develop speech in the nonverbal child. First, any vocalization would be rewarded, then approximations of more specific sounds, and later the sounds are shaped into syllables and words.

Fading is the gradual changing of the stimuli used to elicit a behavior. For instance, the therapist who is developing speech in the child may manipulate the child's lips to assist in the articulation of certain words. The amount of manipulation may be gradually decreased (fading out) or increased (fading in) [48]. The use of prompts or cues assists the child in attending to important aspects of the task [48]. The prompts may be verbal or gestural [48].

Imitation can be taught by guiding the child through the desired action with the guidance faded and imitative behavior shaped [31]. Severely impaired children may only achieve approximations of normal behavior.

GENERALIZATION OF BEHAVIOR CHANGE
When children are taught new skills, the ultimate test of the effectiveness of learning is the child's use of those skills in daily living, adapting newly learned responses to many settings and situations. Severely retarded and autistic children have problems generalizing behaviors learned in one situation to other settings. There is no guarantee that behavior change will be lasting or that newly learned behavior will be

used in all relevant situations [23]. Children grow, develop, and change, and the environment demands change.

The ability to adapt behavior learned in one setting to different settings is called stimulus generalization. Behavior therapists working with severely emotionally and intellectually impaired children will *vary the treatment environment* if they find that the child is emitting the desired response in only one setting. For children who have great difficulty with generalization of stimuli, the therapist might *teach the response in the natural setting,* introducing the many variations of stimuli that might naturally occur. Severely intellectually impaired children will sometimes emit target responses for only the trainer. In that case, *a variety of people* would be included in training sessions, including those who are significant in the child's natural environment [43].

A high ratio of reinforcement may be used to develop new behavior, but if it is unlikely that the natural environment will provide such' a schedule of reinforcement, the therapist will gradually make reinforcement more intermittent or less frequent [43] until it *approximates the naturally occurring schedule of reinforcement.*

Children can be taught to *create their own reinforcement,* to seek praise or attention, and to maintain adaptive behavior. Of course, generalization may occur automatically if the newly learned behavior is so *successful* that it provides its own reinforcement.

Behavior therapists should continually question the generalization of behavior being learned. Does the child understand that the behavior learned in the treatment setting is useful at home? Can the child adapt the frequency, intensity, and duration of a response to the demands of a variety of settings? Has the child had the opportunity to practice new skills so that the behavior change will be lasting? Does the newly learned behavior enhance development, and will it prove useful as the child grows and develops?

PSYCHOSOCIAL DEVELOPMENT

Perhaps the greatest contribution that parents and professionals can make toward the quality of life of the retarded child is in fostering the development of social skills. Learning to get along with other people, to be a congenial companion who respects the rights of others, does more for the child's acceptance by peers and adjustment to the community than any other attributes. In later life, good social skills contribute more to job success of retarded people than do academic skills [25]. In conjunction with learning social adaptation, children must also learn to respect themselves and to develop independence and self-assertion.

Social adaptation refers to the ability to fit in with other people, behaving in a way that is acceptable to one's culture. Self-respect is based on a knowledge of oneself and acceptance of one's strengths and weaknesses. People with self-respect have a sense of their own value. The development of social adaptation and self-respect is a life-long process.

Social skills can be taught, but it is *how* they are taught that either nurtures or injures self-respect. For instance, being independent in toileting is a most critical skill for social adaptation. It frees the individual from a basic dependence on caretakers. Children who are toilet trained have more options for classroom settings and are less likely to be ostracized by nonretarded peers. Toilet training should take place in private, and part of the training is the concept that this is a private function [10]. Children need to learn about privacy, their own right to privacy, and the respect for the privacy of others [10]. They learn this by being given privacy. Retarded people are often not given the privacy they deserve. Frequently others monitor everything they do, enter their rooms without knocking, and supervise them on the toilet and in the shower.

Self-respect is also based on acceptance by others. School is a major social arena for children, and their social adaptation to school is as important as what they learn academically. Gottlieb [16] has identified factors related to social adaptation in school: communication skills, antisocial behavior, physical appearance, and the school environment.

Both verbal and nonverbal communication influence social interactions. Retarded children have more limited vocabularies and make more grammatical errors than their nonretarded peers [16]. They are often oblivious to body language. Children need to learn about the messages their nonverbal behavior communicates. They also need to be taught to be sensitive to the body language of others [16]. Communication skills are fostered for the sake of good social adjustment, as well as for academic achievement.

Physically handicapped children may have impaired or negligible vocal abilities. They can be taught to use communication boards [47] and electronic devices to augment communication. Vanderheiden and Harris-Vanderheiden [47] note that communication aids will not interfere with the development of speech. They may actually facilitate oral communication because children are more relaxed, knowing they can augment their verbal communication with the aid. Nonverbal children, deprived of communication aids, are being deprived of social interaction.

Gottlieb [16] found that inappropriate school behaviors, such as making noises, running, talking aloud, or falling on the floor, have the greatest detrimental effect on the child's social status. Sometimes retarded children are allowed more latitude in their behavior than nonretarded children. This does them no favor. If they do not develop self-control, Dickerson believes one is "adding the handicap of inadequate socialization to the disability of mental retardation" [10].

The structure of the environment can facilitate or impede the acquisition of self-discipline. Gottlieb [16] found that educable children, in free, open classrooms, where they were more apt to display a wide range of behaviors, were less liked by their nonretarded peers. Retarded children are better able to control their behavior in a structured environment where routines are predictable; rules are fair, clear, and consistently applied; and where they know what behavior is acceptable.

The physical appearance of children affects the way others relate to them. Acne can be just as traumatic for retarded adolescents as it is to their peers [11]. Sometimes parents assume that appearance is of little consequence to the child. Yet Drew and colleagues [11] note that "most retarded children strive constantly to be as much like their normal peers as possible. They want nothing to draw any attention to the fact that they are somewhat different from other children. Adverse physical appearance does draw attention and hinders if not precludes social acceptance. Parents and teachers must be aware that how an individual looks usually has a bearing on self-concept."

Eventually, retarded people learn they are different. Dickerson [10] describes the anger and anguish of a retarded adolescent when she realized that her younger brother, whom she called "baby," began to do things that she could not do. Slightly retarded individuals feel frustrated by and anxious about their intellectual deficits. Retarded people can be helped to understand their limitations [10], and they can benefit from psychotherapy if their verbal limitations are taken into account [50].

Learning about sexuality is a developmental process often denied the retarded. When they are young, they are viewed as asexual, and may not learn, for example, to differentiate between showing affection to family members and keeping their distance with strangers [10]. Later, the family may fear the sexuality of adolescents and deny them information about sex or the privacy for sexual experiences. Not everyone supports sex education, let alone the consideration of marriage and child rearing, for retarded people. Yet retarded adults marry and raise families.

Retarded people are not asexual, and they need to be educated about sex. This starts with basic education about body parts and functions. They need to learn the rights and responsibilities of being a sexual person. There are published guidelines for sex education that can help parents and teachers with this subject [10]. Adolescence can be especially difficult. Boys are coping with erections and nocturnal emissions; girls are coping with menstruation. These may occur at just the time they have mastered toilet training [10], and now they need to learn about hygiene and birth control. Dickerson [10] suggests that children should learn the street language associated with sex for their own protection. Even if they are discouraged from using this language at home, they need to recognize what is going on around them and to know when to say "no" to unwanted overtures. Sterilization is a controversial subject, and states have different laws to protect the rights of retarded people. But even when women are protected from unwanted pregnancy, they are not protected from being sexually exploited unless they have been educated [10].

Retarded people also need to learn about the rights of others. "Mildly retarded (people), at least are capable of truly remarkable—almost puritanical—sexual self control both in a hospital and in a community setting" [12]. In their ignorance, however, they may get in trouble for inappropriate sexual behavior. Sexuality is an issue that cannot be ignored, and education starts in childhood.

LIVING ARRANGEMENTS

At some point, institutionalization may be contemplated for the severely retarded child. Large custodial institutions are no longer considered the most appropriate setting for most handicapped retarded of any age. For those who require residential facilities, the trend is toward small, homelike residences in the mainstream of life, with access to community services [2].

Residential placement may be needed for people who require constant monitoring and medical supervision [10]. Sometimes temporary placement in a training institution is indicated for a child who is not progressing well at home. Parents, because of illness, economic hardship, or emotional instability may not be able to give the child required care and training. Some parents overindulge their child, impeding full development of potential. Temporary residential placement can provide training in self-care skills and social adaptation, enabling the child to return to family living at a more functional level [10].

Sometimes the availability of services within the community is a major factor in the decision to place the individual in a residential facility [30]. MacMillan notes "If local physicians are unfamiliar with the unique health problems of the retarded or if special education or vocational training programs are poorly run or available only at a great distance, parents may feel that their child can be better cared for in an institution" [30]. There are many options for residential placement: public and private institutions and foster care and group homes. And, of course, many retarded adults will establish their own homes, living independently and participating in community life.

LIFE AFTER SCHOOL: WORK AND LEISURE

It is possible for the retarded person to be involved in public education from the age of 3 until 21. Attending classes provides social contacts and a structure to daily life that can stop abruptly when the individual leaves school. Life can become very lonely for those who do not have jobs and are dependent on their families for social stimulation. Work skills, leisure-time interests, and social contacts are critical for the quality of life of retarded people. Anticipatory planning is necessary to ensure that developmental experiences do not cease when the individual leaves the educational system. Consideration must be given to residence, jobs, social contacts, and leisure activities. Social workers and vocational rehabilitation counselors can help families and the retarded client identify resources and make choices.

As retarded children grow older, parental concerns do not decrease. Families become anxious about school programs and the child's social adjustment. Parents with adolescent children worry about sexuality and the child's adjustment as an adult. Financial arrangements and guardianship, in the event of the parents' deaths, are additional concerns. Social workers provide information and help. Supplemental Social Security income and Medicaid assistance are available to mentally retarded people over the age of 18 who live in licensed facilities. These are also available for low-income persons who are younger and living at home [10].

Schools usually gear curricula toward developing prevocational skills, and when children reach adolescence, they may be referred for vocational training. But it is an accumulation of work-related life experiences that lays the foundation for work habits and prevocational skills. These are experiences that retarded children may lack unless they are intentionally and systematically provided.

Most children are introduced to work habits by daily contact with workers. They see their parent's concern about getting to work on time or performing household chores according to a routine. Although little conscious attention is paid to these activities, children learn work behaviors from role models in their environment. Retarded children may not absorb this kind of information as automatically as their nonretarded peers. They require specific training in work habits. They need the opportunity to work [34] and this can start with household chores.

Much of the education done in school contributes to prevocational training: the development of time concept, functional reading, learning about when one can socialize and when one must work [34]. But one cannot assume that these skills will be generalized to the work place. Students "must be taught to follow directions, attend to tasks, remember instructions over a period of time, evaluate their own work perfor-mance as to quantity and quality, and ask for help when required. The schools can help students learn to be dependable, punctual, and congenial in a work situation, and thus become better candidates for vocational training and subsequent employment" [10]. Adolescents need to be helped to establish realistic work goals [34]. Retarded people learn best by doing. They need the opportunity to do work and to see people doing the jobs that they might do [34].

The inability to handle leisure time is a common problem for retarded adults [25]. They often have long stretches of unstructured time and they fill it with television or waiting for someone to entertain them. Identification of talents and interests that can be developed for leisure activities starts in childhood. Some retarded children have artistic ability [36] that can be fostered. Others may be athletic or mechanically oriented. Retarded people can fit into activities of the larger community, and getting the child involved in community activities paves the way for community involvement in adulthood. There are also recreational and leisure opportunities specifically designed for retarded people. Retarded people can and do get involved politically. There are self-help groups that give mutual support, social opportunities, and political power [36].

REFERENCES

1. American Psychiatric Association. *Diagnostic and Statistical Manual of Mental Disorders* (3rd ed.). Washington, D.C.: APA, 1980.
2. Anderson, R. M., Greer, J. G., and Dietrich, W. L. Overview and Perspectives. In R. M. Anderson and J. G. Greeg (eds.), *Educating the Severely and Profoundly Retarded.* Baltimore: University Park, 1976.
3. Arena, J. *How to Write an I.E.P.* Novato, CA: Academic Therapy, 1978. P. 37.
4. Baer, D. M., and Stokes T. F. Discriminating a Generalization Technology. In P. Mittler (ed.), *Research to Practice in Mental Retardation, Vol. II: Education and Training.* Baltimore: University Park, 1977.

5. Balla, D., and Zigler, E. Personality Development in Retarded Persons. In N. R. Ellis (ed.), *Handbook of Mental Deficiency, Psychological Theory and Research* (2nd ed.). Hillsdale, N.J.: Erlbaum, 1979. P. 145.

6. Balthazar, E. E. Assessment of Autistic Behaviors in the Severely Retarded. In P. Mittler (ed.), *Research to Practice in Mental Retardation, Vol. II: Education and Training.* Baltimore: University Park, 1977.

7. Bower, A. C. Learning. In J. P. Das and D. Baine (eds.), *Mental Retardation.* Springfield, IL: Thomas, 1978.

8. Budoff, M. The Mentally Retarded Child in the Mainstream of the Public School. In P. Mittler (ed.), *Research to Practice in Mental Retardation, Vol. II: Education and Training.* Baltimore: University Park, 1977.

9. Coleman, J. C., Butcher, J. N., and Carson, R. C. *Abnormal Psychology and Modern Life* (7th ed.). London: Scott, Foresman, 1984.

10. Dickerson, M. U. *Social Work Practice with the Mentally Retarded.* New York: Free, 1981. P. 117.

11. Drew, C. J., Logan, D. R., and Hardman, M. L. *Mental Retardation: A Life Cycle Approach* (3rd ed.). St. Louis: Times Mirror/Mosby, 1984. Pp. 54, 261.

12. Edgerton, R. B. Some Socio-Cultural Research Considerations. In F. F. de la Cruz and G. D La Veck (eds.), *Human Sexuality and the Mentally Retarded.* New York: Brunner/Mazel, 1973. P. 245.

13. Foxx, R. M., and Azrin, N. H. Restitution: A method of eliminating aggressive-disruptive behavior of retarded and brain damaged patients. *Behav. Res. Ther.* 10:15, 1972.

14. Garber, H., and Heber, F. R. The Milwaukee Project. In P. Mittler (ed.), *Research to Practice in Mental Retardation. Vol. I: Care and Intervention.* Baltimore, University Park, 1977.

15. Gottlieb, J. Attitudes Toward Mainstreaming Retarded Children and Some Possible Effects on Educational Practices. In P. Mittler (ed.), *Research to Practice in Mental Retardation, Vol. I: Care and Intervention.* Baltimore: University Park, 1977. P. 39.

16. Gottlieb, J. Observing Social Adaptation in Schools. In G. P. Sacket (ed.), *Observing Behavior, Vol. I: Theory and Applications in Mental Retardation.* Baltimore: University Park, 1978.

17. Grossman, H. J. *Manual on Terminology and Classification in Mental Retardation.* Washington, D.C.: American Association on Mental Deficiency, 1977. Pp. 11, 13.

18. Harris, S. L., and Ersner-Hershfield, R. Behavioral suppression of seriously disruptive behavior in psychotic and retarded patients: A review of punishment and its alternatives. *Psychol. Bull.* 85:1352, 1978. P. 1364.

19. Haywood, H.C. Alternatives to Normative Assessment. In P. Mittler (ed.), *Research to Practice in Mental Retardation, Vol. II: Education and Training.* Baltimore: University Park, 1977.

20. Ingalls, R. P. *Mental Retardation: The Changing Outlook.* New York: Wiley, 1978.

21. Ingram, C. *Fundamentals of Educational Assessment.* New York: Van Nostrand, 1980.

22. Joiner, L. M. *Identifying Children with Special Needs: A Practical Guide to Developmental Screening.* Holmes Beach, FL: Learning, 1978.

23. Kanfer, F. H., and Phillips, J. S. *Learning Foundations of Behavior Therapy.* New York: Wiley, 1970.

24. Katz-Garris, L. The Right to Education. In J. Wortis (ed.), *Mental Retardation and Developmental Disabilities: An Annual Review, X.* New York: Brunner/Mazel, 1978.

25. Kauffman, J. M., and Payne, J. S. *Mental Retardation: Introduction and Personal Perspectives.* Columbus: Merrill, 1975.

26. Kramer, J. J., Nagel, R. J., and Engle, R. W. Recent advances in mnemonic strategy training with mentally retarded persons: Implications for educational practice. *Am. J. Ment. Defic.* 85: 306–314, 1980.

27. Lawson, M. Memory and Rehearsal. In J. P. Das and D. Baine (eds.), *Mental Retardation.* Springfield, IL: Thomas, 1978. P. 90.

28. Leland, H. Adaptation, Coping Behavior, and Retarded Performance. In P. Mittler (ed.), *Research to Practice in Mental Retardation, Vol. II: Education and Training.* Baltimore: University Park, 1977.

29. Leong, C. K. Language Behavior of Moderately Mentally Retarded Children. In J. P. Das and D. Baine (ed.), *Mental Retardation.* Springfield, IL: Thomas, 1978.

30. MacMillan, D. L. *Mental Retardation in School and Society* (2nd ed.). Boston: Little, Brown, 1982. P. 549.

31. Margolies, P. J. Behavioral approaches to the treatment of early infantile autism: A review. *Psychol. Bull.* 84:249, 1977.

32. Meyers, C. E., Nihira, K., and Zetlin, A. The Measurement of Adaptive Behavior. In N. R. Ellis (ed.), *Handbook of Mental Deficiency, Psychological Theory and Research* (2nd ed.). Hillsdale, NJ: Erlbaum, 1979.

33. Ozer, M. N. Levels of Interaction in the Assess-

ment of Children. In P. Mittler (ed.), *Research to Practice in Mental Retardation, Vol. II: Education and Training.* Baltimore: University Park, 1977.

34. Perry, N. *Teaching the Mentally Retarded Child* (2nd ed.). New York: Columbia University Press, 1974.

35. Philips, I. Psychopathology and Mental Retardation. In F. J. Menolascino (ed.), *Psychiatric Aspects of the Diagnosis and Treatment of Mental Retardation.* Seattle: Special Child, 1971.

36. President's Committee on Mental Retardation. *Mental Retardation: The Leading Edge: Service Programs That Work.* (DHEW publication No. (OHDS) 79–21018.) Washington, D.C.: Government Printing Office, 1978.

37. Reynolds, M. C., and Birch, J. W. *Teaching Exceptional Children in All America's Schools: A First Course for Teachers and Principals.* Reston, VA: Council for Exceptional Children, 1977.

38. Robinson, N. M., and Robinson, H. B. *The Mentally Retarded Child* (2nd ed.). New York: McGraw-Hill, 1976.

39. Rosenthal, R. H., and Allen, T. W. An examination of attention and arousal and learning dysfunctions of hyperkinetic children. *Psychol. Bull.* 85:689–715, 1978 p. 691.

40. Sabatino, D. A. Systematic Procedure for Ascertaining Learner Characteristics. In D. A. Sabatino and T. L. Miller (eds.), *Describing Learner Characteristics of Handicapped Children and Youth.* New York: Grune & Stratton, 1979.

41. Schonebaum, R. M., and Zinober, J. W. Learning and Memory in Mental Retardation: The Defect-Developmental Distinction Reevaluated. In I. Bialer and M. Sternlicht (eds.), *The Psychology of Mental Retardation: Issues and Approaches.* New York: Psychological Dimensions, 1977.

42. Schroeder, S. R., Mulick, J. A., and Schroeder, C. S. Management of Severe Behavior Problems of the Retarded. In N. R. Ellis (ed.), *Handbook of Mental Deficiency, Psychological Theory and Research* (2nd ed.). Hillsdale, NJ: Erlbaum, 1979.

43. Schwartz, A. *The Behavior Therapies: Theories and Applications.* New York: Free, 1982.

44. Siegel, P. S. Incentive Motivation and the Mentally Retarded Person. In N. R. Ellis (ed.), *Handbook of Mental Deficiency, Psychological Theory and Research* (2nd ed.). Hillsdale, NJ: Erlbaum, 1979. P. 3.

45. Sontag, E., Burke, P. J., and York. R. Consider-ations for Serving the Severely Handicapped in the Public Schools. In R. M. Anderson, J. G. Greer, and R. M. Smith (eds.), *Educating the Severely and Profoundly Retarded.* Baltimore: University Park, 1976.

46. Tymchuk, A. J. *Behavior Modification with Children: A Clinical Training Manual.* Springfield, IL: Thomas, 1974.

47. Vanderheiden, G. C., and Harris-Vanderheiden, D. Developing Effective Modes for Response and Expression in Nonvocal, Severely Handicapped Children. In P. Mittler (ed.), *Research to Practice in Mental Retardation, Vol. II: Education and Training.* Baltimore: University Park, 1977.

48. Watson, L. S., Jr. *Child Behavior Modification: A Manual for Teachers, Nurses and Parents.* New York: Pergamon, 1973.

49. Whitman, T. L., and Scibak, J. W. Behavior Modification Research With the Severely and Profoundly Retarded. In N. R. Ellis (ed.), *Handbook of Mental Deficiency, Psychological Theory and Research* (2nd ed.). Hillsdale, NJ: Erlbaum, 1979.

50. Work, H. H. Mental Retardation. In J. D. Noshpitz (ed.), *Basic Handbook of Child Psychiatry, Vol. II: Disturbances in Development.* New York: Basic, 1979.

MENTAL RETARDATION ORGANIZATIONS

American Association on Mental Deficiency (AAMD) 1719 Kalorama Rd. N.W. Washington, DC 20009
phone: (202) 387-1968
Members are professionals and others interested in the mentally retarded. Conducts educational seminars; gives awards; promotes the study of the cause, treatment, and prevention of mental retardation.

Accreditation Council on Services for People with Developmental Disabilities (ACDD) 120 Boylston St., Suite 202 Boston, MA 02116
phone: (617) 426-7909
Works to improve the quality of services for people with developmental disabilities. Assesses and accredits agencies serving mentally retarded.

Association for Retarded Citizens (ARC) P.O. Box 6109 Arlington, TX 76005
phone: (817) 640-0204
Parents and professionals interested in mental retardation.

CHAPTER 4

Infantile Autism

Judith D. Ward

In 1943, the child psychiatrist Leo Kanner [17] described a pattern of psychotic characteristics that had its onset in the first 30 months of life [24]. These characteristics included (1) an extreme isolation, (2) a failure to use language for the purpose of communication, (3) an anxiously obsessive desire for the maintenance of sameness, (4) a poor or absent relation to people and an intense fascination with objects and (5) good cognitive potentialities. He called this syndrome early infantile autism.

Autism is a perplexing disorder. These unusual children withdraw from human contact. Some have remarkable mechanical skills but do not communicate or undertake the simplest self-care activities. They may be strangely quiet and preoccupied by minutiae and suddenly become consumed by panic, for no apparent reason.

Autism occurs in every 2,200 live births and affects more boys than girls (4:1) [11]. The cause is unknown and is probably multiply determined [27]. It is most likely caused by impaired brain function that interferes with language, sequencing, abstraction, and coding functions [24]. The neurophysiologic dysfunction has been attributed to retarded maturation of the nervous system [32], biochemical abnormalities [22], and perinatal infections or complications [32]. Autistic children have a greater than average incidence of intrauterine rubella and phenylketonuria [11]. Many autistic children develop seizures in adolescence [21], and 60 percent of autistic children show abnormal rhythms in electroencephalographic (EEG) studies [12]. In a study of 78 classically autistic children (onset before 30 months old and no overt neurologic or EEG abnormalities), Coleman [11] found that 8 percent had relatives who were autistic and 32 percent had laboratory tests showing metabolic or digestive absorption abnormalities.

CLINICAL MANIFESTATIONS

As autism has been studied, Kanner's symptoms have been classified in a manner that represents greater emphasis on the biologic theories of etiology reflected in sensorimotor and cognitive functioning [33]:

Problems with language and communication
Abnormal sensorimotor responses
Uneven cognitive skills
Peculiarities in relating to people and objects
Resistance to changes in the environment
Other problems

Problems with language and communication range from moderate to severe. Some children are mute. Those who speak may not use language to communicate; words or phrases are repeated in a stereotypical fashion, and the rhythm and pitch of speech are odd. Their language may consist of jargon or slogans; or they may repeat precisely what they have heard (echolalia) in a mechanical, robotlike manner. They may associate a particular phrase with a specific event and repeat the phrase forever afterward in relation to similar events [32]. For example, when an autistic child was given a cookie, his mother asked, "Are your hands clean?" Even a year later, the child said, "Are your hands clean?" whenever he saw a cookie. Children who are capable of more spontaneous speech often reverse pronouns and show other peculiarities of grammar [9].

Nonverbal communication is also severely impaired, and gestures, postures, and facial expression are incongruent with communication.

Some children who cannot use spoken language for communication make their needs known by guiding the arm of an adult to a desired object [32]. Some have been able to learn to use sign language [7]. Families of autistic children have reported incidents of children who have been mute and unresponsive to language who speak in an urgent situation and then revert to their withdrawn, uncommunicative state.

The autistic child's comprehension of language is limited. Some children interpret language in a concrete fashion; others can read words but cannot understand concepts. Children who cannot understand the spoken word may respond to gestures. Older, verbal children are unresponsive to the nonverbal clues associated with communication: facial expression, voice intonation, and gestures [23].

In general, one can expect that autistic children will have *abnormal sensorimotor responses,* but there is much variation in the patterns of response found in each child. Some overreact to auditory stimulation [32] and panic on hearing loud noises. Others appear deaf. Paradoxically, autistic children may be oblivious to loud noises but may respond to certain subtle sounds, such as the opening of the refrigerator door [4]. Autistic children may derive great enjoyment from music or spend hours creating their own auditory stimulation by clicking their tongues or snapping their fingers. They are often fascinated by the movement of objects, ignoring a stationary object, but responding to the same object if it is moving. Responses to visual stimuli may be as varied as those to auditory stimuli. They avoid using a steady, direct gaze, appearing to use peripheral visual fields or looking at objects with brief glances [32].

Some autistic children show an aversion to being touched and a distaste for certain textures [28]. The child who shrinks away from light touch may enjoy roughhousing and pressure touch [32]. Some children ignore painful stimuli and disregard cold temperatures; they show aversion to certain foods, probably because of the texture, and do not appear to feel hunger. The young autistic child may have difficulty chewing and swallowing food, and in some cases, malnutrition may result.

Autistic children seem to ignore auditory and visual stimuli, preferring tactile, kinesthetic, proprioceptive, and vestibular stimuli. This has been described as using near receptors rather than distant sensory receptors [28].

Motor responses are also abnormal. Posture and gait may be odd, although many autistic children move gracefully. Some children have difficulty imitating movements, or they may exhibit repetitive, unproductive movements such as grimacing and hand flapping. Head banging, rocking, fluttering fingers before their eyes are all self-stimulating mannerisms common to autism. These repetitive, unproductive behaviors can be injurious, and they consume the child's waking hours if they are not interrupted by parent or therapist.

Uneven cognitive functioning is typically evident in autistic children's poor language and communication skills, coupled with normal performance on tasks involving fitting and assembly, rote memory, or music. This uneven functioning had led some to believe that the autistic child is a normally intelligent child whose emotional problems interfere with use of this intelligence. However, DeMyer [13] points out that the special skills found in autistic children are not skills reflective of normal or high intelligence but may be the "easiest kinds of tasks for developmentally retarded children to perform." Skills in fitting and assembly do not necessarily imply other types of intelligence.

About three fourths of autistic children have some degree of mental retardation [24] and IQ scores, which are related to symptom severity, can be used to predict a child's future development. Children with IQs below 50 have a poor prognosis [27] and are more likely to develop seizures in adolescence [30]. DeMyer [13] found that children who had IQs over 50 responded best to treatment and even had an increase in IQ over time. (It should be noted that untreated children with IQs over 50 did not show as great an increase of IQ as those who were treated.) Speech is more normal, and social withdrawal is less severe in children with higher IQs [13].

The autistic child's *peculiarities in relating to people and objects* may be evident early in life. In infancy many autistic children do not cry out for attention and are described as good children who can keep themselves occupied for long periods of time. Other autistic children are screamers who have erratic sleeping and eating patterns, and their parents often notice the infant's lack of eye contact and discomfort, or even distress, at being held.

Some children spend their time in aimless wandering, rocking back and forth, flapping their hands before their eyes, or spinning objects [32]. They may play with their own fingers or the hair of another person as if they were objects. Kanner [17] cites an account of a child on a crowded beach who would "walk straight toward his goal irrespective of whether this involved walking over newspapers, hands, feet, or torsos . . . he did not intentionally deviate from his course in order to walk on others, but neither did he make the slightest attempt to avoid them."

Autistic children often become more sociable as they grow older [33]. However, even those who are relatively sociable are handicapped or immature in social skills. They are insensitive to the nuances of social relationships, and their interactions are often inappropriate. Children who have the ability to understand and use language are better able to relate to people [33].

The fascination with objects that can be moved repetitively is a characteristic of autistic children, and their manipulation of objects is often surprisingly dextrous. They may become fascinated by part of an object, such as the wheel on a toy truck, which they will twirl with great absorption but never use as a functional object. They seem to be preoccupied with parts of objects rather than wholes. The movement or noise created through manipulation is of more interest than the purpose of the object.

They treat their own bodies in the same way, fluttering their fingers before their eyes as if mesmerized. Autistic children are unable to engage in symbolic play and do not play imaginative games or make-believe. Collecting and ritualistically arranging objects, and self-stimulation activities predominate in play [32].

Kanner called the autistic child's *resistance to change* "an anxiously obsessive desire for the maintenance of sameness" [17]. Changes in the environment, or even slight modification of routine, can give rise to unhappiness and temper tantrums. These children may demand that activities always be carried out in the same sequence. They will play with the same objects, manipulating them or arranging them in the same order, with ritualistic precision. The introduction of new foods, changes of clothing, or a rearrangement of furniture is met with resistance and alarm. Parents may find themselves slaves to routine and ritual [32].

Erratic sleeping patterns are often part of the clinical picture of autism [32], and these children are hazardous to themselves as they roam unsupervised in the night. Eating patterns can be equally disruptive. They may refuse certain foods because they dislike the texture, or they may never request food and give no indication of hunger.

DIAGNOSIS

It is difficult to diagnose autism before the age of 2, when normal children begin to use language. The diagnosis depends on the observation of classic symptoms and the ruling out of disorders that may share common symptoms. Information about the child's history and environment are important considerations in making the diagnosis. Parents can provide a history of the child's development, behavior, and daily activities. The history is especially necessary in the case of the older, verbal child because autistic symptoms are more subtle after 5 years of age [32].

A complete physical and neurologic examination helps establish a diagnosis. Autism must be differentiated from aphasia, deafness, blindness, mental retardation, and other childhood psychoses. Children with aphasia have language problems and may have secondary emotional problems, but they do not show abnormal sensory reactivity, they relate to people, they can communicate with gestures, and when they acquire speech, it is not atonal or echolalic. It may be difficult to rule out deafness since autistic children are often unresponsive to noise and difficult to test with conventional tests; evoked response audiometry, which records responses directly from the auditory nerve and cortex [33] can be used. Blind children may develop behavioral mannerisms (blindisms) similar to autistic mannerisms. However, both blind and deaf children relate to people and develop an interest in the environment [21]. Mental retardation is associated with a variety of disorders; Some retarded children may show some autistic features but most do not [24]. Although autism was once considered a type of childhood schizophrenia, it is now classified by the American Psychiatric Association as a pervasive developmental disorder [2, 24]. Childhood schizophrenia is rare [3] and differs from autism in a few important ways: Autism occurs within the first 30 months of life, but there is a period of normal development in childhood schizophrenia. Language may be impaired in schizophrenia, but the impairment is more a reflection of a thought disorder than the more basic communication problems found in autism. Schizophrenics suffer from delusions and hallucinations; autistic children do not [2, 11].

A number of behavior scales have been developed for diagnostic and research purposes. The *Childhood Autism Rating Scale* (CARS) [29] is one example. In the CARS the child is rated by direct observation on 15 scales: (1) impairment in human relations, (2) imitation, (3) inappropriate affect, (4) bizarre use of body movement and persistence of stereotypes, (5) peculiarities in relating to nonhuman objects, (6) resistance to environmental change, (7) peculiarities of visual responsiveness, (8) peculiarities of auditory responsiveness, (9) near receptor responsiveness, (10) anxiety reaction, (11) verbal communication, (12) nonverbal communication, (13) activity level, (14) intellectual functioning, and (15) general impressions. The child's age is considered in making each rating and, based on the scores, the child is designated not autistic, mild to moderately autistic, or severely autistic [29]. A diagnosis is never based on one test.

ASSESSMENT

A comprehensive evaluation includes the administration of standardized tests, clinical observations, and information from the parents about the child's development and behavioral characteristics (Table 4-1).

Among the *standardized tests,* IQ tests are important because they predict the child's general functioning. However, more specific assessments of functional abilities are needed to plan treatment. When selecting and administering tests, one must consider the autistic child's wide range of skills that may not be testable on any one standardized test. For example, a 5-year-old may be functioning at an infant level in verbal development, and a 6-year level in some performance areas. A test standardized for this child's chronological age may show the child "untestable" in language areas, while an infant scale would not provide the opportunity to demonstrate areas of superior skill. Freeman and Ritvo [15] report that they screen children before administering tests and then select the tests based on the general level of functioning rather than on chronological age.

It may be difficult to focus the child's attention on the test being administered if the child engages in hand flapping and other unproductive, self-stimulating behaviors that interfere with testing. Behavior therapy techniques are useful in focusing and maintaining the child's attention on the test [15]. Schopler [27] claims that autistic children are seldom untestable: "Even uncooperative autistic children will respond to testing when easier or lower develop-

TABLE 4-1. Assessments for autism

Test	Assesses
Bayley Scales of Infant Development	Cognitive function and motor development
Catell Infant Intelligence Scale	General cognitive and motor development
Gesell Preschool Test	Motor, language, and social development performance on problem solving and developmental tasks
Stanford-Binet Intelligence Scale	
Wechsler Intelligence Scale for Children (WISC)	Intellectual functioning, thought processes, ego functioning
Wechsler Preschool and Primary Scale of Intelligence	Intellectual functioning, though processes, ego functioning
LANGUAGE (SEE CHAPTER 7)	
Carrow Test of Auditory Comprehension of Language	Language comprehension
Peabody Picture Vocabulary Test	Language comprehension
Illinois Test of Psycholinguistic Abilities	Comprehension and expression (see Learning Disabilities Test Appendix)
Carrow Elicited Language Inventory	Imitation
BEHAVIOR SCALES	
AAMD Adaptive Behavior Scales	Adaptive behavior (see Mental Retardation)
Childhood Autism Rating Scale (CARS)	Autistic behavior
SENSORIMOTOR EVALUATIONS	
See Test Appendix of Learning Disabilities chapter for complete description of the following tests: Bruininks-Oseretsky Test of Motor Proficiency Purdue Perceptual Motor Survey Rating Scale Frostig Movement Skills Battery Southern California Sensory Integration Tests	

mental test items are used. If a child responds to an easier item, lack of cooperation or 'untestability' can no longer be the main explanation for his poor test performance." In order to treat the autistic child, the therapist must be able to break through the autistic barrier and communicate with the child. Through *informal observation* of the child, the therapist or teacher seeks to assess the response to the learning environment and to identify the factors that will create an optimum learning environment. What kinds of stimuli elicit responses from the child? The sensory modalities that can be used to communicate and teach new skills need to be identified. A knowledge of the child's sensory preferences is helpful in choosing appropriate reinforcers, and behavior problems can sometimes be explained by the child's aversion to certain types of stimulation.

Some children cannot handle multiple, simultaneous sensory stimulation. If they are required to respond to demonstration with verbal instruction, they may respond only to the visual message or only to the verbal [7]. Some children will not respond at all if given multiple stimulation. Some children who disregard the spoken word will respond to music or to a singing voice. Children who seem to avoid eye contact may, in fact, be observing the therapist with peripheral vision or quick, darting glances. Autistic children may attend to a moving object but will ignore it when it is stationary.

How does the child express needs? Problems with facial expression and the use of words and gestures interfere with communication, and it may take the therapist a long time to become familiar enough with the child to understand the child's needs and fears. The parents are crucial in providing information about communication style; they can often explain "unexplainable" behavior arising in treatment or school sessions. Often, ritualistic behavior, as well as temper tantrums, are the expression of frustration or confusion.

What kind of environment will promote optimum learning? How much extraneous stimulation can the child tolerate in the treatment environment? Are they elements in the environment, such as sudden loudspeaker announcements, that cause panic? Sometimes moving toys or machines precipitate hand flapping or twirling mannerisms that interfere with learning. The child may require individual attention to learn some skills, but many children learn well in small groups.

What kind of reinforcement is needed for learning? Treating the autistic child often requires behavior therapy techniques. Does the child respond to social reinforcement: verbal praise, a hug, a smile? Will certain kinds of stimulation attract attention to a task: bright colors, certain noises, vestibular or proprioceptive stimulation? What foods could be used for reinforcement? What schedule of reinforcement will be necessary?

Before working with the child, the therapist should be aware of any dangerous behaviors that could be expected. Autistic children often show no awareness of danger and appear oblivious to pain or cold. They may bite or pick at themselves or other children. They may wander off, run into traffic; stick fingers into electrical sockets; or turn on all the faucets in the bathroom. Parents are encouraged to describe the worst behavior of the child as well as the best.

TREATMENT

Initially, treatment goals focus on parent support and education, behavioral management of the child, and the development of skills that will give the child access to special or regular education [27]. Children do best if they live at home and receive treatment and education in community programs. Older children with severe behavior problems may require institutional care.

Parents should be involved in formulating treatment objectives. They can identify behaviors that are self-injurious and those that make management in the home most difficult. Work with the parents includes differentiating those behaviors that are most important to modify and those behaviors the parents can tolerate or accept. An analysis of the home environment, including the daily routine, may suggest some changes that can be made in the environment to relieve management problems [26]. Parents have good ideas about methods of managing behavior but not necessarily the confidence to pursue them when they do not work immediately. Schopler [26] notes that parents have usually tried many management procedures with their child but may not have pursued a good technique long enough. When the professional encourages them to try their own method longer, they are often successful.

Programs for autistic children include speech therapists, psychologists, teachers, and occupational therapists, all of whom must be knowledgeable about normal development and have experience using behavior modification techniques. Occupational therapists may use sensory integration procedures along with teaching social and occupational performance skills. Teachers should have experience with special education techniques and teaching methods that account for the child's difficulty with language.

In the early stages of treatment, the roles of the professional team overlap, and coordination and communication of efforts are important. All team members share the following objectives:

I. Develop attending behaviors
   A. Decrease self-injurious and self-stimulating behavior
   B. Eliminate fears
   C. Establish eye contact
   D. Overcome tactile defensiveness
   E. Establish auditory attention
II. Promote and enchance sensory awareness
   A. Near receptors—proprioceptive and kinesthetic
   B. Distance receptors—visual and auditory
   C. Other senses
III. Assess and develop sensory discrimination and motor responses
   A. Proprioceptive and tactile discrimination —gross and fine motor response
   B. Auditory discrimination—vocal response
   C. Visual discrimination—vocal and motor response

IV. Assess and develop the ability to imitate
   A. Gross and find motor activities
   B. Vocalization
V. Assess and develop social skills basic to treatment and eduation
   A. Develop trust in an adult
   B. Develop tolerance of the presence of other children
   C. Learn to participate in program routines

The accomplishment of these objectives will give the child skills on which to base additional learning. They provide the foundation on which language, academic, social, and vocational skills can be built.

THE LEARNING ENVIRONMENT

Autistic children learn best in a *highly structured environment*—one in which the adult determines what the child should be doing, as opposed to an environment in which many choices are provided so the child can be self-directed. Autistic children lack imagination and self-direction and tend to fall back on self-stimulating behaviors when left to their own devices [33].

Initially, the therapy/learning environment excludes extraneous stimuli that may divert the child's attention from the activity. Learning activities are carefully graded, starting with those tasks the child can do easily, followed by new skills taught in small incremental steps. Skills are acquired in sequence along a developmental hierarchy [33].

Structuring the stimuli is as important as structuring the sequence of an activity. Some children do not respond to certain sensory experiences [18], and while they may ignore many stimuli, they "over-register" [4] others. For example, a child may appear oblivious to a three-ring circus while attending, meticulously, to a button on his coat. Strong sensations, which may be painful to others, are often enjoyed by these children.

Other autistic children [18] show averse reactions to stimulation. They dislike being touched, refuse certain foods, and are frightened by noise. These children seem to have problems monitoring the intensity of and modulating the responses to sensation [18]. There is some evidence [5] that these children benefit from sensory integration therapy (see Chapter 5).

Through asssessment procedures, the teacher or therapist identifies those sensory modalities the child is best able to use. Learning activities are adapted to involve stimulation of the sensory systems that function most reliably. In general, the tactile and proprioceptive systems are more reliable than the visual or auditory systems and provide a good starting point [10]. For some, magnification of stimuli helps. These children also respond best to one kind of stimulation at a time, and it is wise to start treatment in an environment where there is little competing stimulation [16]. However, eventually the learning environment must include distractions found in everyday life to ensure that learning may be generalized.

Autistic children learn through work with visible materials that can be manipulated, and simple repetitive activities are best [31]. Therapists and teachers can use materials that have been developed according to Montessori's theories, which isolate sensory stimulation and teach concepts about the physical properties of objects [32]. Activities involving sorting and classifying objects according to color, shape, size, temperature, and smell encourage the child to use these senses [31].

Autistic children learn very slowly. They require repetition and a highly consistent schedule of reinforcement for learning [14]. They may not show a pattern of increased skill as they practice under supervision but instead may seem to be going nowhere, with scattered patterns of errors, just before they master a task [9].

Since the simplest tasks require so much effort, autistic children avoid tasks that are difficult. For difficult tasks they require continuous pacing of prompts that do not allow avoidance of work [14]. If negative reinforcement is being used, it should be used as the child initiates the undesired behavior, not when the child completes the act [32]. With children who cannot imitate, shaping, the rewarding of successive approximations of the desired behavior, is required when teaching a new skill.

MANAGING BEHAVIOR

Children who bite themselves, bang their heads, and engage in other self-injurious behaviors may be seeking stimulation [8]. The brains of some autistic children may only register very strong sensations; thus, normally painful stimuli are perceived as pleasurable to the child [4]. Engaging the child's interest in more productive activities, or providing alternative, harmless, strong stimuli, such as heavy pressure touch, vestibular and proprioceptive stimulation (see Therapy Program in Chapter 5), may decrease or eliminate injurious self-stimulation. *Behavior modification* is also used to eliminate self-injurious behavior; reduce stereotypical gestures that interfere with learning, establish eye contact, maintain attention, and reinforce learning (see Chapter 3).

Behavioral techniques are important tools in the treatment of autism because they can quickly eliminate behaviors that are dangerous to the child or that keep the child from attending to learning activities. Operant conditioning breaks through the autistic barriers quickly and effectively by systematically reinforcing attending behavior and focusing attention on the important aspects of a task (see Chapter 3).

There is some question as to whether the child will be able to generalize the learning that takes place through operant conditioning. Behavioral therapists have developed strategies that attempt to facilitate generalization of learning, but some autistic children may not have the capacity to go beyond rote learning. Behavior therapy will not work unless the expected behavior is within the child's biologic capacity. The therapist cannot expect the mute child to immediately produce complete sentences. Similarly, the physiologic responses of the child must be considered when choosing reinforcements.

When choosing reinforcements, the individual child's problems with sensory processing must be considered. Initially, food may be required as tangible, immediate reinforcement. If this is coupled with praise and hugs, the use of food can be gradually phased out and the child will respond to social rewards. The use of punishment to extinguish self-abusive habits must be done under close supervision with the approval of a human rights committee and the parents [26]. Care should also be taken not to deprive children of stimulation. When preventing self-abusive and isolating behavior, one must provide plenty of appropriate stimulation of all senses [32].

Autistic children show significant improvement through behavior therapy, which is most effective if used by the parents at home as well. Parents benefit from the opportunity to observe the therapist employing these techniques, and they may wish to practice techniques while the therapist observes [27]. It has been found that children who have learned skills in behavior modification programs are best able to maintain these skills if they live at home at the end of treatment; institutionalized children tend to regress after behavior therapy is terminated [19].

LANGUAGE STIMULATION

Many consider the problems with *language,* the communication of concepts through the use of symbols, the central disorder in autism [9, 24]. If individuals do not perceive sensation reliably, they cannot code or classify sensory information. If they cannot classify information, they cannot understand or use symbols for communication. Thus, language depends on skills in sensory discrimination, perceptual constancy, and concept formation. Maturation of the nervous system and the individual's experience of the environment are processes basic to language development [25].

A program to teach communication skills teaches concepts as well as labels. It motivates the children to communicate by helping them recognize that their needs will be met if they communicate them. Language cannot be taught in a vacuum. It requires the coordinated efforts of the speech therapist, parents, teachers, and therapists, in stimulating language and communication.

For some children, teaching communication skills starts at a very basic level, that of learning to respond to sound and the engagement in vocal play. Although autistic children may not show much curiosity about their environment, they will respond to sounds that they have learned to associate with pleasure. The therapist begins treatment with objects that are known to give pleasure: Music is often enjoyed; toys that click and clang, ticking clocks, and other objects that move and make noise can be used to gain the child's attention [10]. Eye contact with the therapist can be encouraged by briefly holding toys at the therapist's eye level before presenting them to the child [6]. To gain the child's attention to sounds or objects that are not intrinsically pleasurable, additional reinforcement, such as food, is needed.

Vocal play is encouraged. Mute autistic children may never have experienced the pleasure that normal infants gain from babbling and cooing. Immediate reinforcement of any sound uttered may be necessary to encourage vocalization. Vocal play may be stimulated through the use of roughhousing, using musical instruments, playing games, and imitating sounds of toys [6].

Encouraging nonverbal imitation can help facilitate vocal imitation. To encourage vocal imitation, at first, the therapist may need to use sounds that are in the child's repertoire, gradually building on these to formulate multisyllable combinations of sounds to imitate [6]. As the child develops the ability to imitate sound and produce words, the therapist works to use the words to label familiar objects and activities, gradually introducing the use of phrases. Withholding desired objects can stimulate the child to use familiar phrases to ask for them.

The most difficult phase of language development is the achievement of spontaneous, novel speech. Autistic children are often echolalic, and they will repeat words and phrases that they have heard. Sometimes these phrases are meaningful to the situation, but they may be completely out of context. Some children may never go beyond conditioned, parrotlike speech. Their understanding of concepts and ability to generalize may be too limited to allow them to communicate maturely. Those working with such children must be prepared to accept these limitations and teach, by rote, words and phrases that will help them make their needs known.

Some autistic children are able to learn sign language. Mute children are obvious candidates for sign language training, and Carr [7] found that mute children may learn to talk through vocal training and simultaneous (speech and sign) communication training. Churchill [9] cautions therapists to remember that the development of language requires more than conditioning: It requires biologic capabilities. "Those few autistic children who appear to progress furthest in language development do so by virtue of inherent developmental factors, rather than training wizardry." Nonetheless, language therapy is a critical area of the therapeutic program for autistic children. Even children who have limited capacity will have a better quality of life if they can communicate on even the most primitive level. Behavior problems decrease and attention spans increase as they begin to understand and communicate with the world around them.

ADDITIONAL CONSIDERATIONS

As autistic children become more responsive to teachers and therapists, they can be encouraged to relate to other children. Cooperation can be stimulated through participation in simple games and musical activities. *Training in social skills and activities of daily living* can commence. Developing the ability to focus attention on a task; to obey simple commands and to take care of, or communicate, toilet needs make these children more welcome at school. The

techniques used to teach mentally retarded children social and self care skills are effective with autistic children.

The same toilet-training methods used for normal children are used to train autistic children. A smaller seat or potty chair can be used with the child who is afraid. It may take a lot of time and patience to toilet train an autistic child [29]. Other self-care skills can be taught by moving the child's hands and limbs through the motions of the activity. Autistic children have trouble with motor planning and imitation. Putting on and buttoning up a jacket is a Mount Everest to a child who has unreliable proprioception, no conception of right-left and up-down, and who does not see the need for the the activity in the first place. Children who have trouble chewing and other oral motor skills may need to have their jaws moved for them to get the feel of the movement.

Finding the appropriate treatment and educational setting for an autistic child is important and can be frustrating. The needs of these children change as they mature. Young children may receive treatment at a medical facility that provides therapy and preschool programs. The setting for the education of school-age children depends on their level of functioning and the resources available. Public schools vary in the special services they offer. There are residential and day programs designed specifically for autistic children and programs that include autistic children along with other handicapped children. The National Society for Children and Adults with Autism (1234 Massachusetts Ave., N.W., Suite 1017, Washington, DC 20005; 202-783-0125) has chapters across the country and can provide parents with listings of programs for autistic people.

REFERENCES

1. American Psychiatric Association. *A Psychiatric Glossary* (4th ed.). Washington, D.C.: APA, 1975.
2. American Psychiatric Association. *Diagnostic and Statistical Manual of Mental Disorders* (3rd ed.). Washington, D.C.: APA, 1980.

3. American Psychiatric Association. *Diagnostic and Statistical Manual of Mental Disorders* (3rd ed., revised). Washington, D.C.: APA, 1987.
4. Ayres, A. J. *Sensory Integration and the Child.* Los Angeles: Western Psychological Services, 1979.
5. Ayres, A. J., and Tickle, L. S. Hyper-responsivity to touch and vestibular stimuli as a predictor of positive response to sensory integration procedures by autistic children. *Am. J. Occup. Ther.* 34:375, 1980.
6. Block, J., Gerten, E., and Kornblum, S. Evaluation of a language program for young autistic children. *J. Speech Hear. Disord.* 45:76, 1980.
7. Carr, E. G. Teaching autistic children to use sign language: Some research issues. *J. Autism Dev. Disord.* 9:345, 1979.
8. Carr, J. The Severely Retarded Autistic Child. In L. Wing (ed.), *Early Childhood Autism: Clinical, Educational and Social Aspects* (2nd ed.) New York: Pergamon, 1976.
9. Churchill, D. W. *Language of Autistic Children.* Washington, D.C.: Winston, 1978. P. 129.
10. Churchill, D. W., Alpern, G. D., and DeMyer, M. K. (eds.), *Infantile Autism: Proceedings of the Indiana University Colloquium.* Springfield, IL: Thomas, 1971.
11. Coleman, M. (ed.), *The Autistic Syndrome.* New York: American Elsevier, 1976.
12. DeMyer, M. K. Introduction to Part II. In D. W. Churchill, G. D. Alpern, and M. K. DeMyer (eds.), *Infantile Autism: Proceedings of the Indiana University Colloquium.* Springfield, IL: Thomas, 1971.
13. DeMyer, M. K. Motor, Perceptual-Motor and Intellectual Disabilities of Autistic Children. In L. Wing (ed.), *Early Childhood Autism: Clinical, Educational and Social Aspects* (2nd ed.). New York: Pergamon, 1976. P. 190.
14. Etzel, B. D., and LeBlanc, J. M. The simplest treatment alternative: The law of parsimony applied to choosing appropriate instructional control and errorless learning procedures for the difficult to teach child. *J. Autism Dev. Disord.* 9:361. 1979.
15. Freeman, B. J., and Ritvo, E. R. Cognitive Assessment. In E. R. Ritvo (ed.), *Autism: Diagnosis, Current Research and Management.* New York: Spectrum, 1976.
16. Handleman, J. S. Generalization by autistic-type children of verbal responses across settings. *J. Appl. Behav. Anal.* 12:273, 1979.
17. Kanner, L. *Childhood Psychosis: Initial Studies and New Insights.* Washington, D.C.: Windston, 1973. Pp. 36, 95.
18. Kinnealy, M. Aversive and nonaversive responses to sensory stimulation in mentally retarded children. *Am. J. Occup. Ther.* 27:464, 1973.
19. McGee, J. P., and Saidel, D. H. Individual Behavior Therapy. In S. L. Harrison (ed.), III Therapeutic Interventions. In J. D. Noshpitz (ed.), *Basic Handbook of Child Psychiatry.* New York: Basic, 1979.
20. Nelson, D. L. Evaluating autistic clients. *Occup. Ther. Ment. Health* 1 (4):1, 1980, 1981.
21. Ornitz, E. M., and Ritvo, E. R. Medical Assessment. In E. R. Ritvo (ed.), *Autism: Diagnosis, Current Research and Management.* New York: Spectrum, 1976.
22. Ritvo, E. R., Rabbin, K., Yuwiler, A., et al. Biochemical and Hematologic Studies: A Critical Review. In M. Rutter and E. Schopler (eds.), *Autism: A Reappraisal of Concepts and Treatment.* New York: Plenum, 1978.
23. Rutter, M. Language Disorder and Infantile Autism. In M. Rutter and E. Schopler (eds.), *Autism: A Reappraisal of Concepts and Treatment.* New York: Plenum, 1978.
24. Rutter, M. and Schopler, E. Autism and pervasive developmental disorders: Concepts and diagnostic issues. *J. Autism Dev. Disord.* 17: 159–186, 1987.
25. Sanders, D. A. A Model for Communication. In L. L. Lloyd (ed.), *Communication Assessment and Intervention Strategies.* Baltimore: University Park, 1976.
26. Schopler, E. Editorial: Treatment abuse and its reduction. *J. Autism Dev. Disord.* 16:99–104, 1986.
27. Schopler, E. Toward Reducing Behavior Problems in Autistic Children. In L. Wing (ed.), *Early Childhood Autism: Clinical, Educational and Social Aspects* (2nd ed.). New York: Pergamon, 1976. Pp. 237–238.
28. Schopler, E., and Reichler, R. J. Psychobiological Referents for the Treatment of Autism. In D. W. Churchill, G. D. Alpern, and M. K. DeMyer (eds.), *Infantile Autism: Proceedings of the Indiana University Colloquium.* Springfield, IL: Thomas, 1971.
29. Schopler, E., Reichler, R. J., DeVellis, R. F. et al. Toward objective classification of childhood autism: Childhood Autism Rating Scale (CARS). *J. Autism Dev. Disord.* 10:91–103, 1980.
30. Schopler, E., Rutter, M., and Chess, S. Editorial: Change of journal scope and title. *J. Autism Dev. Disord.* 9:1, 1979.
31. Taylor, J. E. An Approach to Teaching Cognitive Skills Underlying Language Development. In L.

Wing (ed.), *Early Childhood Autism: Clinical, Educational and Social Aspects* (2nd ed.). New York: Pergamon, 1976.

32. Wing, L. *Autistic Children: A Guide for Parents and Professionals.* Secaucus, N.J., Citadel, 1976.

33. Wing, L. (ed.). *Early Childhood Autism: Clinical, Educational and Social Aspects* (2nd ed.). New York: Pergamon, 1976.

Learning Disabilities

Karen Jacobs and Martha K. Logigian

"I have a problem with learning," complains 15-year-old Jesse. "I have never been able to read and I'm failing math."

Barbara, age 10, describes herself as always having difficulty with "paper-and-pencil tasks."

Mr. Smith notes that his 5-year-old son, Martin, "speaks only a few words and even those aren't clear."

Lisa, age 8, is described by her teacher as "never paying attention or following directions."

Andrew, who is in second grade, is always moving and cannot sit still in class. His mother describes him as being "clumsy."

The individuals briefly described above can all be categorized as learning disabled, a designation encompassing a part of the population that has a broad spectrum of levels of achievement and nonachievement. The current conception of learning disabilities is relatively new, although the existence of such a group of disorders has been recognized for over 80 years. They were initially described by James Hinshelwood (1895), an ophthalmologist; James Kerr (1896), a school physician; and W. Pringle Morgan (1898), a general practitioner [65]. Prior to the early 1960s there was a confusing variety of labels used to describe the child with relatively normal intelligence, who was having learning problems. Such a child was labeled with minimal brain dysfunction (MBD), minimal brain injury (MBI), psychoneurologic learning disorders, perceptually handicapped, educationally handicapped, brain injury, language disorders, psycholinguistic disorder, slow learner, dyslexia, attention deficit disorder, hyperactivity, neurologically handicapped, neurologically impaired, educationally maladjusted, and special learning disorder [36, 65, 83].

DEFINING LEARNING DISABILITIES

The term *learning disability* was first used in 1962 by Samuel A. Kirk in his textbook *Educating Exceptional Children*. He stated, "A learning disability refers to a retardation, disorder,

The authors wish to acknowledge the following individuals for their assistance in writing this chapter: Dr. Elizabeth Wiig, Judy Merrill, Barbara Shapiro, Jane Koomar, and Matthew Gold.

or delayed development in one or more of the processes of speech, language, reading, spelling, writing, or arithmetic resulting from a possible cerebral dysfunction and/or retardation, sensory deprivation or cultural or instructional factors" [68]. Kirk continues that these disabilities "refer to a discrepancy between the child's achievement and his apparent capacity to learn as indicated by aptitude tests, verbal understanding, and arithmetic computation" [68].

Rallying around this newest category of special education, which finally had an educationally oriented term, in 1963 parents in New York founded the Association for Children with Learning Disabilities (ACLD). This group would eventually become the largest organization in the United States concerned with learning disabilities and an important advocate for the learning disabled. A few years after ACLD was formed, professionals officially recognized the term by forming the Division for Children with Learning Disabilities (DCLD) of the Council for Exceptional Children (CEC), the major professional organization concerned with the education of exceptional children.

Since then, a number of definitions have been proposed for learning disabilities with none thus far becoming universally accepted. At best, the definition of learning disabilities can be understood as a broad umbrella definition that includes a number of conditions that were once considered separate and distinct. According to the *FOLD Learning Disabilities Guide,* "efforts to identify and help learning disabled children and adults have sometimes been hampered by the inability of the experts to agree on exactly what learning disabilities are" [102].

In 1969 a definition of learning disabilities was presented to Congress by the National Advisory Committee on Handicapped Children, which served as the basis of the 1969 Learning Disabilities Act and was included in Public Law 94-142, the Education for All Handicapped Children Act of 1975. This definition is probably the most widely used and accepted since

TABLE 5-1. Criteria for determining the existence of a specific learning disability

I. A team may determine that a child has a specific learning disability if
   A. The child does not achieve commensurate with his or her age and ability levels in one or more of the areas listed in *B.* of this section, when provided with learning experiences appropriate for the child's age and ability levels; and
   B. The team finds that a child has a severe discrepancy between achievement and intellectual ability in one or more of the following areas:
      1. Oral expression
      2. Listening comprehension
      3. Written expression
      4. Basic reading skill
      5. Reading comprehension
      6. Mathematics calculation
      7. Mathematics reasoning
II. The team may not identify a child as having a specific learning disability if the severe discrepancy between ability and achievement is primarily the result of
   A. A visual, hearing, or motor handicap
   B. Mental retardation
   C. Emotional disturbance
   D. Environmental, cultural, or economic disadvantage

Department of Health, Education and Welfare, Office of Education. *Fed. Reg.* 42(250), 65083. Dec 29, 1977.

schools that receive federal funds are required to use it (Table 5-1).

In September 1984, the board of directors of ACLD adopted its own definition of specific learning disabilities because "in schools, underachievement is often equated with learning disabilities. Misclassification is too common and public funds are often being used inappropriately" [1]. So as not to add to the confusion already related to the definition of learning disabilities, ACLD's definition is worded such that it does not conflict with the one in Public Law 94-142. Instead the definition emphasizes that the condition persists throughout life and does not "go away" even with special instruction. The ACLD definition is

Specific Learning Disabilities is a chronic condition of presumed neurological origin which selectively interferes with the development, integration, and/or demonstration of verbal and/or non-verbal abilities.

Specific Learning Disabilities exist as a distinct handicapping condition in the presence of average to superior intelligence, adequate sensory and motor systems, and adequate learning opportunities. The condition varies in its manifestations and in degree of severity.

Throughout life the condition can affect self-esteem, education, vocation, socialization, and/or daily living activities [1].

Although a clear consensus definition of learning disabilities continues to be difficult, accurate labeling of an individual is crucial. Gallagher [45] notes that accurate labeling makes it possible to provide differentiated treatment and to obtain resources, particularly state and federal funds. It provides the basis for the search for the cause of learning disabilities.

ETIOLOGY

The etiology of learning disabilities is unclear. However, some frequently hypothesized factors include [29]

Brain damage or dysfunction resulting from birth, perinatal anoxia, head injury, fetal malnutrition, encephalitis, and lead poisoning

Allergies

Biochemical abnormalities or metabolic disorders

Genetics

Maturational lag

Environmental factors (for example, neglect, abuse, inadequate stimulation, disorganized home)

INCIDENCE

It is not surprising that since there is difficulty with a consensus definition of learning disabilities, there would be a lack of agreement concerning the incidence of the condition. According to the United States Department of Education, about 1.75 million or about 4.4 percent of the approximately 40 million children enrolled in public schools have specific learning disabilities [103]. The condition is 5 times more common in boys than girls [102]. In addition, learning disabilities tend to run in families. Another interesting finding, whose significance has not yet been established, is from Geschwind's studies, which revealed that left-handed people were far more vulnerable than right-handed to learning disabilities [51].

Due to the differences in state laws and definitions, the number of children ages 8 to 21 identified as learning disabled varies widely from state to state. For example, in 1980, Maryland identified 5.7 percent of its school children as having specific learning disabilities; Massachusetts identified 1.5 percent [102].

A startling statistic, and one that has impact on both state and national levels, is that 32 percent of those youth that have appeared as dependents in legal settings, many of whom are in state detention homes, are learning disabled. [103]. In addition, 9 in every 100 male adolescents with learning disabilities will probably become delinquent compared to 4 in every 100 nonlearning disabled adolescent males [103].

CHARACTERISTICS OF SPECIFIC LEARNING DISABILITIES

Despite the difficulty in devising a consensus definition and gathering specific incidence figures, there are some assumptions about learning disabilities that are generally accepted. First, there is a significant discrepancy between learning potential and the actual level of learning. Often the learning disabled child has an academic performance profile that is characterized by many ups and downs and inconsistencies. Typically these will be evidenced in any of the following five general areas: spoken language, written language, arithmetic, reasoning, and memory [102]. Herskowitz and Rosman [62] note that a significant gap between school performance and intelligence is generally taken to be two grade levels. For example, Jeremy, a fourth-grade child of normal intelligence who is reading at a first- or second-grade level and performs near grade level in mathematics, as long as reading is not a variable, is learning disabled.

In addition to a significant discrepancy between learning potential and the actual level of learning, deficiencies or developmental delays in some of the cognitive processes used in learning are common in the learning disabled population. This may encompass or share many of the following categories that may be deficient in the learning disabled child. It must be stressed that children with learning disabilities exhibit a wide variety of these qualities, and no one of these characteristics is seen in all learning disabled children [49].

MEMORY DISORDERS

Memory disorders include poor short- and long-term memory. These may include either auditory or visual memory. Auditory memory deficits may be reflected in word finding, recall, and retrieval problems (dysnomia) [107]. For example, an individual with word-finding problems may ask for a pencil by saying, "Could you give me the . . . the thing . . . I need to write this letter with."

MOTOR DISORDERS

Some of the motor disorders that might occur are [33]

1. Hyperactivity: The child is in constant and excessive motion, which may ultimately interfere with his or her ability to selectively attend to stimuli.
2. Hypoactivity: Although not as common as hyperactivity, when observed, the child is slow, lethargic, or sluggish.

3. Poor fine or gross motor coordination: This may be manifested in the child having difficulty throwing a ball, running and skipping, cutting with a scissor, and coloring.
4. General clumsiness or awkwardness: This would include problems with planning new motor tasks (dyspraxia).
5. Poor or slow achievement of motor milestones is occasionally observed.

In addition soft neurologic signs are observed in some learning disabled children. These include [21, 62]

1. Choreiform movements: jerky, rapid, irregular movements usually involving the face and distal extremities
2. Dysdiadochokinesia: impaired ability to perform rapidly and smoothly repeated alternating movements.
3. Finger agnosia: inability to name, recognize, or select one's fingers.
4. Mild dysphasias: mild inability to process language.
5. Ocular apraxia: inability to perform purposeful voluntary ocular movements to command when comprehension and sensorimotor skills are present
6. Strabismus: deviation of the eye
7. End-point nystagmus: involuntary rapid movement of the eyeball
8. Exaggerated associated movements: involuntary movements or reflexive increase of tone
9. Tremor
10. Motor awkwardness
11. Fine motor incoordination
12. Awkward gait
13. Pupillary inequalities
14. Mixed laterality
15. Right-left discrimination confusion
16. Unilateral winking defect
17. Avoidance response to outstretched hands
18. Extinction to double-tactile stimulation
19. Borderline hyperreflexia and reflex asymmetries

Perceptual Disorders

Gearheart and Weishann note that the most common perceptual problems are auditory, tactile, proprioceptive, and vestibular [49]. For example, visual/spatial problems may interfere with accurate copying of letters. Auditory/perceptual problems may influence phoneme discrimination (for example, the *p* sound in pit and the *t* sound in tin) and sequencing (processing the correct order) [107]. Other difficulties may include impairments in the following: discrimination in which the child may be unable to distinguish between two different auditory, visual, or tactile stimuli; recognition of common visual, auditory, or tactile stimuli; orientation to time, space, or distance; body image; discrimination of figure ground or part-whole relations; discrimination of left-right; and eye-hand coordination [84].

Overattention or attention fixation exists when a child cannot shift focus of attention. This child may have as much difficulty learning as one who cannot focus on any task long enough to learn new material. The child may be restless and impulsive with motor and verbal perseveration, particularly perseveration in writing and copying [33].

Psychosocial Problems

Because of repeated failure these children may be at risk to develop poor self-concepts and self-esteem. Gordon [75] stresses that this appears to be one distinct commonality among the learning disabled adolescents. In addition, they can be socially inept, have trouble forming friendships, be less socially accepted, and have difficulty playing with peers. Other characteristics include being easily frustrated, irritable, angry, and having frequent temper tantrums.

Another interesting way of classifying learning disabilities has been done by Silver and Carleton [97]. Table 5-2 delineates their classification to specific learning disabilities into four areas corresponding to the four basic steps of the learning process: input, integration, memory, and output.

ASSESSMENT OF LEARNING DISABILITIES

Although sometimes diagnosed by a physician, the learning disabled child is typically labeled as such in an educational setting. In particular, the educators play a vital role in the diagnosis of learning disability with particular focus on the child's academic performance and classroom social adjustment [33].

When a child is suspected to be learning disabled, assessment is used for confirmation. Most often, the assessment is administered in the educational setting and typically necessitates the need for a multidisciplinary approach. All personnel working with the child (occupational and physical therapists, speech pathologists, educators, psychologists, and social workers) are usually part of the assessment process.

In addition, the assessment has many other purposes including [71, 99]

1. Measuring an individual's abilities along a continuum, against a norm, or in relation to his or her own previous score(s)
2. Gathering data on capabilities that are not available from other sources
3. Determining which skill areas require treatment
4. Measuring changes in capabilities as a result of treatment
5. Providing a mechanism to communicate with other professionals, the student, or the family

Assessment is conceptually composed of four parts [104]:

1. Screening: For instance, discussion with other professionals to determine the need for evaluation or treatment
2. Student-related consultation: The process of sharing relevant information with other professionals concerning students who are not currently referred for therapy
3. Evaluation: Obtaining and interpreting specific data necessary for treatment through
   a. Record review
   b. Interviews

TABLE 5-2. Classification of learning disabilities into four areas of the process of learning

1. **Input**

The process of perceiving and recording information in the brain.

Children and adults with input problems may have trouble seeing and hearing accurately. For example, they may confuse or reverse letters, using 3 for E, or b for d.

Reading, writing, or copying designs may be difficult. They may confuse left and right, skip words and lines in reading, and misjudge depth.

Eye-hand coordination may be affected, causing problems with catching and hitting a ball, jumping rope, and similar activities.

Children and adults with hearing input problems may misunderstand words and respond inappropriately. They may require several repetitions of the same question before they can respond. In a classroom or work situation, sounds may distract them.

2. **Integration**

Sequencing—the ability to put things in proper order—and understanding.

Problems with sequencing often affect spelling. The child or adult may include all the right letters in a word but put them in the wrong order.

Recalling the sequence of events in a story or set of instructions may also be difficult. Children and adults with understanding difficulties may grasp only the literal meaning of words and gestures.

3. **Memory**

Storing and retrieving visual and auditory information.

Children and adults with short-term memory problems may forget verbal instructions before they can carry them out.

Children and adults with long-term memory disabilities forget information that should be stored permanently—their home addresses, for example.

4. **Output**

Language and motor coordination.

Children and adults with language disabilities may grope for words or use the wrong word. They may require several repetitions before responding to a question.

A gross motor disability involves the coordination of large groups of muscles such as those used in riding a bicycle.

A problem with fine motor coordination—the coordination of small movements—often appears as poor, laborious handwriting.

Note: In addition to the learning problems outlined above, children and adults with learning disabilities frequently have behavior problems. These behavior problems are often caused by frustration. Tasks that their peers perform easily are difficult or impossible for them. They may have trouble making friends. Occasionally they seem insensitive because they misinterpret the responses of others. A short attention span and a need to be in constant motion may also accompany learning disabilities.

Source: From L. B. Silver and S. Carleton, Learning disabilities can be helped. *Rx Being Well: The Waiting Room Magazine.* Sept–Oct, 1983.

c. Observations

d. Checklists/inventories

e. Standardized and nonstandardized evaluations/tests

4. Reassessment, or, the ongoing process of determining the need to alter treatment plans as a student progresses

A brief case study may serve as a good example to better clarify the use of assessment. This example is from an occupational therapy viewpoint.

Jennifer is in fourth grade and is suspected to be learning disabled by her parents and teacher. The classroom teacher informs the school guidance counselor of Jennifer's parents' and her own concerns about Jennifer. In turn, the school guidance counselor, with the approval of Jennifer's parents, coordinates the referral for a special-needs assessment of Jennifer under Public Law 94-142. Occupational therapy assessment begins with the screening process. The screening included discussion with Jennifer's classroom teacher where it was determined that Jennifer is having the following problems in regular classroom activities:

1. Difficulty with cutting and coloring
2. Handwriting often labored with spacing problems; letters irregularly shaped and typically poorly organized on the page
3. General clumsiness
4. Difficulty copying letters from the blackboard
5. Restlessness
6. Reading at approximately a second-grade level

Through student-related consultation, the occupational therapist shares information gained from the teachers with additional school personnel (speech therapist, physical therapist, resource room teacher), which results in a referral to occupational therapy. The occupational therapist reviews Jennifer's school and medical records, interviews Jennifer and her parents, observes Jennifer in academic and physical education classes, and uses a therapist-made checklist and two standardized evaluations to aid in the development of a treatment program. Treatment is implemented. The use of standardized evaluation tools occurs throughout treatment to facilitate making appropriate changes in Jennifer's treatment program.

The five evaluation techniques used by the occupational therapist are discussed below. The first four will be described briefly with greater emphasis on standardized and nonstandardized evaluations.

1. Review of medical, educational, and vocational records: Information gathered from

record review can provide basic background information on the learning disabled child. Medical records supply data such as

Birth history (pregnancy, delivery, and neonatal period)
Developmental history
Play history
Health care status
Precautions
Medications or other treatment

Educational records will begin with the child's entry into school to the present, answering questions such as "When were school problems first recognized?" "Did behavior problems interfere with school performance during the early years?" "What testing or remediation has been carried out?" "What have been the effects of intervention?" "What are the child's abilities?"

Vocational records, if applicable, will contain information about the student's work-related habits and skills, job interests, experience, and capabilities.

2. Interviews: Interviews with the student, significant others (family and associates), teachers, therapists, and other school personnel assist in gaining an understanding of the student's performance profile and in establishing realistic objectives for treatment.

Obtaining information about the child's family and home environment can be most helpful, for example, ascertaining whether other family members have had difficulties in school and what the parents' academic and career aspirations for their child are. All too often, parents' expectations for their child are set unrealistically high, thus ignoring the child's limitations, or too low due to a lack of understanding of their child's individual strengths.

3. Observations: "Observation is the key to successful evaluation" [52]. For occupational therapists in particular, a large part of their training is directed toward honing this skill as an objective tool [63]. It requires that the therapist carefully use all senses and record data objec-

tively. Ideally this will occur in an uncontrived situation. As illustrated in Table 5-3, there are a wide variety of observation techniques available to the therapist. Modern technology has made video equipment increasingly more accessible, which allows for the recording of a child's activity and replay at a later time for greater analysis.

4. Checklists: Checklists can be devised by the therapist to represent a simple list of factors or behaviors that are considered important to note. These checklists act as guides that may provide data to support the need for referrals, screenings, or more in-depth evaluation.

5. Standardized and nonstandardized evaluations/tests: Observation is an essential aspect of both standardized and nonstandardized evaluation. These two types of evaluations provide a systematic method to determine a person's performance profile.

"Standardized" implies uniformity of procedure in administering and scoring the test and has the advantage of affording comparison of test results with normative or average performance. In addition, validity and reliability have been established. With nonstandardized evaluations, uniform procedure in administering and scoring the test may be established, but normative data, validity, and reliability have not been determined; therefore results are not comparable [63].

"Learning disability" by definition represents a heterogeneous group of individuals with diverse visual, perceptual, motor, and language abilities—and equally diverse psychological, social, developmental, and academic profiles. This is an important factor when selecting an appropriate evaluation. Typically therapists use many evaluations or portions thereof, and various subtests of an evaluation to fit the individual needs of a student. Thus, not all learning disabled children receive the exact same evaluations. Selection of appropriate evaluation(s) is predicated on information obtained in the first two components of assessment (screening and student-related consultation) and record review, interviews, observations, and checklists/inventories. Thus, an evaluation or subtest(s) or both,

TABLE 5-3. Observational techniques for evaluation

1. Rating scale	18. Personal data sheet	31. Health records
2. Anecdotal records	19. Questionnaires (program-service)	32. Use community agencies
3. Ranking scales		33. Checklists
4. Case study	20. Student daily record	34. Administrative reports
5. Self-appraisal devices	21. Sociometric tests	35. Informed teacher reports
6. Autobiographies	22. Sociometric patterns	36. Student interviews
7. Professional observation	23. Cumulative records	37. Projective techniques
8. Play therapy	24. Student-kept cumulative records	38. Study-habit interview
9. Student conferences		39. Sociodrama/psychodrama
10. Follow-up studies	25. Student-parent conferences	40. Discussion groups
11. Scaled data: graphs, charts, percentiles		41. Role playing
12. Scattergrams	26. Group guidance (orientation-therapeutic)	42. Audio-video devices and feedback
13. Expectancy tables	27. Child study program	43. Computer-assisted devices
14. Projection techniques	28. Attitude observation	44. Gaming
15. Student projects	29. Behavior modification	45. Simulated experiences
16. Token economy	30. Modified test procedure (test, re-test)	46. Student input/contracts
17. Peer evaluation		

Source: From D. E. Brolin and C. Kokaska, *Career Education for Handicapped Children and Youth*. Columbus: Merrill, 1979. P. 284.

of an evaluation may be selected that looks more in depth at areas that appear to be problematic.

The Chapter Appendix provides a selective list of evaluations that may be used by speech pathologists and occupational and physical therapists to assess the learning disabled child. Some of these tests are highlighted throughout the remainder of this chapter.

SPEECH AND LANGUAGE
The speech and language evaluation addresses receptive and expressive language and speech production. These areas may be assessed using the following standardized evaluations: Illinois Test of Psycholinguistic Abilities [69], Detroit Tests of Learning Aptitude [58], Peabody Picture Vocabulary Test-Revised [39], Test of Adolescent Language [60], Clinical Evaluation of Language Function [95], Test of Language Competence [107], Test of Adolescent Language (TOAL) [106], Woodcock Language Proficiency Battery [111], Word Test [66], Expressive One-Word Picture Vocabulary Test [46], Upper-Extension Expressive One-Word Picture Vocabulary Test [47], Token Test for Children [99], and Test of Language Development [85].

A brief case study may serve as a good example of the process used in selecting appropriate speech and language evaluations.

Jim is a 17-year-old learning disabled student who presents with significant language deficits such as word retrieval and memory difficulties and articulation errors, with receptive language skills that are functional in general conversation. Based on this information, the school's speech pathologist selects the following evaluations and subtests of evaluations to assess Jim's language functioning: Peabody Picture Vocabulary Test; Detroit Tests of Learning Aptitude-Subtests: verbal opposites, verbal absurdities, oral commissions, oral directions, and pictorial absurdities; Clinical Evaluation of Language Function Subtests: processing linguistic concepts and spoken paragraphs; Illinois Test of Psycholinguistic Abilities Subtests: auditory association, visual association, grammatic closure; and Expressive One-Word Picture Vocabulary Test.

Results from these evaluations reveal that Jim is functioning as follows:

Vocabulary: 6-year deficit
Auditory association: 8-year deficit
Action-agent (verb): 5-year deficit
Verbal absurdities: 4-year deficit
Oral commissions: 9-year deficit
Oral directions: 4-year deficit
Visual association: 9-year deficit
Pictorial absurdities: 8-year deficit
Expressive one-word vocabulary: 8 to 9 year deficit
Poor ability to integrate individual facts into one main idea
Word retrieval difficulties

For a further discussion of language disorders associated with children who have learning disabilities, see Communication Disorders.

PHYSICAL THERAPY EVALUATION
Physical therapists are interested in evaluating the motor and postural functions of the learning disabled child and efficient use of the body [32]. These areas are most commonly evaluated using tests that include [35]

1. Muscle strength
2. Range of motion
3. Ambulation
4. Reflex integration
5. Postural control

Some standardized evaluations that may be used by the physical therapist are Bruininks-Oseretsky Test of Motor Proficiency [28], Purdue Perceptual-Motor Survey Rating Scale [92], Test of Motor Impairment-Henderson Revised [94], Quick Neurological Screening Test [83], and Test of Motor Proficiency of Gubbay [56].

One of the more commonly used evaluations is the Bruininks-Oseretsky Test of Motor Proficiency [28], a norm-referenced test designed to assess motor functioning in eight areas. The subtests include

GROSS MOTOR SKILLS

Subtest 1. Running speed and agility
Subtest 2. Balance
Subtest 3. Bilateral coordination
Subtest 4. Strength

GROSS AND FINE MOTOR SKILLS

Subtest 5. Upper-limb coordination

FINE MOTOR SKILLS

Subtest 6. Response speed
Subtest 7. Visual motor control
Subtest 8. Upper-limb speed and dexterity

The Bruininks-Oseretsky is an individual test that takes approximately 45 minutes to 1 hour to administer and has been standardized for students 4.6 to 14.6 years. A short form of the test has been devised for use as a screening tool, takes approximately 20 minutes, and includes only the gross motor or fine motor subtests.

OCCUPATIONAL THERAPY EVALUATION

The occupational therapist has similar concerns as the physical therapist for the postural basis of movement but stresses fine motor abilities, sensory integration, and visual/spatial and perceptual functions [21]. In addition, occupational therapists are interested in assessing the work-related behaviors, habits, and skills of the learning disabled child.

All of the previously mentioned standardized evaluations used to assess motor performance by physical therapists may also be used by the occupational therapist. Other evaluations used by occupational therapists that may assess additional skill areas include Frostig Movement Skills

Test Battery [86], Miller Assessment of Pre-schoolers [79], Meeting Street School Screening Test [57], Southern California Sensory Integration Tests [19], Bender Gestalt Test for Young Children [70], Developmental Test of Visual Motor Integration [26], Developmental Test of Visual Perception [44], Basic Motor Ability Tests-Revised [5], McCarthy Scales of Children's Abilities [76], Illinois Test of Psycholinguistic Abilities [69], Goodenough-Harris Drawing Test [54], The Pediatric Assessment System for Learning Disorders [74], and Jacobs Prevocational Skills Assessment [63].

The Pediatric Assessment System for Learning Disorders [74] is a neurodevelopmental examination divided into three age bands:

1. The Pediatric Examination of Educational Readiness (PEER) is given to children 4 to 6 years and is composed of a general health assessment, observation of dressing/undressing during a physical examination, and a developmental attainment component. The latter component consists of 29 tasks delineated into the following categories:

Orientation, e.g., identify body parts
Gross motor, e.g., stand on one foot (10 seconds)
Visual fine motor, e.g., manipulates sticks
Sequential, e.g., finger opposition
Linguistic, e.g., spatial directions
Preacademic learning, e.g., write letters, name symbols

2. The Pediatric Early Elementary Examination (PEEX) is given to children 7 to 9-years old and consists of the following major sections: developmental attainment, neuromaturation, general health, task analysis, and associated behavioral observations.

3. The Pediatric Examination of Education Readiness at Middle Childhood (PEERAMID) is given to children 9 to 15 years and older with specific neurodevelopmental areas and items such as minor neurologic indicators, fine motor

function, selective attention, language, and gross motor function.

In addition, the Aggregate Neurobehavioral Student Health and Educational Review System (Anser) is a supplemental test to be used in conjunction with the PEER, PEEX, and PEERAMID. It is composed of a series of questionnaires to be completed by parents, school personnel, and children ages 9 and older to assess the development, behavior, and health of a child suspected of having a specific learning disability or behavior disorder, or both.

WORK-RELATED ASSESSMENT

Vocational assessment for the learning disabled is an area in which little work has been done. To date, there is no standard, well-validated battery of tests on which to base decisions for vocational programming [75]. This lack of information was the impetus for developing an evaluation to be used for the learning disabled child, particularly the adolescent. The Jacobs Prevocational Skills Assessment (JPSA) was devised to assess a student's performance in specific work-related skills, behaviors, and habits [63]. These areas include fine motor coordination; eye-hand coordination; motor planning; figure-ground; sorting; classification/sequencing; decision making; problem solving; organizational skills; use of tools; ability to follow visual, written, and verbal directions; conceptual skills; task focus and behavioral observations. The JPSA is a standard evaluation composed of 15 simulated work tasks:

1. Quality control
2. Filing
3. Carpentry assembly
4. Classification
5. Office work
6. Telephone directory
7. Factory work
8. Environmental mobility
9. Money concepts
10. Functional banking
11. Time concepts
12. Work attitudes
13. Body scheme
14. Leather assembly
15. Food preparation

The JPSA is administered individually and is completed after approximately 1 to 2 hours; it has been found to be a useful screening instrument and should be used in conjunction with other evaluations.

SENSORY INTEGRATION ASSESSMENT

Sensory integration [9, 18] refers to the ability of the brain to organize and interpret sensory stimuli for an adaptive response. It contributes to the development of adequate perception, language, cognition, academic skills, emotional maturation, and behavior control. Figure 5-1 provides a schematic representation of sensory integration that suggests that sensory information is integrated via the central nervous system to produce a functional end product. The latter is a necessary component for successful learning and interaction with the environment.

When the brain is not processing the flow of sensory impulses appropriately, such as in sensory integrative dysfunction, accurate information about self or the environment is not received. Thus, children with this problem may be unable to direct their behavior effectively. Without efficient sensory integration, learning is difficult, and the individual often feels uncomfortable when moved or touched and cannot easily cope with ordinary demands and stress. Children with a learning disability may exhibit problems with sensory integration.

The evaluation process for children suspected of having sensory integrative dysfunction primarily involves the use of the Southern California Sensory Integration Tests (SCSIT) [10, 19, 20], Southern California Postrotary Nystagmus Test [13], measurements of postural and ocular responses, and indices of lateralization (Fig. 5-2). The Illinois Test of Psycholinguistic Abilities (ITPA) [69], Flowers-Costello

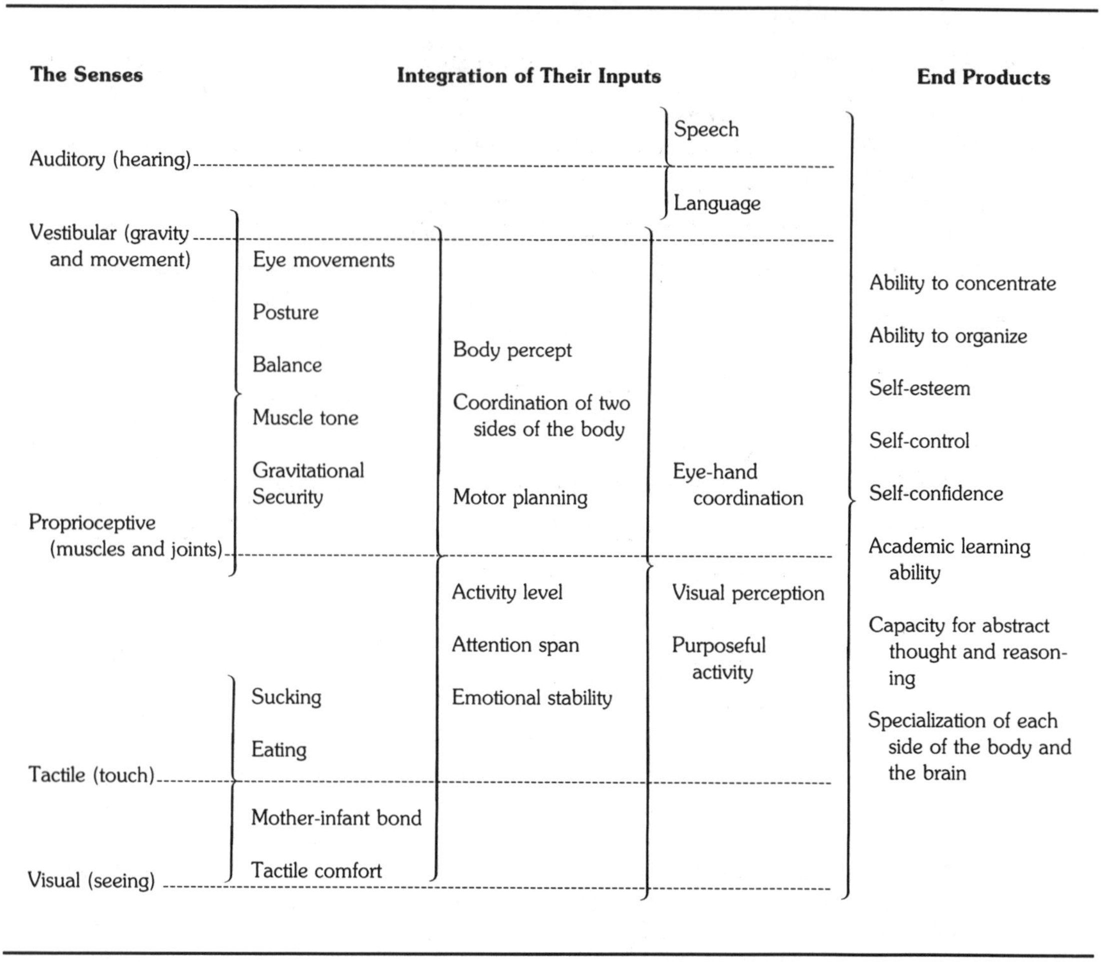

The Senses   **Integration of Their Inputs**   **End Products**

Auditory (hearing) — Speech / Language

Vestibular (gravity and movement)

Eye movements
Posture
Balance
Muscle tone
Gravitational Security

Body percept
Coordination of two sides of the body
Motor planning

Proprioceptive (muscles and joints)

Activity level
Attention span
Emotional stability

Eye-hand coordination

Visual perception
Purposeful activity

Sucking
Eating
Mother-infant bond
Tactile comfort

Tactile (touch)

Visual (seeing)

End Products:
Ability to concentrate
Ability to organize
Self-esteem
Self-control
Self-confidence
Academic learning ability
Capacity for abstract thought and reasoning
Specialization of each side of the body and the brain

FIG. 5-1. The senses, integration of their inputs, and their end products. (Copyright © 1979 by Western Psychological Services. Reprinted from A. J. Ayres, *Sensory Integration and the Child* by permission of the publisher, Western Psychological Services, 12031 Wilshire Boulevard, Los Angeles, California 90025, U.S.A.)

Test of Central Auditory Abilities (FCTCAA) [41], and a dichotic listening test, among others, are also recommended parameters of assessment.

COGNITIVE AND MEDICAL EVALUATIONS
Intellectual performance is most commonly evaluated using any of the following tests: the Wechsler Intelligence Scale for Children-Revised (WISC-R) [105] and the Woodcock Johnson Psycho-Educational Battery (WJPEB) [110]. The WISC-R is standardized on students 6 to 16.11 years and is administered individually (approximate testing time—50 to 75 minutes). The WJPEB has been standardized for ages 3 to 80 and is administered individually. Its

Name: _____ Hand: R L Test date: yr ___ mo ___ day ___
                                                      Birth date: yr ___ mo ___ day ___
Parents: _____ Age: yr ___ mo ___ day ___

Address: _____ Telephone: _____

Familial handedness: _____ Referred by : _____

1. Hyperactivity, distractibility:
   3—normal activity
   2—slt. hyperactivity
   1—def. hyperactivity
2. Tactile defensiveness:
   3—no responses
   2—1 or ? response
   1—2 responses or def.
3. Muscle tone:
   3—normal hyportonic
   2—sl. hypotonic
   1—def. hypotonic
   R–L differences ____

4. Eye dominance: *Eye*   *Hand*
   Sights eye through ring of examiner's fingers at 6 in.   R L
   Sights eye through hole in paper   R L
   Sights eye through different objects: cone, telescope, kaleidoscope, etc. R L   R L
                                                                           R L   R L
   Independent eye closure (optional, circle if adequate)   R L   R L

5. Eye movements:

	Across midline	Pursuits in general	Convergence	Quick Localization
	3—normal	3—normal	3—normal	3—normal
	2—slt. irreg.	2—slt. irreg.	2—slt. irreg.	2—slt. irreg.
	1—def. poor	1—def. poor	1—def. poor	1—def. poor
R–L differences	_____	_____	_____	_____

6. Ability to perform slow motions: 3—smooth   2—slt. irreg.   1—jerky, too fast _____

7. Diadochokinesia:

	Right ___ times	Left ___ times	Both simul.
	3—normal	3—normal	3—normal
	2—slt. defic.	2—slt. defic.	2—slt. defic.
	1—def. poor	1—def. poor	1—def. poor

8. Thumb-finger touching:

	Right ___ times	Left ___ times	Both simul.
	3—normal	3—normal	3—normal
	2—slt. defic.	2—slt. defic.	2—slt. defic.
	1—def. poor	1—def. poor	1—def. poor

FIG. 5-2. An evaluation of sensory integrative dysfunction, measuring postural and ocular responses and indices of lateralization. (Adapted from A. J. Ayres, 1977.)

FIG. 5-2. (CONTINUED)

9. Tongue to lip movement:

	Right ___ times	Left ___ times	Both simul.
	3—normal	3—normal	3—normal
	2—slt. defic.	2—slt. defic.	2—slt. defic.
	1—def. poor	1—def. poor	1—def. poor

10. Co-contractions, arm, shoulder, neck:
    3—normal
    2—slt. deficiency
    1—def. deficiency

11. Postural Insecurity, supine position:
    3—normal
    2—slt. deficiency
    1—def. deficiency

12. Postural background movements:
    3—normal
    2—slt. deficiency
    1—def. deficiency

13. Equilibrium reactions, prone position:
    3—normal
    2—slt. deficiency
    1—def. deficiency

14. Equilibrium reactions, quadruped position:
    3—normal
    2—slt. deficiency
    1—def. deficiency

15. Equilibrium reactions, sitting:
    3—normal
    2—slt. deficiency
    1—def. deficiency

16. Schilder's arm extension posture:

Choreoathetosis	Post changing arms	Trunk rotation	Head resist	Discomfort
3—normal	3—normal	3—normal	3—normal	3—normal
2—slight	2—slight	2—slight	2—slight	2—slight
1—definite	1—definite	1—definite	1—definite	1—definite

    a. Arm raised: R   L
    b. Elbow hyperextended: R   L

17. Prone extension position:

    3—holds 20 or more sec with moderate exertion
    2—holds to 10 sec, or 20 sec with great exertion
    1—unable, or holds 0–9 sec

18. Symmetrical TNR, quadruped position; head flexed and extended:

    3—no change in joint flexion or extension
    2—slight change in joint position
    1—definite change in joint position

19. Asymmetrical TNR:
    a. Quadruped position

    3—no flexion on passive head turning
    2—slight flexion on passive head turning
    1—definite flexion or head resistance

    b. Reflex: inhibiting posture

    3—can assume and maintain balance
    2—can assume only with great difficulty
    1—cannot assume

FIG. 5-2. (CONTINUED)

20. Flexed supine position:

3—holds 20 or more sec with moderate exertion
2—holds to 10 sec or 20 sec with great exertion
1—unable to, or holds 0–9 sec

21. Hopping/Jumping:

Right	Left	Both simul.
3—normal	3—normal	3—normal
2—slt. irreg.	2—slt. irreg.	2—slt. irreg.
1—def. irreg.	1—def. irreg.	1—def. irreg.

22. Skipping:

3—normal
2—slt. irreg.
1—def. irreg.

23. Walking beam: Lead foot   R   L

4 in. wide   Forward _____ Backward _____

2 in. wide   Forward _____ Backward _____

Comments and directions for clinical observations

---

1. Hyperactivity, distractibility: Observe during testing and clinical observations, and later in treatment.
2. Tactile defensiveness: Observe during testing, especially tactile tests and clinical observations.
3. Muscle tone: Check for hyperextension in elbow and wrist, and observe during treatment. Can also palpate muscles for tone. Check for right/left differences.
4. Eye preference: Offer cone, tube, kaleidoscope, etc., at midline. Observe which is used to sight with, and also which hand reaches for object.
   Independent eye closure (optional): Observe if child can close each eye independently.
5. Eye pursuits: Use a pencil or other appropriate object; hold about 8–10 in. from the child's eyes and move the pencil diagonally and horizontally. Observe for midline problems. (Dr. Ayres does this test without the child's glasses.) For convergence, bring the pencil close to the eyes; check eyes together and independently by first covering one eye then the other. Observe for right/left differences. Can also ask child, "Which eye do you like best?"
6. Ability to perform slow motions (optional): Directions: "Watch me doing this, then do it with me. Don't go too fast, don't go too slow." Examiner starts with shoulders abducted at 90° and hands touching shoulders. Slowly extend elbows, then flex elbows and return fingertips to touch shoulders.
7. Diadochokinesia (rapid forearm rotation): The child and the examiner are seated facing each other, arms are flexed, resting on laps. Examiner demonstrates rapid supination and pronation, then asks the child to imitate and says, "Do it fast." Count the times the palms slap the thighs in 10 sec. Observe for incoordination. Compare right and left scores.
8. Thumb-finger touching: Thumb touches each finger in sequence from index to little, and then back in sequence to index finger, repeating several times. Observe speed, coordination, and right/left differences.
9. Tongue to lip movement: Examiner demonstrates, then asks child to do the same. Observe coordination and ability to touch the sides of the mouth, upper and lower lips with tongue.
10. Co-contraction: The examiner sits facing the child. Child should not stabilize against the back of the chair. Directions: "Squeeze my thumbs; don't let me push you; don't let me pull you." Allow some elbow flexion and give the child a chance to build up tone. Can also test one arm at a time and palpate. For neck co-contraction, the examiner places a hand on top of the child's head and says, "Freeze like a statue." The examiner pushes down slightly and attempts to move the head slightly back and forth and from side to side. Do not expect as much of the neck muscles as the arms.
11. Postural insecurity: Test the child supine on an unstable surface (e.g., ball, vestibular ball); move the surface. Note the degree of fearfulness.

FIG. 5-2. (CONTINUED)

12. Postural background movements: Observe during testing, especially on Kinesthesia and Motor Accuracy, and during clinical observations. Observe how easily the child adjusts posture to complete a task.

13, 14, 15.

Equilibrium reactions and protective extension: Test in several different positions and on different surfaces (ball, vestibular board, etc.)

16. Schilder's arm extension posture:
    a. Examiner tells the child, "Put your feet together, arms out, spread your fingers apart, close your eyes, and (if possible) count to twenty." Observe if choreoathetoid movements are present, if the child hyperextends at the elbows, or tries to stabilize with hands together. Check if one arm rises or lowers.
    b. Examiner tells the child to keep arms in front while examiner moves child's head. Observe for lowering or turning of arms, inadequate tonic background, resistance to head turning. Check for right/left differences.

17. Prone extension position: Ask the child to assume the position. Demonstrate and/or place child in the position if necessary. If positioning or demonstration is needed, allow the child to rest and then reassume position. Have child count out loud to avoid a stabilizing effect by holding breath. Position: Child is prone, arms abducted, elbows flexed, legs extended with knees not touching mat.

18. Symmetrical tonic neck reflex: Child is in the quadruped position. The examiner flexes and extends the child's head and observes for changes in joint position and trunk posture.

19. Asymmetrical tonic neck reflex:
    a. The child is in the quadruped position. Make sure elbows are not locked. The examiner turns the head to the right and the left and observes the amount of elbows flexion as head is turned.
    b. The child is placed in the reverse ATNR position (hand on hip, opposite leg raised, head turned toward the side of the flexed arm). Observe the effect of the ATNR on equilibrium, noting if the child can assume and maintain this position.

20. Flexed supine position: Ask the child to assume the position or place child in the position (arms crossed on chest, ankles crossed, flexion at neck, hips, and knees). Observe how long and how well the child can maintain this posture. Let child rest, then ask child to reassume the position and apply resistance at head and knees to see if child can hold it. Expect very little of 6 years and under. Children 8 years and older can be expected to hold for 20–30 sec.

21, 22, 23.

Balance reactions are assessed during several different activities while standing.

---

three parts take the following amount of time to administer: Part I, 60 to 90 minutes; Part 2, 30 to 45 minutes; and Part 3, 15 to 30 minutes [110]. The WJPEB's subtests are miniature learning tasks. Both evaluations are typically administered by the school psychologist. In addition, the McCarthy Scales of Children's Abilities [76] is frequently used and may be administered by an occupational therapist.

The following reading and arithmetic achievement tests are commonly used: Reading achievement: Durrell Analysis of Reading Difficulty [40], Gates-McKillop Reading Diagnostic Test [48], Gray Oral Reading Test [55],

Monroe Reading Aptitude Test [82], Spache Diagnostic Reading Scales [100], and Woodcock Reading Mastery Tests [109], Arithmetic achievement: Key Math Diagnostic Arithmetic Test [34] and Stanford Diagnostic Mathematics Test [25].

Finally, the physician may evaluate the child suspected of being learning disabled. However, according to the American Psychiatric Association's *Diagnostic and Statistical Manual of Mental Disorders (DSM III)*, the physician may diagnose a child with any of the following labels: attention deficit disorder, developmental reading disorder, developmental arithmetic disorder, developmental language disorder, and mixed specific developmental disorders [33, 108]. Some evaluations that may be used by the physician to diagnose a child with a suspected learning disability include [62]

1. Electroencephalography (EEG)
2. Thyroid function tests
3. Skull x rays
4. Cranial computed tomography (CT) scan
5. Adrenal function tests
6. Lumbar puncture
7. Brain electrical activity mapping (BEAM)
8. Positron emission tomography (PET)

TREATMENT

Just as the assessment of a learning disabled child needs to be multidisciplinary, this is also critical for effective treatment. Since the management of this child takes place most commonly in the school setting, the approach needs to take into consideration the educational, psychological, social, physiologic, and medical needs of the child and include all personnel working with him or her.

Treatment techniques can be conceptualized along a continuum: At one end are the sensorimotor or somatic therapies and at the other end are the academic or cognitive methods.

SENSORIMOTOR APPROACH

A sensory integrative approach is a frequently used sensorimotor intervention strategy for children with learning disabilities. Its theory is built on four postulates [9, 12, 18]:

1. The brain functions as a whole and that integration of the parts is required for optimal function of the whole. Thus, it is hypothesized that sensory input enhances sensory integration and improves the efficiency of the nervous system.
2. The evolution of the brain comprised a series of hierarchic stages. New structures evolved and provided more complex activity, yet they remained dependent on older structures. For the cortex to function adequately, integrating structures in the brain stem have to function optimally.
3. There is plasticity in the central nervous system, that is, the nervous system can be influenced to change, especially through the use of particular sensory stimulation.
4. Through the use of sensory stimulation, an adaptive response is elicited, thus actively promoting sensory integration.

According to Ayres [18], of the sensory systems, the vestibular system is the one that unifies the brain. It forms a person's relationship to gravity and the environment. The vestibular system interprets the orientation of the head and body so that the information from the eyes can be understood. (Is it the object in front of us, or are our eyes moving?) It tells us if the head is moving or tilted and is able to provide information about the rest of the body through the interaction of gravity and movement receptors with muscle and joint sensations. The vestibular system maintains a stable visual field by adjusting eye and neck muscles to compensate for head and body movements [89].

In response to spinning, reflex eye muscle contractions are elicited through activation of the semicircular canals, that is, nystagmus (rapid back and forth eye movement) is the normal reflex response to vestibular stimulation. The duration of postrotary nystagmus provides a measure of the efficiency of the vestibular system [13, 18]. Current research [14, 17, 30, 37, 38, 101] has associated a depressed post rotary nystagmus with learning and language problems in children. DeQuiros [38] identified vestibuloproprioceptive disintegration, a disorder found among learning disabled children. These children demonstrated vestibular hyporeflexia in response to caloric stimulation. Ayres [18] suggested that if this situation occurs, the vestibular nuclei are not receiving adequate vestibular stimulation or are not processing it properly. On the other hand, if the child exhibits a hyperreflexive response to rotary motion, the vestibular system may be overresponding and not inhibiting the vestibular stimulation adequately.

The vestibular system's influence on academic learning was noted by Kephart [67] when he recognized the significance in the child's relationship to gravity. Frank and Levinson [43] and DeQuiros [37] suggest that problems with vestibular processing are reflected in difficulties with reading and writing and thus interfere with academic achievement and emotional development.

Within the area of sensory integration, several syndromes of dysfunction have been identified [6, 8, 9, 11, 15, 16] including problems in vestibular-bilateral integration, dyspraxia, tactile defensiveness, left-hemisphere dysfunction, and right-hemisphere dysfunction. In addition, several other domains of sensorimotor and language dysfunction have been suggested relative to sensory integration including gravitational insecurity [15, 16, 18, 96].

Vestibular Dysfunction
Disorders involving the vestibular system include vestibular-bilateral disorder (underreactive vestibular system) and gravitational insecurity (overreactive vestibular response).

A child with a vestibular-bilateral disorder often appears normal and healthy, yet in school has difficulty learning to read, write, and do mathematics. Gross movements may be clumsy as well as activities calling for the coordinated use of both sides of the body such as in baseball.

Clark [31] identifies the following parameters as indicative of the vestibular-bilateral syndrome:

1. Depressed nystagmus
2. Poor bilateral development and lateralization as indicated by eye, hand, ear dominance patterns and the ratio on the dychotic listening test
3. Poor oculomotor control

4. Poorly integrated postural mechanisms (particular difficulty in assuming prone extension)

Researchers [16, 32, 87] have suggested that low scores on the following SCSIT correlate with vestibular processing dysfunction: Standing Balance (eyes open and closed) Motor Accuracy (when raw scores are similar), Bilateral Motor Coordination Space Visualization Contralateral use, and other right-left test scores. The latter two parameters are examples of indications that expected patterns of cerebral hemisphere specialization have not developed and of poor bilateral integration [9]. In addition, other test scores correlated with vestibular dysfunction include a low ratio on dichotic listening, low reading scores (from standardized reading tests), inconsistent visual/spacial perception scores, and inadequate language development [9, 16, 18].

Another disorder of the vestibular system is manifest in gravitational insecurity. This disorder appears to involve the inability of the brain to modulate stimulation from the otoliths (gravity receptors). On evaluation these children often exhibit hyperactive nystagmus. In addition, there is an excessive emotional reaction to vestibular sensations, such as being placed in an unusual position or being moved by another person. Proprioceptive impulses may be inadequate for postural security, and the child demonstrates a dyskinesia [18].

The child with this disorder is extremely fearful of falling even when there is no danger of falling. This can be observed in the child's reluctance to use playground equipment or lack of enjoyment in being lifted from the ground. These children may develop manipulative behavior and become uncooperative due to the fear of novel situations and in an attempt to reduce adult physical contact [18].

Developmental Dyspraxia
Developmental dyspraxia, or its more extreme form, apraxia, is a disorder of sensory integra-

tion that interferes with the ability to motor plan or execute nonhabitual tasks. Motor planning involves the organization of tactile, vestibular, and proprioceptive sensations interacting with the environment through movement. The dyspraxic child has great difficulty motor planning and appears awkward and clumsy.

Parameters of the syndrome include

1. Depressed or prolonged nystagmus
2. Low scores on the Imitation of Postures test
3. Somatosensory deficits as demonstrated by low scores on the SCSIT somatosensory tests (FI, Graph, LTS, MFP)
4. Supine flexion tends to be more involved than prone extension [31]
5. Problems in manipulatory play and gross and fine motor activities

Other signs of dysfunction can include inadequate lateralization development, left-hemisphere dysfunction, visual/spatial problems, and a CML score that is better than CMLX [31]. Other SCSIT that tend to load with this syndrome are BMC, DC, MAC, and SBO [31]. The dyspraxic child may also exhibit an emotional lability and generally have difficulty coping with life situations [18].

Tactile Defensiveness
Tactile defensiveness suggests an imbalance in the tactile system. It presents as a tendency to react aversively and emotionally to sensory stimulation (hypersensitivity to touch). It is characterized by hyperactivity and distractability [18, 32].

Tactile defensive behavior is identified primarily through clinical observation. The Sensory History has been found useful in identifying this problem [72] and although the SCSIT may not discriminate for this syndrome, the child's cumulative reaction to the SCSIT tactile tests can be an indicator of this behavior. Additionally, Bauer [23, 24] has developed the Tactile Sensitivity Behavioral Responses Checklist

to rate defensive responses by children given the SCSIT, KIN and Tactile Perception Tests.

Left-Hemisphere Dysfunction
Difficulties with auditory and language skills and somatosensory deficits affecting the right side of the body in conjunction with normal visual/spatial abilities are associated with left-hemisphere dysfunction [32]. Children with this syndrome exhibit auditory processing and language deficits, hemisphere discrepancies, vestibular dysfunction, and often have problems with reading achievement [16]. Other parameters indicative of this syndrome include [31]

1. Poor auditory language scores on the ITPA and FCTCAA
2 Low right/left ear ratio on the dichotic listening test
3. Poorer scores with the right than left hand on tactile and motor tests, with the right hand less dextrous than the left
4. A definite gap between language and visual test scores

In language development, there appears to be a strong association of auditory and language function. Children with language deficits who demonstrate a depressed postrotary nystagmus and poor postural reactions appear to make appreciable gains with sensory integrative therapy [14, 21]. However, those with a prolonged postrotary nystagmus along with signs of unilateral cerebral dysfunction suggest a problem with higher cortical structures. Those with adequate vestibular and somatosensory function language deficits indicate the involvement of other neurolinguistic mechanisms that interfere with speech mechanisms [16].

Right-Hemisphere Dysfunction
Deficits in visual form and space perception and somatosensory problems on the left side of the body in children who demonstrate normal lan-

guage development are indicative of right-hemisphere dysfunction [32]. Key signs of this syndrome include

1. Unilateral disregard of the left side of the body and space with underuse of the left hand
2. Somatosensory scores lower on the left than right side (DTS, MFP, GRA, CMLX)
3. Errors on the left side of SU as well as poor scores on visual perception tests (FG, VSM, VC, MAC, DC, RLD [left-sided items], SU, the latter with more errors on the left side)
4. CMLX, RLD, SBO, right arm superior on rotation

With this disorder, visual and auditory test scores tend to cluster in two distinct groups with visual functions more impaired [32]. Postrotary nystagmus is average or prolonged, the latter suggests a right cerebral hemisphere dysfunction rather than a vestibular disorder.

THERAPY PROGRAM

Sensory integrative therapy is designed to meet the needs of each child. There is no "cookbook" approach. However, there are general concepts on which therapeutic intervention is based. Therapy involves providing specific sensory input (vestibular, proprioceptive, and tactile stimulation) while enabling an adaptive response from the child. Thus, the therapist controls the physical and social environment of the child's developmental level, eliciting an adaptive response that is within the child's capacity [9]. The child meanwhile is self-directed, an active participant, who appears to be playing. "The therapist tries carefully to balance structure and freedom in a way that leads to constructive exploration" [4]. Finally, throughout the sensory integrative program, the therapist is careful to follow a developmental sequence.

The therapy program for children with sensory integrative dysfunction requires the professional judgment of a trained clinician. Proce-dures involve substantial sensory stimuli, and discretion in their use is critical to minimize risks. Possible side effects include peripheral changes such as flushing or sweating, depressed heart or respiration rate, and seizure activity.

To help understand sensory integrative therapy, the following treatment plan of a child with a vestibular-bilateral disorder is presented. It is interesting to note that children with vestibular-bilateral syndrome, one parameter of which is hyporeactive nystagmus, appeared to benefit more from sensory integrative therapy than from a traditional approach [14].

In general, the sensory integrative therapy program proceeds in the following sequence:

1. Tactile stimulation: It must be remembered that touching the skin can have both a positive and negative effect on the nervous system. The child's response to stimuli must be respected. Light touch such as from soft clothing can itch and feel intolerable to some children. Often deep pressure (touch pressure) can be more soothing. Activities can include rolling up in a blanket, rubbing with a terry cloth towel, and allowing the child to be barefoot on carpeted surfaces or in a sandbox.

2. Vestibular stimulation: The child should experience vestibular stimulation in as many different head positions and motions as possible, to stimulate all vestibular receptors. Depending on the response of the child, this can include passive stimulation given while the child is lying or seated in a net hammock. If the child is threatened by this, the spinning can be done actively by the child using hands on the floor to push off. Active involvement facilitates an adaptive response and balances the inhibitory/excitatory aspects of the stimulation [9]. Vestibular and proprioceptive stimulation can be incorporated into a variety of activities. In general, response to slow vestibular stimulation is inhibiting and fast stimulation is stimulating. A rocking chair and playground equipment are excellent sources of vestibular and proprioceptive stimulation. Carrying a child and allowing the child to

push objects can provide touch-pressure and proprioceptive impulses.

3. Motor control: Using neurophysiologic procedures and activities to elicit a more mature level of response, the sensory integration (SI) program encourages the integration of primitive postural reflexes. Particular attention is given on developing supine flexion and prone extension postures [98]. Activities can include riding a scooter board, bolster swing, or net hammock. Those activities that encourage the assimilation of the tonic-neck reflex (TNR) and activation of the neck-righting reflex should also be included, if problems exist on this level of reflex maturation. These can be rolling in a blanket or barrel, or positioning on a rocking board. Subsequently, attention is given to developing more mature postural reactions through activities that elicit equilibrium reactions. Following a developmental sequence of prone, quadruped, sitting, and standing, activities can include the use of the therapeutic ball, equilibrium board, or platform swing. Obstacle courses can be set up in a variety of positions, with or without the use of the scooter board. Games such as hopscotch, jump rope, or bean bag relay help to encourage higher-level equilibrium reactions. Many of these activities [2] also encourage extraocular muscle control, muscle co-contraction, bilateral coordination, and interhemispheral integration [98]. (See the Suggested Readings for citations with specific procedures for a sensory integration program.)

VOCATIONAL TRAINING

Along the range of treatment techniques is a focus on the development of work-related skills, behaviors, and habits, frequently referred to as "prevocational and vocational skill training." Although a beneficial technique for all learning disabled children, it is particularly crucial for the lower-functioning child. Work-related programming focuses on the development of an occupational role and the development of appropriate work-related skills, behaviors, and habits. Some of these may include cooperative behav-

ior, task focus, motivation, reliability, and independence. Frequently these behaviors are underdeveloped in the learning disabled child because of limited or lack of exposure to the world of work and limited career expectations for them on the part of parents and society [63].

Several authors support the need to initiate work-related programming at an early age [53,63,75]. Activities should be presented in a developmental fashion and include ones that foster career awareness and explore vocational capabilities and interests. In addition significant prevocational and career education should be initiated as early as possible, certainly by junior high school [53]. Gerber reinforces the need for work-related programming at an early age by stating, "At the secondary level, there is a lack of vocational direction and skill development and a limited amount of time left for preparation" [50]. Furthermore, Lynch and colleagues note that, "Training materials and work performance requirements should increasingly approximate actual industrial demands and training should move from the school to the actual work site as soon as possible" [75].

The choice of techniques is often governed by the student's potential for future academic achievement, for example, going to college [106]. For the student functioning at a high level of performance, the educational and therapeutic focus is typically geared toward academic or cognitive methods. While the student performing at a lower level may receive the same type of academic or cognitive training as a child, as an adolescent the focus becomes functional, and compensatory strategies are reinforced.

ACADEMIC PROGRAMS

This section focuses on the adolescent learning disabled student.

The majority of learning disabled students will be in regular schools leaving their regular classrooms to receive resource room assistance. An effective model has been the language-based program where all areas of training are designed to build a student's vocabulary and understanding of language and to improve ability to communicate more effectively (written and oral). This has been particularly successful when coupled with a small class size, individualized remediation, and multimodel techniques.

However, Lynn believes that the best education for learning disabled children is offered by private schools [102]. The Learning Prep School (LPS) located in West Newton, Massachusetts is presented as an example of one such school.

The school is composed of 200 students ranging in age from 15 to 22 years with moderate-to-severe learning disabilities. LPS offers a language-based life-centered curriculum of academic and vocational education and a work/study component for the older students. In addition, students receive Adaptive Physical Education (APE), career education, and human adjustment classes, and when appropriate, therapeutic intervention such as occupational, physical, speech, and language therapy and counseling. To round out its rigorous program, LPS provides special events and social activities. The average amount of time a student attends the school is variable, depending on the student's individual needs. However, completion of the program may lead to a high school equivalency diploma [63].

One of the primary goals of LPS is to develop behaviors and skills important for future vocational tasks and job placement (Fig. 5-3).

FIG. 5-3. Learning Prep School student attending a vocational workshop. (Food service photograph courtesy of Kristina Eagan-Mast.)

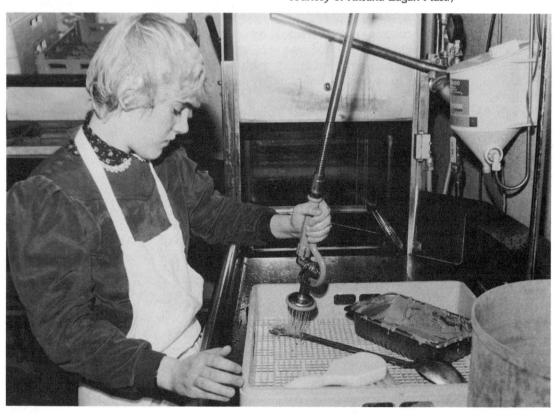

The achievement of this goal is evidenced in the fact that approximately 50 percent of the students enrolled will be competitively employed following graduation. The other 50 percent will enter various types of rehabilitation workshops [64].

The following discussion of therapeutic intervention that is offered at LPS is presented as a model of the type of treatment that has been found beneficial to an adolescent learning disabled population.

Occupational Therapy
Occupational therapy is an essential component of the success of the school's programming; therapists function as liaisons between instructors and vocational and academic administrators. In actuality they become consultants to personnel who may not have expertise in tasks and job analysis, adaptive and assistive equipment, techniques of work simplification, and activities of daily living. "In addition, the therapist uses information from the JPSA to assist staff in developing teaching strategies based on the student's learning style. The therapist also functions as a role model, working side by side with several students or individually with one who may need extra attention" [63].

The majority of direct treatment is offered in the form of task groups. These include a series of learning experiences that will enable the student to make appropriate vocational decisions and develop work-related habits, skills, and behaviors necessary for eventual employment. At present, the following task groups are offered:

1. Establishing and maintaining a school library
2. Developing and managing a school store
3. Organizing and producing a school yearbook
4. Performing the duties of a lunchroom cashier
5. Establishing and running a "cookie-gram" company
6. Engaging in an arts and crafts group and selling these items at the biannual arts and crafts fairs
7. Being an employee of the work center, which entails performing varied subcontract work (Fig. 5-4)

Physical Therapy
Typically for the young child, this strategy addresses motor and postural functions and efficient use of the body. Both occupational and physical therapy approaches often include techniques of sensory integration, neurodevelopmental treatment, sensorimotor stimulation, developmental motor skill training, and physical fitness. These categories are far from mutually exclusive, either in theory or in practice, and most therapists use a combination of two or more approaches [29].

Speech and Language Therapy
This intervention assists students in developing various strategies so that they may communicate more effectively. These may include listening strategies and verbal planning. For the young child, therapy often focuses on articulation and language remediation. For the older student, speech and language therapy is geared toward helping the student to develop strategies to deal with functional situations.

Specific examples may serve to exemplify these strategies. A student with word-finding problems is frequently taught to describe the word he or she cannot remember or give other clues to the listener rather than just calling something a "thing-a-ma-jig" or expecting the listener to guess at what is referred to. The student with verbal-planning problems (difficulty organizing what he or she wants to say) is taught the common sensory strategy of taking time to "stop and think" before starting to speak [73].

Role-playing activities may be used during therapy sessions to help students gain facility with everyday social skills needed for survival. These may include [73]

Verbalizing a request for information
Verbalizing a request for repetition
Verbalizing a request for clarification

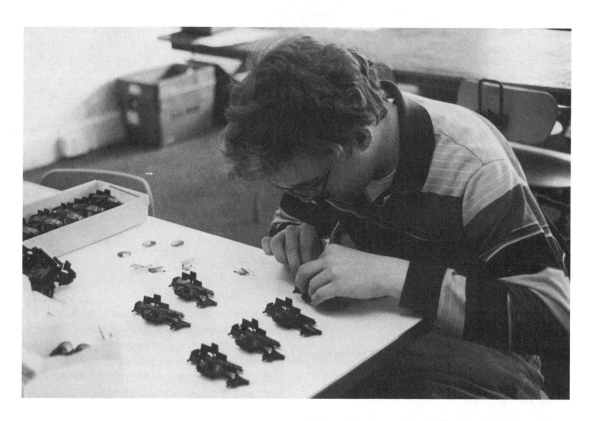

FIG. 5-4. Learning Prep School student performing subcontract work at the school's work center.

Verbalizing a request for assistance

Verbalizing and responding to a complaint or compliment

Relating the steps of an event in proper sequence

Psychological Counseling

For the older child/adolescent, disability awareness and coping with the normal stresses of adolescence and the additional ones that learning disabilities place on them may be the focus of supportive therapy. This may occur in either individual or group settings and is frequently conducted by the school psychologist or mental health counselor. Psychological therapy is frequently for the treatment of associated affective disorders, depression, and anxiety [62].

Environmental, Technologic, and Medical Interventions

A quiet place to study with minimal visual and auditory distractions will benefit the child with a learning problem [62]. Consistency between the school and home environment is particularly important. Table 5-4 outlines some important steps in fostering independence in the learning disabled student.

Devices such as tape recorders, dictating machines, calculators, typewriters, and computers are often valuable compensatory strategies for the learning disabled student. For example, the student with reading difficulties may use prerecorded materials to supplement textbooks and other printed material. An important resource in this area is the Library of Congress, Division for the Blind and Physically Handicapped, which

TABLE 5-4. Steps to independence for an LD child . . . Nonnie's thoughts for parents

Establish house rules early and stick to them consistently.

Parents must be models to their children.

Do not meekly submit to temper tantrums and impulsive behavior. This teaches them to be even more demanding.

Assign appropriate responsibilities gradually. Explain each task specifically. *Check* to see the task is finished before assigning another chore.

Teach directions by repetition and reinforcement using landmarks, drawings, and diagrams. (Patience is of the essence.)

Encourage children to make their own doctor, tutor, etc. appointments. (Using a phone, clock, and phone book is essential.)

Explain how to make lists, label drawers, put objects in the same place, follow routines. Devise ways to help the individual child learn to memorize by demonstration and visual models.

Do not shower the LD child with gifts and privileges he or she has not earned because you feel sorry for the child or guilty. Give them jobs in the house to earn their allowance.

Be fair in giving appropriate rewards or punishments.

Use patience and repetition to teach LD children to concentrate on one thing at a time, to listen without interrupting, to hold eye contact, and to think about the other person.

Teach children to be emotionally and physically responsible for their own actions.

Encourage hobbies early for good use of leisure time.

Do not take over when a child is frightened about trying some new task. Help him or her try a small part of the task and point out the skills necessary to complete it successfully.

What have you done to overprotect your child today?

Source: Reprinted from *Their World* magazine with permission of the editor, Julie Gilligan. *Their World* is the annual publication of Foundation for Children With Learning Disabilities, 99 Park Avenue, New York, N.Y. 10016. Founder and President, Carrie Rozelle.

has developed a Talking Books program that produces specially designed record players and cassette machines and a bimonthly bulletin listing available books and magazines at no cost.

The personal computer has become an important tool for the learning disabled student and is being found more both at school and home. Computers are fast, multisensory, and give the student immediate reinforcement. They also allow for infinite repetition of a task and can be adjusted with respect to student's response. Pertinent computer software is evolving rapidly that has been designed specifically for the learning disabled individual. One such example is a 10- to 15-hour program developed by the Minnesota Association for Children and Adults with Learning Disabilities (MACALD) [80] entitled "Good For Me," which has been designed to further the social and emotional development of the learning disabled adolescent [80].

A number of drugs are used by physicians for the treatment of attention deficits, which may be an aspect of the child's learning disability. Medications frequently prescribed include dextroamphetamine (Dexedrine), methylphenidate (Ritalin), and magnesium (Cylert). For disorders of movement involving spasticity or dystonia, diazepam (Valium) and trihexyphenidyl (Artane) are used, respectively, to help improve motor function involved in speech and in handwriting [62].

REFERENCES

1. ACLD Newsbriefs. Pittsburgh: ACLD, Jan/Feb, 1985.
2. *Activities for the Remediation of Sensorimotor Dysfunction in Primary School Children.* Title III ESEA Project, Goleta, CA: Goleta Union School District, 1973.
3. Anastasi, A. Goodenough-Harris Drawing Test. In O. K. Buros (ed.), *Mental Measurements Yearbooks.* Highland Park, NJ: Gryphone, 1972.
4. Anderson, L. E. (ed.). *Helping the Adolescent with the Hidden Handicap.* Los Angeles: California Association for Neurologically Handicapped Children, 1970.
5. Arnheim, D. D., and Sinclair, W. A. *The Clumsy Child.* St. Louis: Mosby, 1979.

6. Ayres, A. J. Patterns of perceptual-motor dysfunction in children: a factor analytic study. *Percept. Mot. Skills* 20:335, 1965.

7. Ayres, A. J. Deficits in sensory integration in educationally handicapped children. *J. Learn. Disabil.* 2:160, 1969.

8. Ayres, A. J. Improving academic scores through sensory integration. *J. Learn. Disabil.* 5:338, 1972.

9. Ayres, A. J. *Sensory Integration and Learning Disorders.* Los Angeles: Western Psychological, 1972.

10. Ayres, A. J. *Southern California Sensory Integration Tests.* Los Angeles: Western Psychological, 1972.

11. Ayres, A. J. Types of sensory integrative dysfunction among disabled learners. *Am. J. Occup. Ther.* 26:13, 1972.

12. Ayres, A. J. *The Development of Sensory Integrative Theory and Practice.* Dubuque, IA: Kendall/Hunt, 1974.

13. Ayres, A. J. *Southern California Postrotary Nystagmus Test.* Los Angeles: Western Psychological, 1975.

14. Ayres, A. J. The Effect of Sensory Integrative Therapy on Learning Disabled Children, The Final Report of a Research Project. Pasadena, CA: Center for the Study of Sensory Integrative Dysfunction and the Valentine-Kline Foundation, 1976.

15. Ayres, A. J. Cluster analyses of measures of sensory integration. *Am. J. Occup. Ther.* 31(6):362, 1977.

16. Ayres, A. J. *Interpreting the Southern California Sensory Integration Tests.* Los Angeles: Western Psychological, 1978.

17. Ayres, A. J. Learning disabilities and the vestibular system. *J. Learn. Disabil.* 11(1):30, 1978.

18. Ayres, A. J. *Sensory Integration and the Child.* Los Angeles: Western Psychological, 1980.

19. Ayres, A. J. *Southern California Sensory Integration Tests.* Los Angeles: Western Psychological, 1980.

20. Ayres, A. J. *Southern California Motor Accuracy Test, Revised 1980.* Los Angeles: Western Psychological, 1980.

21. Ayres, A. J., and Mailloux, Z. Influence of sensory integration procedures on language development. *Am. J. Occup. Ther.* 35:6, 1981.

22. Baker, H. J., and Leland, B. *The Detroit Tests of Learning Aptitude.* Indianapolis: Bobbs-Merrill, 1967.

23. Bauer, B. A. Tactile-sensitive behavior in hyperactive and nonhyperactive children. *Am. J. Occup. Ther.* 31:7, 1977.

24. Bauer, B. A. Tactile sensitivity: development of a behavioral responses checklist. *Am. J. Occup. Ther.* 31:6, 1977.

25. Beatty, L., Madden, R., and Gardner, E. *Stanford Diagnostic Arithmetic Test.* New York: Harcourt Brace Jovanovich, 1966.

26. Beery, K., and Buktenica, N. *Developmental Test of Visual Motor Integration.* Chicago: Follett, 1967.

27. Brolin, D. E., and Kokasks, C. *Career Education for Handicapped Children and Youth.* Columbus: Merrill, 1979.

28. Bruininks, R. H. *Bruininks-Osteretsky Test of Motor Proficiency.* Circle Pines, MN: American Guidance, 1978.

29. Cermak, S. A., and Henderson, A. *Learning Disabilities in Neurological Rehabilitation.* St. Louis: Mosby, 1985.

30. Cheek, C. W. Electronystagmosgraphy in children with specific learning disabilities. *Dissertation Abstracts International* 31:217A, 1970, 1971.

31. Clark, F. A. Data classification for SCSIT. Los Angeles: University of Southern California Press, 1978.

32. Clark, F. A., and Shuer, J. A clarification of sensory integrative therapy and its application to programming with retarded people. *Mental Retard.* 16(3):227, 1978.

33. Clark, P. N., and Allen, A. S. *Occupational Therapy for Children.* St. Louis: Mosby, 1985.

34. Connolly, A., Natchman, W., and Pritchett, E. Key Math *Diagnostic Arithmetic Test.* Circle Pines, MN: American Guidance, 1973.

35. Denckla, M. B., Rudel, R. G., Chapman, C., et al. Motor proficiency in dyslexic children with and without attentional disorders. *Arch. Neurol.* 42:228, 1980.

36. Dennis, S. The predictive diagnostic validity of the ITPA. *Dissertation Abstracts International* 40:5786A, 1980.

37. deQuiros, J. B. Diagnosis of vestibular disorders in the learning disabled. *J. Learn. Disabil.* 9:39, 1976.

38. deQuiros, J. B. Vestibular-proprioceptive Integration: Its Influence on Learning and Speech in Children. In *Proceedings of the 12th International American Psychologic Congress, Lima, Peru, 1966.* Mexico City: Editorial Trillas, 1967.

39. Dunn, L. M., Dunn, L. M., Robertson, G. J., et al. *The Peabody Picture Vocabulary Test-Re-*

vised. Circle Pines, MN: American Guidance, 1981.

40. Durrell, D. D. *Durrell Analysis of Reading Difficulty.* New York: Harcourt Brace Jovanovich, 1955.
41. Flowers, A., Costello, M. R., and Small, V. *Flowers-Costello Test of Central Auditory Abilities.* Dearborn, MI: Perceptual Learning, 1970.
42. Franham-Diggory, S. *Learning Disabilities—a Psychological Perspective.* Boston: Harvard University Press, 1978.
43. Frank, J., and Levinson, H. Dysmetric dyslexia and dyspraxia. *J. Am. Acad. Child Adolesc. Psychiatry* 12:690, 1973.
44. Frostig, M. *Developmental Test of Visual Perception.* Palo Alto: Consulting Psychologists, 1963.
45. Gallagher, J. J. Learning disabilities and the near future. *J. Learn. Disabil.* 17:9, 1984.
46. Gardner, M. F. *Expressive One-Word Picture Vocabulary Test.* Novato, CA: Academic Therapy, 1979.
47. Gardner, M. F. *Upper-Extension Expressive One-Word Picture Vocabulary Test.* Novato, CA: Academic Therapy, 1983.
48. Gates, A. T., and McKillop, A. S. *Gates-McKillop Reading* Diagnostic Test. New York: Teachers College, 1982.
49. Gearheart, B. R., and Weishann, M. W. *The Exceptional Student in the Regular Classroom.* St. Louis: Mosby, 1984.
50. Gerber, P. J. Learning Disabilities and Vocational Education: Realities and Challenges. In B. P. Lynch, W. E. Diernan, and J. A. Stark, (eds.), *Prevocational and Vocational Education for Special Needs Youth: A Blueprint for the 1980s.* Baltimore: Brookes, 1982.
51. Geschwind, N., and Behan, P. Left-handedness: association with immune disease, migraine and development learning disorder. *Proc. Natl. Acad. Sci. U.S.A.* 1982.
52. Gilfoyle, E. M. (ed.). *Training: Occupational Therapy Educational Management in Schools.* Rockville, MD: American Occupational Therapy Association, 1980.
53. Goldstein, H. *The Social Learning Curriculum.* Columbus: Merrill, 1974.
54. Goodenough, F. L., and Harris, D. B. *Goodenough-Harris Drawing Test.* New York: Psychological Corporation, 1963.
55. Gray, W. S. *Gray Oral Reading Tests.* Indianapolis: Bobbs-Merrill, 1963.
56. Gubbay, S. S. *The Clumsy Child.* Philadelphia: Saunders, 1975.

57. Hainesworth, P. K., and Siqueland, H. L. *Meeting Street School Screening Test.* East Providence, RI: Crippled Children and Adults of Rhode Island, 1969.
58. Hammill, D. D. *The Detroit Tests of Learning Aptitude* (2nd ed.). Austin, TX: Pro-Ed, 1985.
59. Hammill, D. D., and Bryant, B. R. *The Detroit Tests of Learning Aptitude—Primary.* Austin, TX: Pro-Ed, 1986.
60. Hammill, D. D., Brown, V. L., Larsen, S. C., et al. *Test of Adolescent Language.* Austin, TX: Pro-Ed, 1980.
61. Harris, D. B. Review of Bender-Gestalt Test for young children. *Child Dev.* (abstract) 39:165, 1965.
62. Herskowitz, J., and Rosman, N. P. *Pediatric, Neurology and Psychiatry—Common Ground.* New York: Macmillan, 1982.
63. Jacobs, K. *Occupational Therapy: Work-Related Programs and Assessments.* Boston: Little, Brown, 1985.
64. Jacobs, K., Mazonson, N., Pepicelli, K., et al. Work Center: a School-Based Program for Vocational Preparation of Special Needs Children and Adolescents. In *Occupational Therapy in Health Care.* New York: Haworth, 1985, 1986.
65. Johnson, D. J., and Myklebust, H. R. *Learning Disabilities—Educational Principles and Practices.* New York: Grune & Stratton, 1967.
66. Jorgensen, C., Barrett, M., Huisingh, R., et al. *The Word Test.* Moline, IL: Lingui, 1981.
67. Kephart, N. C. *The Slow Learner in the Classroom.* Columbus: Merrill, 1960.
68. Kirk, S. A. *Educating Exceptional Children.* Boston: Houghton Mifflin, 1962.
69. Kirk, S. A., Mccarthy, J. M., and Kirk, W. D. *Illinois Test of Psycholinguistic Abilities.* Champaign-Urbana: University of Illinois Press, 1968.
70. Koppitz, E. M. *The Bender Gestalt Test for Young Children.* New York: Grune & Stratton, 1963.
71. Kronick, D. *What About Me? The Id Adolescent.* Novato, CA: Academic Therapy, 1975.
72. Larson, K. A. The sensory history of developmentally delayed children with and without tactile defensiveness. *Am. J. Occup. Ther.* 36:9, 1982.
73. Lauck, K., and Merrill, J. Speech and Language. In K. Gray, and B. D. Klane (eds.), *The Link.* West Newton, MA: Learning Prep School, 1985.
74. Levine, M. D. *The Pediatric Assessment System for Learning Disorders.* Cambridge: Educators Publishing, 1980–1985.

75. Lynch, K. P., Kiernan, W. E., and Stark, J. A. (eds.). *Prevocational and Vocational Education for Special Needs Youth: A Blueprint for the 1980s.* Baltimore: Brookes, 1982.

76. McCarthy, D. *The McCarthy Scales of Children's Abilities.* New York: Psychological Corporation, 1972.

77. McLoughlin, J. A., and Lewis, R. B. *Assessing Special Students: Strategies and Procedures.* Columbus: Merrill, 1981.

78. Menkes, J. H. *Textbook of Child Neurology.* Philadelphia: Lea & Febiger, 1974.

79. Miller, L. J. *The Miller Assessment of Preschoolers.* Littleton, CO: Foundation for Knowledge in Development, 1981.

80. Minnesota Association for Children and Adults with Learning Disabilities, Suite 494-N, 1821 University Ave., St. Paul, MN 55104.

81. Mitchell, J. V., Jr (ed.). *The Ninth Mental Measurements Yearbook,* vol 2. Lincoln: University of Nebraska Press, Buros Institute of Mental Measurements, 1985.

82. Monroe, M. *Monroe Reading Aptitude Test.* Boston: Houghton Mifflin, 1935.

83. Mutti, M. A., Sterling, R. M., and Spalding, N. V. *The Quick Neurological Screening Test.* Novato, CA: Academic Therapy, 1978.

84. Myers, P. I., and Hammill, D. D. *Learning Disabilities Basic Concepts, Assessment Practices, and Instructional Strategies.* Austin, TX: Pro-Ed, 1982.

85. Newcomer, P. L., and Hammill, D. D. *The Test of Language Development.* Austin, TX: Pro-Ed, 1977.

86. Orpet, R. E. *Frostig Movement Skills Test Battery.* Palo Alto: Consulting Psychologists, 1972.

87. Ottenbacher, K. Identifying vestibular processing dysfunction in learning disabled children. *Am. J. Occup. Ther.* 32(4):217, 1978.

88. Paraskevopoulos, J., and Kirk, S. *The Development and Psychometric Characteristics of the Revised Illinois Test of Psycholinguistic Abilities.* Champaign-Urbana: University of Illinois Press, 1969.

89. Parker, D. E. The vestibular apparatus. *Sci. Am.* 243(5):118, 1980.

90. Preston, J. M. Review of the Illinois Test of Psycholinguistic Abilities—Revised. In D. J. Keyser and R. C. Sweetland (eds.), *Test Critiques: Vol. I.* Kansas City: Test Corporation of America, 1984.

91. Reynolds-Lynch, K. Prevocational and Vocational Assessment in Occupational Therapy. In M. Kirkland and S. C. Robertson (eds.), *Planning and Implementing Vocational Readiness in Occupational Therapy.* Rockville, MD: American Occupational Therapy Association, 1985.

92. Roach, E. G., and Kephart, N. C. *Purdue Perceptual-Motor Survey Rating Scale.* Columbus: Merrill, 1966.

93. Salvia, J., and Yaseldyke, J. E. *Assessment in Special and Remedial Education.* Boston: Houghton Mifflin, 1978.

94. Scott, D. H., Moyes, F. A., and Henderson, S. E. *Test of Motor Impairment—Henderson Revised.* Ontario: Brook Educational, 1984.

95. Semel, E. M., and Wiig, E. H. *Clinical Evaluation of Language Function.* Columbus: Merrill, 1980.

96. Shuer, J., Clark, F., and Azen, S. P. Vestibular function in mildly mentally retarded adults. *Am. J. Occup. Ther.* 34(10):664, 1980.

97. Silver, L. B., and Carleton, S. Learning disabilities can be helped. *Rx: Being Well,* Sept/Oct 1983.

98. Silverzahn, M. Sensory Integrative Theory. In H. L. Hopkins and H. D. Smith (eds.), *Willard and Spackman's Occupational Therapy* (6th ed.). Philadelphia: Lippincott, 1983.

99. Simoni, F. D. *The Token Test for Children.* Allen, TX: Developmental Learning Materials, 1978.

100. Spache, G. D. *Diagnostic Reading Scales.* Monterey: California Test Bureau, 1963.

101. Stilwell, J. M., Crowe, T. K., and McCallum L. W. Postrotary nystagmus duration as a function of communication disorders. *Am. J. Occup. Ther.* 32(4):222, 1978.

102. *The FOLD Learning Disabilities Resource Guide.* New York: Foundation for Children with Learning Disabilities, 1985.

103. *Their World.* New York: Foundation for Children with Learning Disabilities, 1985.

104. *Uniform Terminology for Reporting Occupational Therapy Services.* Baltimore: American Occupational Therapy Association, 1979.

105. Wechsler, D. *Wechsler Intelligence Scale for Children—Revised.* New York: Psychological Corporation, 1974.

106. Wiig, E. H. Personal communication, 1986.

107. Wiig, E. H., and Secord, W. *Test of Language Competence.* Columbus: Merrill, 1985.

108. Williams, J. B. W. (ed.). *Diagnostic and Statistical Manual of Mental Disorders* (3rd ed.). Washington, D.C.: American Psychiatric Association, 1980.

109. Woodcock, R. W. *Woodcock Reading Mastery Tests.* Circle Pines, MN: American Guidance, 1974.

110. Woodcock, R. W., and Johnson, M. B. *Wood-

cock-Johnson Psycho-Educational Battery. Allen, TX: Teaching Resources, 1977.
111. Woodcock, R. W., and Johnson, M. B. *Woodcock Language Proficiency Battery.* Allen, TX: Developmental Learning Materials, 1981.

SUGGESTED READING

LEARNING DISABILITIES

Lynn, R. *Learning Disabilities: An Overview of Theories, Approaches and Policies.* New York: Free, 1979.

SENSORY INTEGRATION

Bhatara, B., Clark, D. L., and Arnold, L. E. Behavioral and nystagmus response of a hypokinetic child to vestibular stimulation. *Am. J. Occup. Ther.* 32:311, 1978.

Chee, F. K. W., Kreutzberg, J. R., and Clark, D. L. Semicircular canal stimulation in cerebral palsied children. *Phys. Ther.* 58:1071, 1978.

Clark, D. L., Kreutzberg, J. R., and Chee, F. K. W. Vestibular stimulation influence on motor development in children. *Science* 196:1228, 1977.

deQuiros, J. *Neuropsychological Fundamentals in Learning Disabilities.* San Rafael, CA: Academic Therapy, 1978.

EVALUATIONS

Buros, O. *Personality Tests and Reviews II.* Highland Park, MD: Gryphon, 1975.

Meyers, C. E., Nihira, K., and Zetlin, A. The Measurement of Adaptive Behavior. In N. R. Ellis (ed.), *Handbook of Mental Deficiency, Psychological Theory and Research* (2nd ed.). Hillsdale, NJ: Erlbaum, 1979.

A SELECTIVE LIST OF EVALUATIONS USED BY OCCUPATIONAL AND PHYSICAL THERAPISTS AND SPEECH PATHOLOGISTS

Test	Author(s)	Source	Age	Administration	Administrator OT PT SP
AAMD Adaptive Behavior Scale, 1974	K. Nihira, R. Foster, M. Shellhaas, and H. Leland; American Association on Mental Deficiency	American Association on Mental Deficiency, 1719 Kalorama Rd., N.W., Washington, DC 20009	3–12, 13 and over	Individual: 20–25 min for children 25–30 min for adults	Can be administered by informants who know the individual's daily behavior well
Basic Motor Ability Tests— Revised (BMAT-Revised) (1979) [5]	D. D. Arnheim and W. A. Sinclair	D. D. Arnheim and W. A. Sinclair, *The Clumsy Child*, St. Louis; Mosby, 1979	4–12 yr	Individual: 15–20 min. Group; 30 min	X

124

Description	Construction & Reliability	Comments

Adaptive behavior scale for mentally retarded, emotionally maladjusted, and developmentally disabled individuals
 	
Ten behavioral domains
  1. Independent functioning
  2. Physical development
  3. Economic activity
  4. Language development
  5. Numbers and time
  6. Domestic activity
  7. Vocational ability
  8. Self-direction
  9. Responsibility
 10. Socialization
Maladaptive behavior
  1. Violent and destructive
  2. Antisocial
  3. Rebellious
  4. Untrustworthy
  5. Withdrawal
  6. Stereotyped and odd mannerisms
  7. Inappropriate interpersonal manners
  8. Unacceptable vocal habits
  9. Unacceptable or eccentric habits
 10. Self-abusive
 11. Hyperactive tendencies
 12. Sexually aberrant
 13. Psychological disturbances
 14. Use of medication
	Norms based on 4014 institutionalized retardates aged 3–69 yr
	Interrater reliability: Part I subscales 0.071–0.93, mean 0.86; Part II subscales 0.37–0.77, mean 0.57
		There is a public school version of the AAMD Adaptive Behavior Scale for TMR, EMR, EH (special class and learning disabled and regular class children).

The BMAT-Revised is composed of 11 tests:
  1. Bead stringing
  2. Target throwing
  3. Marble transfer
  4. Back and hamstring stretch
  5. Standing long jump
  6. Face down to standing
  7. Static balance
  8. Basketball throw for distance
  9. Ball striking
 10. Target kicking
 11. Agility run
	Standardized on 1563 children, however this information is incomplete. Test-retest reliability coefficient of 0.93 has been reported.	The BMAT—Revised is structured to allow individual tests to be used independently. Cermak and Henderson note that "Use of the test as a whole or in part could be a valuable part of an evaluation program." (29)

Test	Author(s)	Source	Age	Administration	Administrator		
					OT	PT	SP
The Bender Gestalt Test for Young Children (1964) [70]	E. M. Koppitz	Grune & Stratton, Inc., 111 Fifth Ave., NY, NY 10003	5–10 yr	Individual: 7–15 min.	X*		
Bruininks-Oseretsky Test of Motor Proficiency (1978) [28]	R. H. Bruininks	American Guidance Service, Inc., Circle Pines, MN 55014	4.6–14.6 yrs	Individual: 45 min–1 hr	X	X	
Clinical Evaluation of Language Functions (CELF) (1980) [95]	E. M. Semel and E. H. Wiig	Charles E. Merrill Publishing Co., 1300 Alum Creek Dr., Columbus, OH 43216	K–12th grade	Individual screening test: 15–20 min each. Diagnostic Battery: 1 hr, 20 min.			X

126

Description	Construction & Reliability	Comments
The Bender Gestalt Test for Young Children is an adaptation of the Bender Visual Motor Gestalt Test. The test is used to assess visual motor functions and possible neuropsychological impairment. The Bender Gestalt consists of nine designs that are presented to the student individually. The student is given an unlimited amount of time to reproduce each successive design on a sheet of paper.	Harris notes that "Although many measures of association are presented in terms of chi square, the scoring method appears to predict school achievement in the primary grades about as well as the Lee-Clark Reading Readiness Test or the Metropolitan Readiness Test (about the order of a correlation of .60)" [35] Reliabilities on the Bender Gestalt Test for Young Children tend to be fairly high for scores of .88–.96. Test-retest reliability over 4 mo was .54–.66.	The Bender Gestalt Test is most typically used by psychologists.
The test evaluates motor functioning in eight areas: 1. Running speed and agility 2. Balance 3. Bilateral coordination 4. Strength 5. Upper-limb coordination 6. Response speed 7. Visual motor control 8. Upper-limb speed and dexterity	Standardized on 765 subjects. Test-retest reliability coefficients for subtests ranged from .50–.89	A 15–20-min short form can be used for screening
CELF includes two main components: Screening Tests and Diagnostic Battery, which give a more in-depth assessment. Screening Tests assess both processing and production of oral language. There are two levels: Elementary for K–4th grade Advanced for 5th–12th grade CELF Diagnostic Battery was developed "to provide differentiated measures of selected language functions in the areas of phonology, syntax, semantics, memory, and word finding and retrieval" [95] Thirteen subtests include *Processing subtests* 1. Processing word and sentence structure 2. Processing word classes 3. Processing linguistic concepts 4. Processing relationships and ambiguities	Both the Screening Tests are standardized on 1400 students ages K–12th grade. Reliability of screening tests by test-retest method is adequate. Validity coefficients range from .46–.62 when compared to the ITPA and DTLA. Diagnostic Battery is standardized on 159 students (K–12th grade). Reliability based on test-retest methods and coefficients ranged from .56–1.00 with most subtests at .80 level or above. Validity was assessed by comparison to the ITPA and DTLA. Most coefficients were in the .40–.60 range.	Weaknesses include: 1. Questionable procedures for establishing norms and cut-off scores 2. Uneven reliability across grade levels 3. Little evidence of the types of validity and reliability most appropriate for screening measure [81]

Test	Author(s)	Source	Age	Administration	Administrator		
					OT	PT	SP
The Detroit Tests of Learning Aptitude (2nd ed.) (DTLA-2) (1985) [58]	D. D. Hammill	Pro-Ed, 5341 Industrial Oaks Blvd., Austin, TX 78735	6–17 yr	Individual: 120 min			X
Developmental Test of Visual Motor Integration (VMI) (1967) [26]	K. Beery and N. Buktenica	Follett Publishing Co., 1010 W. Washington Blvd., Chicago, IL 60607	2–15 yr	Individual or group: 10–15 min	X		

5. Processing oral directions
6. Processing spoken paragraphs
Production subtests
7. Producing word series
8. Producing names on configurations
9. Producing word association
10. Producing model sentences
11. Producing formulated sentences
Supplemental subtests
12. Processing speech sounds
13. Producing speech sounds

The DTLA-2 is the revised version of the 1967 DTLA. This version contains 20 scores, 11 from the following subtests [58]: Word opposites Sentence imitation Oral directions Word sequences Story construction Design reproduction Object sequences Symbolic relations Conceptual matching Word fragmentation Letter sequences and 9 composite Scores from Verbal aptitude Nonverbal aptitude Conceptual aptitude Structural aptitude Attention-enhanced aptitude Attention-reduced aptitude Motor-enhanced aptitude Motor-reduced aptitude Overall aptitude	Standardized on 1532 children in 30 states. Reliability of internal consistency on subtests was .80s–.90s and on composite was .90s; Test-retest coefficients of .80s on subtest and .80s–.90s on composite manual contains information on the evidence of content, criterion-related, and construct validity.	In 1986, D. D. Hammill and B. R. Bryant developed the DTLA-Primary for children 3 and one-half–9 yr. [59] Standardized on 1676 children in 36 states Reliability of internal consistency was .89–.95. Test-retest was .77–.88. The DTLA-Primary manual reports evidence of content, criterion-related, and construct validity.
The VMI is a test of eye-hand coordination. According to the manual, the VMI "was devised as a measure of the degree to which visual perception and motor behavior are integrated in young children." [26]	Norm-referenced standardized test that has been standardized on a sample of 1000 children. The manual provides limited information on reliability.	The VMI is difficult to score, although relatively easy to administer. It is useful as an adjunct to other evaluations.

Test	Author(s)	Source	Age	Administration	Administrator		
					OT	PT	SP
Developmental Test of Visual Perception (DTVP) (1963) [44]	M. Frostig	Consulting Psychologists Press, 577 College Ave., Palo Alto, CA 94326	4–8 yr	Individual or groups: 45 min–1 hr	X		

The VMI consists of 24 geometric forms in a space provided below each form. Testing is discontinued when the student fails three forms in a row. Forms are arranged in an age-graded sequence. The manual provides pass/fail criteria for scoring.

The DTVP was devised to test visual perceptual ability relevant to school performance. The DTVP is divided into the following five subtests:

1. *Eye-motor coordination* consists of the drawing of continuous straight, curved, or angled lines between boundaries of various width, or from point to point without guide lines

2. *Figure-Ground* involves shifts in perception of figures against increasingly complex grounds. In addition, intersecting and "hidden" geometric forms are used

3. *Constancy of Shape* (Form Constancy) involves the recognition of certain geometric figures that are presented in various sizes, shadings, textures, and positions in space, and their discrimination from similar geometric figures. The following figures are used: circles, squares, rectangles, ellipses, and parallelograms

4. *Position in Space* involves the discrimination of reversals and rotations of figures presented in series

5. *Spatial Relationships* (Relations) involves the analysis of simple forms and patterns consisting of angles and various length lines. The student is required to copy these items using dots as guide points [26, 29]

Standardized on more than 2100 students, although the manual admits that the sample was not representative. Salvia and Yaseldyke note that "Individual subtests of the DTVP lack the necessary reliability and validity to be used in diagnostic prescriptive teaching" and "performance on the DTVP must be interpreted with considerable caution". [93]

The DTVP should be used with other evaluations and not in isolation.

Test	Author(s)	Source	Age	Administration	Administrator		
					OT	PT	SP
Expressive One-Word Picture Vocabulary Test (EOWPVT) (1979) [46]	M. F. Gardner	Academic Therapy Publications, 20 Commercial Blvd., Novato, CA 94947-6161	2–12 yr	Individual. Although not a timed test, total administration is 10–15 min/level.			X
Frostig Movement Skills Test Battery (1972) [86]	R. E. Orpet	Consulting Psychologists Press, Inc., 577 College Ave, Palo Alto, CA 94326	6–12 yr	Individual: 25 min. Group (3–4): 45 min.	X		
Goodenough-Harris Drawing Test (1963) [54]	F. L. Goodenough and D. B. Harris	The Psychological Corporation, 757 3rd Ave., NY, NY 10017	3–15 yr	Individual and group: 10–15 min	X		
Illinois Test of Psycholinguistic Abilities (ITPA) (1968) [69]	S. A. Kirk, J. M. McCarthy, and W. D. Kirk	University of Illinois Press, 54 E. Gregory Dr., P.O. Box 5081, Sta. A, Champaign, IL 61820	2.4–10.3 yrs	Individual: 45–60 min	X		X

Description	Construction & Reliability	Comments
The EOWPVT was designed to obtain a basal estimate of the child's verbal intelligence. It consists of 110 line drawings that are presented individually, with the child asked to identify it in one-word descriptions. The drawings are categorized into the following four areas of language: 1. General Concepts (common characteristics) 2. Grouping (plurals) 3. Abstract Concepts (a single characteristic of a number of items or objects) 4. Descriptive Concepts (only one or two items on this test were identified by a participle, for example "cutting tools" [46].	Standardized on 1607 children. Reliability was determined by the split-half method from a coefficient of .87–.96 with a median reliability of .94. These appear adequate. Criterion-related validity is correlated with the Peabody Picture Vocabulary Test-Revised (PPVT-R) at .67–.78.	The EOXPVT can be administered to bilingual children. Line drawings appear dated and are generally mediocre, although recognizable. The EOXPVT is a useful compliment to the Peabody Picture Vocabulary Test-Revised, McCarthy Screening Test, or the Bender Gestalt Test.
The test is designed to evaluate the sensorimotor development and motor skills of children. Twelve subsets are included in the following five areas: 1. Hand-eye coordination 2. Visually guided movement 3. Flexibility 4. Strength 5. Balance	Published as an experimental edition. Validity has not been established; reliability is inadequate based on available information.	Scale scores should be considered only approximate.
The Goodenough-Harris Drawing Test is a revision and extension of the Goodenough Intelligence Test. Student is asked to draw a picture of a man, woman, and himself or herself. Anastasi notes that the test "focuses on the child's accuracy of observation and on the development of conceptual thinking, rather than on artistic skill." [3]	Standardized on 2975 children. Test-retest reliabilities were reported as .60–.70. Interscorer reliabilities are .80–.96 and correlations with Stanford Binet are .36–.65. There are 73 scorable points for the draw-a-man and 71 scorable points for the draw-a-woman.	Test should be used with other screening tests to make a complete battery that can be used to select children who should receive more thorough evaluation.
The ITPA is a diagnostic tool used to "delineate areas of difficulty in communication. . ." [69]. It is composed of 10 required and 2 supplementary subtests: Auditory Reception	Standardized on 962 children. Internal consistency coefficients range from .60–.96 with a median of .88, except for one coefficient of .45 for subtest	Frequently the entire battery is not administered, and subtests such as Grammatic Closure, Auditory Association, Auditory Reception, and Verbal

Test	Author(s)	Source	Age	Administration	Administrator		
					OT	PT	SP
The Jacobs Prevocational Skills Assessment (1985) [63]	K. Jacobs	K. Jacobs. *Occupational Therapy: Work-Related Programs and Assessments.* Boston: Little Brown, 1985.	9–18 yr	Individual: 1–2 hr	X		
The McCarthy Scales of Children's Abilities (MSCA) (1972) [76]	D. McCarthy	The Psychological Corporation, 757 3rd Ave., NY, NY 10017	2.5– 8.5 yr	Individual: 45 min– 1 hr	X		

Description	Construction & Reliability	Comments
Visual Reception Auditory Association Visual Association Verbal Expression Manual Expression Grammatic Closure Visual Closure Auditory Sequential Memory Visual Sequential Memory Auditory Closure (Supplementary) Sound Blending (Supplementary)	Sound Blending (age level 8.7–9.1 yr) Five month test-retest reliability coefficients for 4–, 6–, 8–yr olds ranged from .28–.90 with a median of .71 for subtests, .87–.93 for composite scores, and .86–.91 on psycholinguistic quotients. Dennis [36] found in a study of predictive validity that subtests, Visual Sequential Memory, and Auditory Association predicted best for learning disabled children. Preston [90] notes that studies such as Dennis' "provide evidence for validity of various subtests".	Expression are given as useful measures of oral language. In 1985 J. J. McCarthy provided an appendix to the ITPA technical manual with a complete lisiting of validity studies [76].
The Jacobs Prevocational Skills Assessment is composed of 15 tasks that assess an individual's performance in specific work-related skills, behaviors, habits. The 15 simulated work tasks include quality control, filing, carpentry assembly, classification, office work, telephone directory, factory work, environmental mobility, money concepts, functional banking, time concepts, work attitudes, body scheme, leather assembly, and food preparation.	A standard instrument that is not yet normed.	Originally developed for a learning disabled adolescent population and has adapted version for the head injured and psychiatrically disabled.
The McCarthy Scales of Children's Abilities consist of 18 tests grouped into the following six areas: 1. Verbal 2. Perceptual-performance 3. Quantitative 4. Composite (general cognitive index GCI) 5. Memory 6. Motor	Standardized on a sample of 1032 children. Internal consistency coefficients for General Cognitive Index averaged .93. The mean reliability coefficient for the other five areas range from .79–.88.	Frequently therapists administer particular subtests rather than the entire battery. Also available is the McCarthy Screening Test, which is an adaptation of this instrument. The screening is not a diagnostic tool and is infrequently used.

Test	Author(s)	Source	Age	Administration	Administrator OT	PT	SP
Meeting Street School Screening Test (1969) [57]	P. K. Hainesworth and H. L. Siqueland	Crippled Children and Adults of Rhode Island, Inc., Meeting Street School, 667 Waterman Ave., East Providence, R.I. 02914	4–7.6 yr	Individual: 20 min	X		

Description	Construction & Reliability	Comments

The General Cognitive Index (GCI) is based on 15 of the 18 tests and provides a cognitive level in relation to chronologic age. The 18 tests are

1. Block building
2. Puzzle solving (timed)
3. Pictorial memory (timed)
4. Work knowledge
5. Number questions
6. Tapping sequence
7. Verbal memory
8. Right/left orientation
9. Leg coordination
10. Arm coordination
11. Imitative action
12. Draw a design
13. Draw a child
14. Numerical memory
15. Verbal fluency (timed)
16. Counting and sorting
17. Opposite analogies
18. Conceptual grouping

Description	Construction & Reliability	Comments

Meeting Street School Screening Test was designed to assist in identifying cerebral or neurologic impairment in children 4–7 ½ yr. Three subtests compose the screening and include
 	
1. *Motor patterning*
   Gait patterns
   Clap hands
   Hand patterns
   Follow directions I
   Touch fingers
2. *Visual-perceptual-motor*
   Block taping
   Visual matching
   Visual memory
   Copy forms
   Follow directions II
3. *Language*
   Repeat words
   Repeat sentences
   Counting
   Tell-a-story
   Language sequencing
From these subtests the therapist is able to identify children in need of further evaluation [57].
	Standardized on 500 children. Reliability for entire test is 0.85; subtests between 0.75 and 0.85
	The manual reviews various predictive validity studies.
		Test can be used for screening large numbers of children. In addition, the same authors have developed "Early Identification in Preschool Children," a version of the Meeting Street School Screening Test for children aged 4–4 ½.

Test	Author(s)	Source	Age	Administration	Administrator		
					OT	PT	SP
The Miller Assessment of Preschoolers (MAP) (1981) [79]	L. J. Miller	Foundation for Knowledge in Development (KID Foundation), 1901 West Littleton Blvd., Littleton, CO 80120	2.9–5.8 yr	Individual: 20–30 min (including scoring)	X		
The Peabody Picture Vocabulary Test-Revised (PPVT-R) (1981) [39]	L. M. Dunn, G. J. Robertsons, and J. L. Eisenberg	American Guidance Service, Inc., Publishers Building, Circle Pines, MN 55014	2.6–4.0 yr	Individual: approximately 10 min			X

Description	Construction & Reliability	Comments
MAP was designed to determine school readiness and potential learning difficulties. MAP consists of 27 items and a series of structured observations. These items are delineated into the following five performance areas: 1. *Foundations:* Items generally found on standard neurologic examinations and sensory integrative neurodevelopmental tests 2. *Coordination:* Gross, fine, and oral motor abilities and articulation 3. *Verbal:* Cognitive language abilities, including memory, sequencing, comprehension, association, following directions, and expression 4. *Nonverbal:* Cognitive abilities such as visual figure-ground, puzzles, memory, and sequencing 5. *Complex tasks:* Tasks requiring an interaction of sensory motor and cognitive abilities [29, 79].	Standardized on 1200 preschool children. Test-retest reliability on 90 children, 81% of their scores remained stable. Internal consistency coefficient was .798. Interrater reliability based on 40 children was .98. Several validity studies are cited in the manual.	MAP was developed by an occupational therapist and is a fairly new tool that shows promise as a useful screening instrument.
The PPVT-R was designed as a measure of receptive language and has replaced the original PPVT (1959). The PPVT-R retains many of the best features of its predecessor. The PPVT-R consists of two parallel forms (L and M) and allows for a verbal and nonverbal response. The PPVT-R contains 350 items.	Standardized on a sample of 4200 children and 828 adults. Internal consistency .66–.81 using the split-half method. Reliability as .71–.91 from the standardized sample. Concurrent validity was established against the PPVT coefficients of the concurrence and ranged from .53–.87, with a median of .72 on raw scores. These indicate an adequate to high degree of concurrence. No predictive validity data are available.	This is a useful replacement to the original revision with an expanded age range 2.6–4.0 yr

A SELECTIVE LIST OF EVALUATIONS USED BY OCCUPATIONAL AND PHYSICAL THERAPISTS AND SPEECH PATHOLOGISTS (Continued)

Test	Author(s)	Source	Age	Administration	Administrator OT	PT	SP
The Pediatric Assessment System for Learning Disorders (1980–1985) [74]	M. D. Levine	Educators Publishing Service, Inc., 75 Moulton St., Cambridge, MA 02238	3–12+ yr	Individual: 40 min to administer each (PEER, PEEX, and PEERAMID)	X		

Description	Construction & Reliability	Comments

The Pediatric Assessment System for Learning Disorders is a neurodevelopmental examination that is divided into three age groups:
1. The Pediatric Examination of Educational Readiness (PEER) is administered to children aged 4–6 and is composed of a general health assessment, observation of dressing/undressing during a physical examination, and a developmental attainment component. The latter component consists of 29 tasks delineated into the following categories:
  a. Orientation
  b. Gross motor
  c. Visual fine motor
  d. Sequential
  e. Linguistic
  f. Preacademic learning
2. The Pediatric Early Elementary Examination (PEEX) is administered to children aged 7–9 and consists of the following major sections:
  Developmental attainment
  Neuromaturation
  General health
  Task analysis
  Associated behavioral observations
3. The Pediatric Examination of Educational Readiness at Middle Childhood (PEERAMID) is administered to children 9–15 yr and older and is composed of items such as: minor neurologic indicators, fine motor function, sleective attention, language and gross motor function. In addition, the Aggregate Neurobehavioral Student Health and Educational
	No information about reliability and validity are provided in the manuals. No overall rating system, although certain components can be scored.	There are many portions of this assessment that can be useful for occupational therapists.
		
		According to the manual, PEEX is "more comprehensive than a developmental screening test, but it does not yield a total or definitive evaluation of development in any particular area." [46] PEEX generates a functional profile.
		
		According to the manual, "The PEERAMID should never be used in isolation; it should be part of a multifaceted evaluation. . . ." [46]. The Anser System is a supplemental test to be used with objective standardized evaluations and should not be used in isolation.

Test	Author(s)	Source	Age	Administration	Administrator OT	PT	SP
Purdue Percep-tual-Motor Survey Rating Scale (1966) [92]	E. G. Roach and N. C. Kephart	Charles E. Merrill Publishing Co., 1300 Alum Creek Dr., Columbus, OH 43216	6–10 yr	Individual: 30 min–1 hr	X	X	
The Quick Neurological Screening Test (QNST) (1978) [83]	M. A. Mutti, H. M. Sterling, and N. V. Spalding	Academic Therapy Publications, 20 Commercial Blvd., Novato, CA 94947	5+ yr	Individual: 20 min	X	X	

Review (Anser System) is a supplemental test to be used in conjunction with the PEER, PEEX, and PEERAMID. It is composed of a series of questionnaires to be completed by parents, school personnel, and children 9 and older to assess the development, behavior, and health of a child suspected of having a specific learning disability or behavior disorder or both.

The Purdue Perceptual-Motor Survey measures fine and gross motor and perceptual skills. Five subtests include

1. Balance and postural flexibility
2. Body image and differentiation
3. Perceptual motor match
4. Ocular control
5. Visual achievement forms (developmental drawings or form perception)

Standardized on 200 children; however, a test-retest reliability of .95 was based on only 30 children. Reliability has not been established. "Overall, the standardization of the test is poor." (11)

Hammill and Bartel note that this test is better used as a structured informal device, rather than as a standardized instrument. (29)

The QNST is a screening tool to identify children suspected of having a learning disability. The following tasks are adapted from developmental assessments and pediatric neurologic examinations:

Hand skills
Figure recognition and production
Palm form recognition
Eye tracking
Sound patterns
Finger nose
Thumb and finger circle
Double simultaneous stimulation of hand and cheek
Rapid reversing, repetitive hand movements
Arm and leg extension
Tandem walk
Stand on one leg
Skip
Left-right discrimination
Behavior irregularities

QNST has not been formally standardized. Norms are not given. Incomplete data are reported on reliabilities of .81 and .71

QNST should be used as an adjunct to clinical observation. QNST tests motor function primarily.

Test	Author(s)	Source	Age	Administration	Administrator		
					OT	PT	SP
Southern California Sensory Integration Tests (SCSIT) (1980) [10, 13, 20]	A. J. Ayres	Western Psychological Services, 12031 Wilshire Blvd., Los Angeles, CA 90025	4–8 yr	Individual: 1 ¼– 1 ½ hr, examiner certification recommended	X	X	
Test of Adolescent Language (TOAL) (1980) [60]	D. D. Hammill, V. L. Brown, S. C. Larsen, and J. L. Wiederholt	Pro-Ed, 5341 Industrial Oaks Blvd., Austin, TX 78735	11– 18.5 yrs	Group: 1–3 hr, 2 of its 18 subtests must be administered individually	X		X

Description	Construction & Reliability	Comments
The SCSIT was devised to identify sensory integrative dysfunction in learning disabled children. SCSIT is composed of 17 tests that were derived from either neurologic or psychological tests. The tests are 1. Space visualization (SV) 2. Figure-ground perception (FG) 3. Position in space (PS) 4. Design copy (DC) 5. Motor accuracy-revised (MAC-R) 6. Kinesthesia (KIN) 7. Manual form perception (MFP) 8. Finger identification (FI) 9. Graphesthesia (GRA) 10. Localization of tactile stimuli (LTS) 11. Double tactile stimuli (DTS) 12. Imitation of postures (IP) 13. Crossing the midline (CML) 14. Bilateral motor coordination (BMC) 15. Right-left discrimination (RLD) 16. Standing balance—eyes open (SBO) 17. Standing balance—eyes closed (SBC) In addition, complete interpretation requires the use of a test of postrotary nystagmus (vestibular function) and a series of clinical observations.	The SCSIT have been revised and restandardized. Currently, test-retest reliability coefficients show moderate reliability. Cermak and Henderson note that "The tests have been criticized on this basis as well as on the lack of study of criterion related validity" [29]	Certification in administration and interpretation of the SCSIT are essential for appropriate use. Cermak and Henderson note, "The tests are a vehicle by which a clinician can gain insight to a child's problems and plan a remediation program. They are not designed to be used in monitoring change with treatment. [29] Occasionally physical therapists use the SCSIT.
The TOAL assesses various aspects of oral and written language. There are eight subtests: 1. Listening/Vocabulary 2. Listening/Grammar 3. Speaking/Vocabulary 4. Speaking/Grammar 5. Reading/Vocabulary 6. Reading/Grammar 7. Writing/Vocabulary 8. Writing/Grammar	Standardized on over 2700 students. The majority of reliability coefficients fell above .80. Validity was tested, and most correlation coefficients were below .80.	TOAL is one of the few tests that evaluates language in adolescents.

Test	Author(s)	Source	Age	Administration	Administrator OT	PT	SP
Test of Language Competence (TLC) (1985) [107]	E. H. Wiig and W. Secord	Charles E. Merrill, Inc., 1300 Alum Creek Dr., Columbus, OH 43216	9–21 yr	Individual: 35–45 min– 1 hr			X
The Test of Language Development (TOLD) (1977) [85]	P. L. Newcomer and D. D. Hammill	Pro-Ed., 33 Perry Brooks Bldg., Austin, TX 78701	4–8.11 yr	Individual: 35–40 min			X

Description	Construction & Reliability	Comments

The TLC is a strategic situational measure of language competence (74) composed of 4 subtests:
    Understanding ambiguous sentences
    Making inferences
    Recreating sentences
    Understanding metaphoric expressions
In addition the TLC includes a supplemental task, "Remembering Word Pairs," which is not routinely used but may be given to the student who "shows significant areas of weakness on the TLC subtests. In that case, performance on the 'Remembering Word Pairs' task can be used to validate the presence of a generalized language disability that cuts across auditory memory" [107].
	Standardized on 1796 students ages 9–19 yr. Reliability coefficient of .78 and construct validity correlations range was from .29–50. The manual notes criterion-related validity was assessed using "a priori classification of students by a related variable, in this case the classification of students as language-learning disabled (LLD) or normally achieving (non LLD)" [107].	"TLC was not designed to provide in-depth assessment at the level of phonology. . . . The results of the TLC should be complemented by administration of standardized measures of receptive vocabulary development and by an analysis of a spontaneous speech sample" [107]. Wiig suggests that the Test of Adolescent Language (TOAL) [60] is a feasible complement to the TLC [106]. The TLC fills the void for a needed assessment to measure "language competence" in older children and adolescents.

The TOLD assesses phonology, syntax, and semantics—components of receptive and expressive language. There are seven subtests:
I. *Principal subtests*
  A. Semantics (the study of meaning in language)
    1. Picture Vocabulary (receptive)
    2. Oral Vocabulary (expressive)
  B. Syntax (the study of word order and inflections)
    1. Grammatic Understanding (receptive)
    2. Sentence Imitation (expressive)
    3. Grammatic Completion (receptive and expressive)
II. *Supplementary Subtests*
  A. Phonology (the sound system of language)
    1. Word Discrimination (receptive)
    2. Word Articulation (expressive)
	Standardized on 1014 children. Split-half method of reliability was used and appears adequate. Concurrent validity coefficients range in the .70s and .80s.	According to the TOLD manual, "The results yielded by the TOLD will focus attention upon the specific areas of language in which the child is unable to perform as well as his peers do. . . . However, before a remedial program is planned, it will be necessary to determine through informal assessment, including criterion-referenced testing, and possibly diagnostic teaching, the specific skills within an area which are in need of remediation" [85].

Test	Author(s)	Source	Age	Administration	Administrator		
					OT	PT	SP
Test of Motor Impairment-Henderson Revised (1984) [94]	D. H. Scott, F. A. Moyes, and S. E. Henderson	Brook Educational Publishing, Ltd., P.O. Box 1171, Guelph, Ontario, Canada N1H6N3	5–12 yr	Individual: 20–40 min	X	X	
Tests of Motor Proficiency of Gubbay (1975) [56]	S. S. Gubbay	S. S. Gubbay. *The Clumsy Child,* Philadelphia: Saunders, 1975	8–12 yr	Individual: 2–5 min	X	X	
The Token Test for Children (1978) [99]	F. D. Simoni	DLM Teaching Resources, P.O. Box 4000, 1 DLM Park, Allen, TX 75002	3–12 yr	Individual			X

Description	Construction & Reliability	Comments
The test is a version of the Bruininks-Oseretsky Test of Motor Proficiency, designed to differentiate the child with motor impairment from the normal child. Test consists of eight categories: 1. Manual dexterity 1 2. Manual dexterity 2 3. Manual dexterity 3 4. Ball skills 1 5. Ball skills 2 6. Static balance 7. Dynamic balance 1 8. Dynamic balance 2 There is a single item in each category for the four age groups (5–6, 7–8, 9–10, and 11–12 yr) assessed.	Standardized on 923 children. "A number of studies of reliability and validity used the 1972 version as well as the current revision." (29)	This revision is much clearer than the former version.
Tests of Motor Proficiency of Gubbay compose a quick screening tool for the identification of developmental dyspraxia (the clumsy child). This instrument is composed of eight items: 1. Whistle through pursed lips 2. Skip forward five steps 3. Roll ball with foot around objects 4. Throw tennis ball, clap hands, then catch tennis ball 5. Tie one shoelace with double bow 6. Thread 10 beads 7. Pierce 20 pinholes in graph paper 8. Posting box: fit six shapes in appropriate slots [11] Items 1 and 2 are scored pass/fail; item 4 is the number of claps; the remaining items are scored.	Nonstandardized. Percentile values are reported for each age level (8–12 yr).	Tests of Motor-Proficiency of Gubbay is described in Gubbay, *The Clumsy Child* and must be purchased or constructed. This is a quick screening to be used in conjunction with teacher questionnaires.
This test is based on an adaptation by Noll, Berry, and Whitaker of the TOKEN Test originally devised by De Renzi and Vignolo. This original test consisted of 20 "tokens" differentiated by color (red, white, blue, green and yellow), shape (square and round), and size (small and large). The present version evaluates	Standardized on 1304 children aged 3–12.6 yr. The manual provides no reliability or validity. However previous research with various adaptations of the original TOKEN test may assist in inferring a tenuous validity of sorts [99].	"The author provides no reliability, validity, or adequate and useful norm for the Token Test for Children. While the test may provide the experienced speech and language pathologist with a basis for making clinical

Test	Author(s)	Source	Age	Administration	Administrator OT	PT	SP
Upper-Extension Expressive One-Word Picture Vocabulary Test (EQWPVT) (1983) [47]	M. F. Gardner	Academic Therapy Publications, 20 Commercial Blvd., Novato, CA 94947-6191	12–15.11 yr	Individual: 5–10 min (although not a timed test) Small group: (responses are written)			X
Woodcock Language Proficiency Battery (1980–1981) (WLPB) [111]	R. W. Woodcock and M. B. Johnson	DLM Teaching Resources, P.O. Box 4000, 1 DLM Park, Allen, TX 75002	3+ yr	Individual: 45 min, entire battery approximately 15 min/subtest			X

Description	Construction & Reliability	Comments

receptive language and consists of 61 verbally presented items (commands) arranged in five parts of increasing difficulty. For example, item 1: "Touch the red circle." Item 61: "Before touching the yellow circle pick up the red square."

inferences regarding aspects of a child's receptive language, the user is cautioned against using the Token Test for Children as a norm-reference measure" [81].

The purpose of the Upper-Extension EOWPVT is to assess a basal estimate of verbal intelligence for students 12.0–15.11 yr. (The EOWPVT assesses ages 2–12). It is composed of 70 items (pictures) arranged progressively more difficult, which fall into the following five language-processing categories:

1. General concrete concepts (common characteristics and common elements)
2. Groupings (plural)
3. Abstract concepts (a single characteristic common to a number of items or objects)
4. Descriptive concepts (items identified by a participle, i.e., noun ending in "ing")
5. Letter symbols and geometric and other meaningful forms [47].

Standardized on 465 students. Reliability was determined by the split-half method and ranged from a coefficient of .89–.94 with a median reliability of .92. Criterion-related validity with the Peabody Picture Vocabulary Test-Revised ranged from .69–.80, median .74. Correlations with the WISC-R Vocabulary Subtest ranged from .74–.84, median .83.

Can be administered to a bilingual student (English/Spanish)

Woodcock Language Proficiency Battery is an oral and written language and reading proficiency battery consisting of eight subtests from the Woodcock-Johnson Psycho-Educational Battery. These subtests include

1. *Oral Language*-picture vocabulary, antonyms-synonyms, analogies
2. *Reading*-letter-word identification, word attack
3. *Written Language*-dictation, proofing

Administration of this entire battery provides a general index of overall language function.

Standardized on 4732 subjects. Reliability and validity studies appear to be thorough.

"Given the superior standardization procedures, the versatility of the test in terms of its applications, and the academic significance of the language functions measured, the WLPG is highly recommended as an assessment tool" WLPG has been found to be a useful tool in collecting longitudinal data for determining the long-term effects of treatment.

Test	Author(s)	Source	Age	Administration	Administrator		
					OT	PT	SP
The WORD Test (1981) [66]	C. Jorgensen, M. Barrett, R. Huisingh, and L. Zachman	Lingui Systems, Inc., 1630 5th Ave., Suite 806, Moline, IL 61265	7+	Individual: 30–40 min			X

Description	Construction & Reliability	Comments
The WORD Test was designed to assess expressive vocabulary and semantic abilities. It is composed of 6 tasks: 1. Associations 2. Synonyms 3. Semantic absurdities 4. Antonyms 5. Definitions 6. Multiple definitions	Norms established on children age 7–11.11 yr. Validity established by the method of internal consistency.	The WORD Test provides a standardized analysis of each student's specific areas of strengths and weaknesses.

6 Attention Deficit Disorder/Hyperactivity

Judith D. Ward

Attention deficit disorder (ADD) is a syndrome found in 3 percent of preadolescent children [1]. It has been recognized for almost 30 years and is identified by a variety of names: hyperactivity, hyperkinesis, hyperkinetic impulse disorder, and minimal brain dysfunction. The American Psychiatric Association has recently classified the syndrome as attention deficit hyperactivity disorder, or if hyperactivity is not evident, undifferentiated attention deficit disorder [2]. Here, the terms *attention deficit disorder* (ADD) and *hyperactivity* will be used interchangeably.

Children with attentional deficits have trouble at home, at school, and even at play. Wender [42] describes two severe classic cases:

Thomas ". . . was referred by his school public health nurse with the following complaints: "Disruptive classroom behavior, a discipline problem at home. Outbursts of misbehavior—seems to lack self-control, especially when not under direct supervision of teacher (hits other children for no reason, rolls on floor, jumps off of chairs). Even under teacher's direct supervision he talks out, makes facial grimaces. He gets out of his seat frequently. Even during his 'quiet' moments he seems tense, cracks his knuckles, plays with buttons on his clothes, can't sit still. Has no close friends at school; seems to reject other children's attempts to make friends. Has above average ability but not working up to that level now."

Eight-year-old Michael ". . . cries a lot, especially when told he cannot do something, when told he must come in from play, and also at mealtimes, because he does not want to eat . . . . He does not play well with the neighborhood children . . . he always wants to fight, wrestle, and poke people . . . he finds it difficult to play any game that isn't all activity . . . . He had nightly enuresis and had never been trained.

Not all children are as severe or as hyperactive as Thomas and Michael. Although the hyperactivity appears to be the most outstanding symptom of both boys, they also illustrate other problems. In school Thomas was not achieving at the level expected for his intelligence and he had trouble with social relationships; Michael had emotional lability and nighttime bed wetting.

The primary problems of children with ADD are their inability to sustain attention and control their impulses. The attentional difficulties interfere with completion of school work and household tasks. These children cannot keep themselves entertained at play for prolonged periods, and they do not seem to listen to others. Their impulsivity results in careless school work and irritability or aggression toward others. Barkley [5] considers the hyperactive child's noncompliance as a primary problem that most often prompts referral for help.

The American Psychiatric Association's *Diagnostic and Statistical Manual of Mental Disorders (DSM III-R)* [2]* provides the following criteria for diagnosing attention deficit hyperactivity disorder in children:

A. A disturbance of at least 6 months during which at least eight of the following are present:
   1. Often fidgets with hands or feet or squirms in seat (in adolescents, may be limited to subjective feelings of restlessness)
   2. Has difficulty remaining seated when required to do so
   3. Is easily distracted by extraneous stimuli
   4. Has difficulty awaiting turn in games or group situations

* Reprinted with permission from the *Diagnostic and Statistical Manual of Mental Disorders* (3rd ed. rev.). Washington D.C.: American Psychiatric Association, 1987.

   5. Often blurts out answers to questions before they have been completed
   6. Has difficulty following through on instructions from others (not due to oppositional behavior or failure of comprehension), e.g., fails to finish chores
   7. Has difficulty sustaining attention in tasks or play activities
   8. Often shifts from one uncompleted activity to another
   9. Has difficulty playing quietly
   10. Often talks excessively
   11. Often interrupts or intrudes on others, e.g., butts into other children's games
   12. Often does not seem to listen to what is being said to him or her
   13. Often loses things necessary for tasks or activities at school or at home (e.g., toys, pencils, books, assignments)
   14. Often engages in physically dangerous activities without considering possible consequences (not for the purpose of thrill-seeking), e.g., runs into street without looking
B. Onset before the age of 7
C. Does not meet the criteria for a pervasive developmental disorder

DEVELOPMENTAL CHARACTERISTICS
ADD arises in childhood but may not be recognized until the child starts school and is required to attend to academic tasks. Those children who show symptoms of the disorder in infancy are difficult babies [33] who sleep irregularly. They do not like to be cuddled [41] and will squirm and twist when bathed, fed, or diapered. Some cry a lot and cannot be comforted.

All toddlers are normally busy, curious, and self-assertive. Hyperactive toddlers are more driven than busy, more impulsive and destructive than curious, and more irritable and frustrated than assertive. They are dangerous to themselves because they seem to have no fears [41]. Children with extreme forms of hyperactivity may be asked to withdraw from nursery school because they are unable to sustain attention for school activities and cannot play with their peers [41].

The diagnosis of ADD is most often made in middle childhood. The academic setting requires children to sit still, listen, organize information, and cooperate with others. These activities are difficult for hyperactive children. Although they have average or higher intelligence, some have learning disabilities (see Chapter 5). Others have trouble in school because they cannot concentrate on their work or because their behavior problems disrupt the class. When their academic achievement does not reflect their intellectual potential [41], parents and teachers may attribute this to carelessness or laziness.

Many hyperactive children are smaller than their peers, and some show other signs of physical immaturity [5]. Some are uncoordinated. Their handwriting is sloppy, and they are clumsy at sports. They seem to trip over their own feet and are rough on their toys and clothes. Fifty percent of hyperactive children have problems with bed wetting and twenty-five percent with encopresis [5]. Some parents report that the children are unresponsive to physical punishment, and they ignore bumps, bruises, and hard knocks [5, 42]. It is not known if there is a physiologic basis for this stoicism or if they just do not pay attention to pain.

Hyperactive children are often rejected by their peers because they disrupt play activities and intrude on others during school work. Wender [42] calls them unsuccessful extroverts because they are able to make friends easily but cannot keep them. Parents and teachers are frustrated by the children's unresponsiveness to social demands and emotional lability. They are unpredictable—happy one minute and irritable the next.

Rejected by peers and misunderstood by adults, it is no surprise that older ADD children have poor self-esteem. Failure in many situations leads to a decrease in motivation and can become a vicious cycle leading to antisocial behavior in adolescence. Twenty-five to fifty percent of these adolescents are referred to the courts for theft or truancy [41]. Those who were overactive as children appear to be less so in adolescence. They are better able to channel their activity but are always busy with something. Impulsivity and poor peer relationships become important problems in adolescence [41].

ETIOLOGY

The etiology of ADD is unknown, and it is likely that there is no single cause [15, 36]. There is evidence of constitutional or genetic components in some cases, although adequate studies to confirm this are needed [15,20]. Hyperactivity runs in families [15, 33], and twin studies suggest a genetic influence on activity level [33]. ADD is more common in boys (1:5) than girls (1:9) [41].

There is a higher-than-average frequency of minor, congenital physical anomalies in children with ADD [15]. Some have mild-to-moderate electroencephalogram (EEG) abnormalities [1, 15], but only about 5 percent of hyperactive children have diagnosable neurologic disorders [1]. There may be a subgroup of young hyperactive children who are affected by food additives and salicylates [15, 39], and the use of restricted diets for these children continues to be studied [24].

Children with aggressive behavior are more likely to come from low socioeconomic status families who demonstrate aggressive or lax parenting [19, 25, 26]. Psychogenic theories do not attribute ADD solely to parental practices but propose that the stress of caring for a demanding, restless, fretful child [33], coupled with family problems, may have an adverse effect on parental attitudes, which exacerbate the difficulties.

Studies of brain dysfunction due to biochemical abnormalities or problems with the excitatory and inhibitory systems within the central nervous system are inconclusive [36], but these theories seem the most promising for ultimately explaining ADD.

ATTENTION, AROUSAL, AND INHIBITION

Douglas and Peters [10] contend that ADD would be more accurately described as attentional impulsivity disorder, and they attribute the difficulties to three related processes:

1. Investment of attention and effort
2. Modulation of arousal
3. Inhibition of impulses

Attention, arousal, and inhibition are all interrelated components of information processing. Attention is the process by which an individual receives, selects, and processes information about the environment [31, 32]. Arousal is the physiologic and psychological state of readiness to process information [12]. Attention and arousal are intricately related: Arousal activates attention and attention increases arousal [31].

"Inhibition is the neural process in which one part of the nervous system prevents another part from overreacting to sensory input . . . " [3]. Modulation is "the process of increasing or reducing a neural activity to keep that activity in harmony with all the other functions of the nervous system" [3].

Hyperactive children obviously have problems with attention, but the nature of the problem is not clear. Parents and teachers complain that they do not listen, are careless with school work, do not follow directions, do not obey, and do not pay attention. However, the same children who have trouble sustaining attention in the classroom can watch TV for hours [33]. An important goal of research in ADD is identifying which aspects of attention are impaired.

In their own research and in extensive review of clinical, educational, and research literature, Douglas and Peters [10] have tried to identify more clearly the attentional deficits of hyperactive children. Most of the research has focused on sustained and selective attention [10].

Selective attention is the ability to focus on stimuli that are important to a task while ignoring irrelevant stimuli. An individual is considered distractible if performance deteriorates in the presence of irrelevant stimuli [5, 10]. Children with ADD have been described as distractible, unable to filter out extraneous stimuli. Although children with ADD pay more attention to extraneous stimuli than normal children, Douglas and Peters conclude that this does not interfere with performance. Because hyperactivity increases in stimulus-reduced environments, Douglas and Peters speculate that attention to extraneous events may be due to the ADD child's need for stimulation rather than an inability to screen out irrelevant stimuli.

Sustained attention refers to the alertness of the individual, the cognitive equivalent of physiologic arousal [32]. Sustained attention involves arousal, orienting toward relevant stimuli and vigilance. Tests of sustained attention include reaction-time tasks and tasks where the individual must maintain alertness while waiting to respond to a specific stimulus.

Hyperactive children have trouble with sustained attention. They have trouble with vigilance tasks and those tasks where they must organize their efforts, use self-discipline to stick to the task and refrain from impulsive responding [9]. Brown's [6] description of ADD children is that they "make decisions too rapidly, fail to pause to consider possible alternatives, fail to reflect on possible consequences of a decision, and seize on the first response that comes to mind." Douglas [9] notes that the problems with concentration reflect the children's impulsivity and are closely related to difficulties with levels of *arousal*.

Stimulus-seeking behavior may be due to underarousal of the central nervous system [9, 10] where excessive activity is a compensatory behavior to increase proprioceptive input [29, 32]. Douglas [9, 10] and Peters [10] propose that ADD children have a narrow range of arousal within which they can function and that their arousal patterns are labile. In addition, these children have trouble modulating the level of arousal to meet situational or task demands [9, 10, 32].

ADD children act without thinking and take risks that other children would not. They "fly off the handle" easily, and they are not good problem solvers. These are all characteristics of *impulsivity*. This *lack of behavioral inhibition* may be due to an imbalance of autonomic and central nervous system excitatory/inhibitory mechanisms, a reflection of the children's cognitive style [29], or both. The impulsive behavior has consequences in *every* aspect of the children's life, and because it interferes with problem solving, Douglas and Peters [10] believe it may handicap cognitive development: "Their inclination against looking and listening carefully or reflecting upon their experiences in a thoughtful manner would impede the establishment of rich, subtle, and complex schemata, which in turn, would impair the effective deployment of perceptual and cognitive operations and the cycle would be continuously repeated." This inability to "stop, look, and listen" [9] becomes an important consideration in social and academic learning.

DIAGNOSIS AND ASSESSMENT
The diagnosis of attention deficit disorder is based primarily on direct and indirect observation of the child's everyday behavior and on tests that rule out other disorders (see diagnostic criteria earlier in this chapter). There is no laboratory test that identifies ADD, and it is difficult to differentiate hyperactive children from normally active children or those with conduct disorders. The procedures for diagnosis and assessment include interviews, observation, the use of behavioral rating scales, and psychometric tests [4] (Table 6-1).

The DSM III-R [2] diagnostic criteria for attention deficit hyperactivity disorder describe specific behaviors in everyday situations (see discussion earlier in this chapter). It is difficult for the physician to observe these characteristics during a clinical interview of the child because these children are typically quieter, less impulsive, and more attentive in a one-to-one encounter with a strange adult. Thus, an *interview* of those who are familiar with the child's daily behavior is a more important source of information than an interview with the child.

Parents, and if possible, teachers are relied on for much of the information about the child's behavior. The interview provides a developmental, medical, and academic history. Current behavior is discussed, exploring specific social interactions, activities, and the characteristics of the environment. Teachers know the child's interaction with peers, in large groups, and on the playground, and they can provide information about academic and task behaviors.

Behavioral rating scales cover a wide array of problems that are too unwieldy to cover in an interview [5]. Scales designed for use by parents and teachers identify and rate behavior that can be compared to ratings of normal peers [5]. Rating scales are also useful later for assessing the effects of treatment, but as Barkley [5] points out, they are not helpful in formulating treatment strategies because they describe behavior but do not identify the antecedents or consequences of that behavior. Rating scales cannot take the place of direct observation for evaluating the environmental influences on the child's actions.

Direct observation provides important information about the children in their everyday environments. Parents, teachers, or therapists use diaries or structured forms for recording target behaviors and their antecedents and consequences. The frequency, duration, and products of behaviors are noted [5]. These data are used to identify which environments trigger undesirable behaviors or promote positive ones. If it is impossible to document observation in the natural environment, an analogous environment is created, in which the therapist observes parent-child interaction, free play, and task behaviors [5].

Intelligence tests measure intellectual capacity and rule out mental retardation. Achievement

TABLE 6-1. Diagnosis and assessment: Attention deficit disorder

Method/instrument	Purpose	Information obtained	Comments
MEDICAL EXAMINATION	Rule out medical causes of behavior problems		Not helpful in treatment planning [5] Periodic exams when medication used in treatment [5]
INTERVIEW Parent	Contributes to diagnosis Contributes to assessment for treatment planning	Demographic Behavioral, developmental, medical history Family interactions Child's current social behavior [5] Child's strengths and weaknesses	
Child		Child's perception of problem Observation of depression and low self-esteem [5]	Child's behavior in a one-to-one interview does not usually reflect typical behavior [5]
Teacher		Academic performance Behavior with peers and in groups [5]	
DIRECT OBSERVATION Natural or analogous environment (done by parent, teacher or clinician) Observation schedules Diaries	Assessment for treatment planning Assess effects of treatment	Recording frequency, duration, intensity of target behaviors Identify antecedents and consequences of social interactions	Very costly [5,35]
BEHAVIOR RATING SCALES	Scales with normative data used in diagnosis Assess effectiveness of treatment [5]	Attention, activity level, sociability, excitability, perseverance, aggression Conduct and personality problems Behaviors related to play, meals, TV, school [35]	Cover wide array of problems faster than an interview [5]
Connors Parent Symptom Questionnaire [7]			Rating by parents
Connors Teacher Questionnaire [8]			Rating by teacher
Greenberg Hyperactivity Rating Scale [38]			Rating by teacher
Werry-Weiss-Peters Home Activity Rating Scale [5, 34]			Rating by parents or by interview of parents

160

INTELLIGENCE AND ACHIEVEMENT TESTS	Rule out mental retardation Compare child's abilities to demands of environment Educational planning	General intelligence Academic achievement	A profile comparing intelligence, achievement, and performance tests identifies learning disabilities [5] Administered by teachers and psychologists
Intelligence tests WISC Stanford Binet McCarthy Scales of Childrens Abilities Achievement tests Peabody Individual Achievement Tests Wide Range Achievement Tests [5]			
PERFORMANCE TESTS	Educational and treatment planning	Perceptual motor skills	A profile comparing intelligence, achievement, and performance tests identifies learning disabilities [5]
Bender Visual Motor Gestalt Test		Visual motor perception	Requires attention to detail, indirect measure of attention, and impulsivity [35] Administered by psychologist
Marianne Frostig Developmental Test of Visual Perception		Visual perception	Requires reflection, attention to detail, indirect measure of attention, and impulsivity [35] Administered by teacher, occupational or physical therapist
Goodenough-Harris Human Figure Drawing Test Southern California Sensory Integration Tests		Cognitive development Sensory integrative function	Indirect measure of attention and impulsivity [35] Administered by occupational and physical therapists
MEASURES OF COGNITIVE STYLE	Diagnosis Treatment planning	Reflection/impulsivity Field independence/dependence	Field independence/dependence influences attention/distractibility [35]
Matching Familiar Figures Test Embedded Figure Test			

tests show academic performance. It is not unusual for there to be a discrepancy between IQ and performance in children with ADD. Educational tests are also used to identify specific learning disabilities and the child's cognitive style.

Assessment of ADD children is multidisciplinary and broad because the disorder pervades every aspect of life [5]. Social workers; psychologists; educators; and physical, occupational, and speech therapists may all be part of the evaluation team. The goal of assessment is to produce a profile of the child in which psychosocial, cognitive, and academic strengths and weaknesses are specified. The environment is examined to determine which factors contribute to behavioral problems and which enhance performance. A treatment plan is formulated in which objectives for medical, academic, and behavioral intervention are specified.

TREATMENT

Except in extreme cases of antisocial behavior, children with attention deficits are treated in their natural environment. They continue in school, some receiving special education services and therapy through the school system. Ideally, their families take an active part in behavioral management with the help of professionals. The physician monitors progress and prescribes medication when appropriate.

MEDICATION

A common treatment of ADD is the use of psychostimulant *medication:* methylphenidate hydrochloride (Ritalin), magnesium pemoline (Cylert), and the amphetamines. Between 1 and 2 percent of school-age children take stimulant medication [5]. Although the precise action of stimulant drugs is not known, they are thought to enable the cerebral cortex to screen out distracting stimuli thus increasing concentration and attention [4]. Attributed to improved concentration is a decrease in impulsivity; irrelevant motor activity; aggression; and noisy, disruptive behavior [5]. About 75 percent of hyperactive children improve with stimulant medication. Twenty-five percent worsen or remain unchanged [4].

The use of stimulant medication for the treatment of hyperactivity is a well-established practice, and the effects of stimulants have been studied for more than 30 years. The short-term effects of stimulants are positive. They improve the child's behavior, allowing for better school performance, better social interaction, and a more confident child. The people around the child react more positively to improved behavior, so the child's life is easier [5, 30].

The most common side effects of stimulants are insomnia and decreased appetite. Less than 50 percent of children on medication will experience weight loss and irritability. Some will have headaches and abdominal pains [5]. The side effects are dose related and may disappear after a few weeks on medication or by lowering the dosage. Physicians usually discontinue medication during school vacations when demands on the child are less. The drug-free periods allow for considerable gains in weight and height that may be suppressed while on stimulants [4, 43].

There is concern about increased blood pressure found in some children on stimulants. Although the increase is slight, it is not known what the long-term effects are on the cardiovascular system [43]. Stimulant-induced psychosis has been noted in some studies, but these symptoms disappear when the drug is discontinued [5]. Barkley [5] has seen some children develop tics when on methylphenidate, and those with a prior history of tics have developed Tourette's syndrome in response to stimulants. These are irreversible symptoms, and Barkley urges that children with a history of tics or highly anxious children not be given stimulant drugs.

Tricyclic antidepressants or neuroleptics have been used with children who have a negative response to psychostimulants [40]. The use of these drugs with children has not been adequately studied, and psychostimulants remain the drug treatment of choice for ADD [43].

The fear of future drug abuse by children who have been treated with stimulant medication is often expressed by parents. Barkley [5] contends that just the opposite occurs: These children are often anxious to stop taking medication.

Although the improvements in attention and concentration are dramatic while the child is being treated with psychostimulant medication, follow-up studies [4] comparing the functioning of children who have received drug treatment and those who have not show that medication does not have a long-term effect on the outcome of the disorder. Medication does not cure the attention deficits but rather helps children better manage their behavior and adapt to academic and social demands. Probably the greatest drawback in using medication is the risk that additional measures will not be taken to help the child educationally and psychologically. Some do not recommend medication until other measures have been tried [30].

BEHAVIOR THERAPY

Except for drug treatment, *behavior therapy,* when consistently employed, is the most effective means of improving the behavior of hyperactive children [5]. Behavior therapy focuses on the social environment of the child. It can be used in conjunction with drug treatment, and the techniques can be implemented by parents, teachers, and others in the child's environment.

Graziano [13] calls behavior therapy "controlled learning." It is based on the principles of operant conditioning and social learning theory. *Operant conditioning* is learning that occurs when specific behaviors are emitted in the expectation of certain consequences. Operant conditioning occurs naturally all the time. Children learn to do things that will please their parents (social reinforcement). Individuals engage in behaviors that are unpleasant if the satisfaction of the consequences outweighs the unpleasantness of the act. In therapy, the environment and the consequences of targeted behaviors are carefully controlled in order to improve the functioning of the child.

A consequence of a behavior that affects the frequency, intensity, quality, or duration of a behavior is a reinforcer. *Positive reinforcement* is the pleasurable consequence of an action, and it tends to increase the frequency or duration of the action. A *negative reinforcer* strengthens behavior that serves to avoid or weaken unpleasant consequences. *Punishment* is an aversive consequence that serves to weaken or eliminate the behavior that produces it.

In behavior therapy, the choice and implementation of reinforcers are of critical importance. The therapist must know the child's likes, dislikes, values, and physical and intellectual capacities. A reinforcer must be meaningful to the child, and it must be applied in a manner that will accelerate learning.

The nature of the action being solicited will also determine the quality and quantity of the reinforcer required. A task that is unpleasant or frustrating requires more frequent reinforcement than a task that contains its own reinforcing elements. The initiation of new behaviors requires stronger, more frequent or intense reinforcement than the maintenance of behavior.

The *schedule of reinforcement* is also important. A reinforcement schedule is the pattern in which reinforcement is applied [23]. Continuous reinforcement is the application of reinforcement to *every* targeted response. Intermittent reinforcement is where the correct response is sometimes reinforced. The ratio of reinforcement is the ratio of responses to reinforcement [16, 37]. Continuous reinforcement is on a $1:1$ ratio. People learn more quickly if reinforcement is continuous [37], and this may be required to develop difficult skills or for new learning. Behavior can be maintained with intermittent reinforcement.

Hyperactive children display a number of

characteristic responses to reinforcement that must be considered when implementing a behavior modification program.

Initially, continuous rewards or punishments are more effective than intermittent ones. Later, as positive behaviors become established, one can gradually diminish the frequency of reinforcement [5]. Care must be taken when diminishing the frequency of reinforcement of some tasks. Based on her research, Douglas [9] reports that with continuous positive reinforcement of complex cognitive tasks, hyperactive children did as well as normal children, but when a partial schedule of reinforcement was instituted, they performed more poorly than controls. She attributes this poor performance to frustration and disruption when ADD children failed to receive expected reinforcement.

Immediate positive attention and praise increase the frequency of desired behavior in hyperactive children; however, parents are at a disadvantage in using praise because hyperactive children are less responsive to parental praise than normal children are, and they are more responsive to praise from novel adults than from their parents [5]. Families may need to learn additional reinforcement methods if praise is not working.

There is some evidence to suggest that positive reinforcement increases arousal and may lead to impulsive responding. While positive reinforcement may serve to heighten arousal and improve involvement in dull repetitive tasks, randomly administered praise on more complex tasks appears to cause deterioration of function in hyperactive children [9]. Douglas [9] interprets this response: "It is possible that the praising statements increased arousal without providing the specific cues to guide attentional processes, which hyperactive children require and which are provided by contingent reinforcement."

The relationship of reinforcement and arousal needs more study, but it seems to be important to monitor the child's state of arousal in response to any treatment approach.

PARENTAL AND FAMILY INVOLVEMENT

Parents can effectively implement behavioral strategies when given proper training. Parent training may be in groups or individually. Dubey and Kaufman [11] describe their approach to teaching behavioral methods to parents of hyperactive children. They work with groups of parents in "classlike" sessions held once a week for 10 weeks. In these 2-hour sessions parents learn environmental and behavioral analysis, how to set behavioral goals, and how to implement behavior modification techniques. They are provided with an instructional manual and are given assignments to carry out at home between sessions. The homework always involves written documentation that can be read by the instructors and used as a basis for discussion in subsequent classes.

Parent training is not only therapeutic for the child but helps the parents gain a real sense of competence. Even the most skillful parent cannot help feeling helpless and frustrated when bringing up a hyperactive child. Parents need to know that the problem is not their fault and that they can learn management strategies to alleviate some of the problems [5, 27].

Training families is not without problems. Sometimes parents disagree with the practices of behavior therapy. They view positive reinforcement as bribery. Or, they attribute the child's problems to basic personality attributes, which they feel cannot be changed [28].

Consistency is an important element in behavior therapy and requires the cooperation of parents, siblings, and teachers. Parents who have marital problems or who do not agree on child-rearing practices may not be able to provide the consistency required to effectively carry out a program [28]. A parent who has always been impulsive when dealing with the child will have to learn new ways of responding in addition to learning behavioral techniques [28].

Parents who do not have the time to adequately monitor the child at home or siblings who overmonitor the child can undermine the

164

program. Teachers may not have the time required to spend with one child's problems. Classmates or siblings may reinforce undesirable behavior [28].

Barkley [5] suggests that when parents first learn behavioral techniques, they should implement these with a target behavior that will be relatively easy to manage so they will gain confidence for some of the more difficult behaviors. He also warns that many behaviors of the ADD child are obtrusive, and parents are likely to choose a negative behavior as a target. The choice of target behaviors requires careful analysis and consideration. It is easy to focus on the most annoying behaviors. Negative behaviors may be the result of deficient positive behaviors. Barkley advises that "the therapist must continually guard against the temptation to design programs simply for the reduction of inappropriate, negative behaviors, without giving equal if not more time to designing positive programs aimed at increasing the more appropriate, actively social forms of child behavior" [5].

Parents should be taught to keep records on target behaviors. Records provide information on which the therapist can evaluate the home program. Record keeping not only helps clarify approaches but also documents subtle progress that might go unnoticed and that will help parents recognize their successes [5].

COGNITIVE BEHAVIOR MODIFICATION AND
SELF-CONTROL

Hyperactive children need the external controls that behavior therapy provides in order to feel more secure about their own competence. But the ultimate goal of treatment is the development of purposeful control over their own behavior. *Cognitive behavior modification* is a behavior therapy approach that addresses the development of self-control. The strategies the children learn can be applied in social situations and in the development of academic and complex problem-solving skills.

In a review of studies of behavior modification with hyperactive children, Keogh and

Barkett [17] concluded that behavioral techniques that focus on changing specific social behaviors will not necessarily enhance educational competencies. For example, children whose disruptive classroom behavior is the target for change may show improvement in classroom behavior but not an improvement in academic performance. For academic achievement to improve, specific academic behaviors must be the target for intervention.

Hyperactive children have trouble with tasks that demand concentration, self-direction, and self-sustained effort [10]. Douglas and her collegues have identified the kind of tasks that are difficult for ADD children [9, 10]

1. Dull, long repetitive vigilance and reaction-time tasks
2. Visual, auditory, or haptic perceptual tasks that require careful analysis of cues
3. Complex problem-solving and memory tasks where they have to consider, rehearse, and evaluate relevant information and knowledge

Douglas [9] attributes these difficulties to problems with the modulation of arousal: the inability to inhibit impulsive responses and problems with sustaining attention and effort. This nonreflective cognitive style seriously hampers academic and social learning and can have serious consequences in the child's life when active problem solving is required [9].

Cognitive behavior modification addresses cognitive style. It teaches children to think about how they think (metacognition). Children are taught to observe, monitor, and control their own behavior—to plan and think before they act. This is done through a combination of verbal mediation, modeling, and contingency management techniques.

Verbal mediation is the process where children talk themselves through a task [21]:

"What am I to do?" (problem definition)
"How will I do it?" (problem approach)
"What is important? What do I do first?" (focusing attention)

"Am I right?" "Go slowly." (coping statements)

"Good job." (self-reinforcement)

Verbal mediation training is based on the theory that voluntary motor behavior (rule-governed behavior) is directed by speech. Normally, children first learn to control their behavior, through the verbal direction of others. As speech develops, they regulate their own behavior by talking aloud to themselves. And finally, the verbalization becomes covert and automatic [21, 22].

Hyperactive children have deficiencies in rule-governed behavior, and the purpose in learning verbal mediation is to reflectively guide their own actions instead of reacting impulsively [5]. To use verbal mediation, children must have the neurologic capacity to acquire language and the physical ability to follow commands [5].

Modeling is an important component of cognitive training. The therapist or the child's peers demonstrate the task, verbalizing self-instruction and cognitive strategies. Contingency management techniques are used to reinforce learning, especially at the beginning of training, to keep motivation high.

Douglas [9] describes a three-level program that teaches *cognitive self-management:*

Level I   Helping the child understand the nature of the deficits
Level II   Strengthening the child's motivation and capacity to deal with the problem-solving role
Level III Teaching specific problem-solving strategies

Before ADD children can benefit from learning self-control strategies, they must understand the nature of their problems and be motivated to change [9]. In the level I phase the trainer encourages the children to think of recent events where they got into trouble because they acted without thinking. ADD children are not introspective and do not understand that their problems with attention and impulsivity contribute to their problems in school and at home. Douglas and her colleagues describe the problems to the children in language they can understand. For example, to explain attention and arousal, "We point out that, if they are not fully 'awake', they will not be 'sharp' enough to solve problems; we remind them, too, that they sometimes have the opposite problem, that is, they get too excited to think clearly" [9]. Although the children in level I may not completely understand the concepts, the trainers stress that they can help them modify these deficits. Then the children are introduced to the cognitive training.

In level II the children's motivation for self-management is strengthened by success experiences. Activities are graded for difficulty and individualized for each child's abilities. The children are taught how to identify the demands of the task, how to assess their own knowledge, and how to evaluate their work. Active learning and independence are rewarded, and the children are reminded of behaviors and attitudes that interfere with problem solving [9].

Specific problem-solving strategies are taught in Level III. The children learn to scan, to focus on important attributes of a task, and to organize their work. They are taught to use mnemonic devices, rehearsal techniques, and how to inhibit impulsive responses [9].

Cognitive self-control training is a relatively new approach in the education of hyperactive children. Most of the work in this area has been done by trained therapists, with small groups of children, in research settings [5]. There is no recipe for cognitive training. The therapist must be sensitive to the child's problems and creative in developing strategies for overcoming difficulties.

OTHER TREATMENT APPROACHES

Those familiar with the theories of *sensory integration* can see that many of the problems associated with ADD could be attributed to sensory integration dysfunction. The learning and social/emotional problems associated with deficits in attention, arousal, and inhibition can be explained by examining the tactile, vestibular, and proprioceptive functions of the nervous system. Ayres [3] says, "The organization of a child's brain can be seen in his attention span and activity level."

The vestibular system modulates the nervous system. The vestibular nuclei and the reticular core of the brain bring together all kinds of sensory input. The vestibular system sends sensory impulses into the reticular arousal system and helps to keep the level of arousal balanced. An underactive vestibular system contributes to hyperactivity and distractibility because it does not adequately modulate neural activity. The proprioceptive system processes body and gravity sensations, modulates the vestibular system, and helps to organize the nervous system [3].

Tactile stimulation can have either a facilitory or inhibitory effect on the nervous system. Some hyperactive and distractible children may be tactilely defensive. They overreact to some kinds of tactile sensory input, which causes emotional irritability and distractibility, which interferes with learning and social relationships [3].

In sensory integrative therapy, the physical or occupational therapist uses activities that provide vestibular, tactile, and proprioceptive stimulation to enhance the functioning of the nervous system [3] (see discussion in Chapter 5).

There has been considerable public interest in the effect of *diet* on hyperactivity. Some parents have reported dramatic improvements in their children on diets that exclude naturally occurring salicylates, artificial colors and flavors, and some preservatives [24].

In 1982 the National Institutes of Health held a consensus development conference to examine the scientific evidence relating to diet and hyperactivity. They concluded that a small proportion of children show less evidence of hyperactivity on restricted diets and further research was recommended [24].

A restricted diet is not advocated for all hyperactive children [5, 24, 39]. It appears to be more effective in young children [5, 39], and diet should not take precedence over consideration of more traditional approaches [5, 24].

OUTCOME

Clinicians and researchers are concerned about the factors that influence the outcome of ADD. Studies suggest that children of similar ages, IQs, levels of hyperactivity, and attentional problems show different outcomes in adolescence depending on the degree of aggression they exhibit at referral [26]. The more aggressive the child is at referral, the worse the adjustment is in adolescence [5]. Aggression is correlated with aggressive family interactions and socioeconomic status (SES) [18, 19, 26]. Children who come from stable middle-class homes, whose parents are firm and accepting in their interactions with their children, do better academically, socially, and occupationally than those from chaotic, low SES families [5, 18].

Hechtman and colleagues [14], in their study of 76 young adults who had a history of hyperactivity, found that the former hyperactive subjects completed less education than controls and had more car accidents. However, as adults, many of the high school drop outs attended night school and made up their educational deficits. The hyperactives did not differ from controls in job status or job satisfaction. Impulsivity and restlessness seemed to persist into adulthood but "even though [adult] hyperactive subjects continue to have problems, they do not load the psychiatric or antisocial population. Few showed serious psychopathology" [14].

ADD is the most widely studied childhood disorder [5], yet there is much to learn about its causes and treatment. It involves a complex interaction of biologic, psychological, and social factors presenting challenges to parents, teachers, therapists, and researchers.

REFERENCES

1. American Psychiatric Association. *Diagnostic and Statistical Manual of Mental Disorders* (3rd ed.). Washington, D.C.: APA, 1980.
2. American Psychiatric Association. *Diagnostic and Statistical Manual of Mental Disorders* (3rd ed.—revised). Washington, D.C.: APA, 1987. Pp. 52–53.
3 Ayres, A. J. *Sensory Integration and the Child.* Los Angeles: Western Psychological, 1979. P. 63.
4. Barkley, R. A. A review of stimulant drug research with hyperactive children. *J. Child Psychol. Psychiatry* 18:137–165, 1977.
5. Barkley, R. A. *Hyperactive Children: A Handbook for Diagnosis and Treatment.* New York: Guilford, 1981. P. 242.
6. Brown, R. T. Impulsivity and psychoeducational intervention in hyperactive children. *J. Learn. Disabil.* 13:19–24, 1980. P. 19.
7. Connors, C. K. Rating scales for use in drug studies with children. *Psychopharmacol. Bull.* (special issue: Pharmacotherapy of Children). 24–84, 1973.
8. Connors, C. K. Teacher rating scale for use in drug studies with children. *Am. J. Psychiatry.* 126:884–888, 1969.
9. Douglas, V. I. Treatment and Training Approaches to Hyperactivity: Establishing Internal or External Control. In C. K. Whalen and B. Henker (eds.), *Hyperactive Children: The Social Ecology of Identification and Treatment.* New York: Academic, 1980. P. 305.
10. Douglas, V. I., and Peters, K. G. Toward a Clearer Definition of the Attentional Deficit of Hyperactive Children. In G. A. Hale and M. Lewis (eds.), *Attention and Cognitive Development.* New York: Plenum, 1979. P. 224.
11. Dubey, D. R., and Kaufman, K. F. Training Parents of Hyperactive Children in Behavior Management. In M. Gittelman (ed.), *Strategic Interventions for Hyperactive Children.* Armonk, NY: Sharpe, 1981.
12. Eysenck, M. W. *Attention and Arousal: Cognition and Performance.* New York: Springer-Verlag, 1982.
13. Graziano, A. M. Some Implications of Behavior Modification Concepts: The New Therapists. In A. M. Grazino (ed.), *Behavior Therapy With Children.* Chicago: Aldine, 1971.
14. Hechtman, L., Weiss, G., Perlman, T., et al. Hyperactive Children in Young Adulthood: A Controlled Prospective, Ten-year Follow-up. In M. Gittelman (ed.), *Strategic Interventions for Hyperactive Children.* Armonk, NY: Sharpe, 1981. P. 196.
15. Johnson, J. A. The etiology of hyperactivity. *Except. Child.* 47:348–353, 1981.
16. Kanfer, F. H., and Phillips, J. S. *Learning Foundations of Behavior Therapy.* New York: Wiley, 1970.
17. Keogh, B. K., and Barkett, C. J. An Educational Analysis of Hyperactive Children's Achievement Problems. In C. K. Whalen and B. Henker (eds.), *Hyperactive Children: The Social Ecology of Identification and Treatment.* New York: Academic, 1980.
18. Loney, J. Hyperkinesis comes of age: What do we know and where should we go? *Am. J. Orthopsychiatry* 50:28–42, 1980.
19. Loney, J., and Milich, R. The role of hyperactive and aggressive symptomatology in predicting adolescent outcome among hyperactive children. *J. Pediatr. Psychol.* 4:93–112, 1979.
20. McMahon, R. C. Biological factors in childhood hyperkinesis: A review of genetic and biochemical hypotheses. *J. Clin. Psychol.* 37:12–21, 1981.
21. Meichenbaum, D. Application of Cognitive-Behavior Modification Procedures to Hyperactive Children. In M. Gittelman (ed.), *Strategic Interventions for Hyperactive Children.* Armonk, NY: Sharpe, 1981.
22. Meichenbaum, D., and Goodman, J. Training impulsive children to talk to themselves. *J. Abnorm. Psychol.* 77:115–126, 1971.
23. Mikulas, W. L. *Behavior Modification: An Overview.* New York: Harper & Row, 1972.
24. National Institutes of Health Consensus Development Conference. NIH consensus development conference: Defined diets and hyperactivity. *Clin. Pediatr. (Phila)* 21:627–630, 1982.
25. Paternite, C. E., and Loney, J. Childhood Hyperkinesis: Relationships between Symptomatology and Home Environment. In C. K. Whalen and B. Henker (eds.), *Hyperactive Children: The Social Ecology of Identification and Treatment.* New York: Academic, 1980.
26. Paternite, C. E., Loney, J., and Langhorne, J. E. Relationships Between Symptomatology and SES-Related Factors in Hyperkinetic/MBD Boys. In B. B. Lahey (ed.), *Behavior Therapy with Hyperactive and Learning Disabled Children.* New York: Oxford University Press, 1979.

27. Phillips, D. R., and Wright-Saunders, M. H. Behavior Therapy with Hyperactive Children. In M. Gittelman (ed.), *Strategic Interventions for Hyperactive Children.* Armonk, NY: Sharpe, 1981.
28. Pollack, E., and Gittelman, R. Practical Problems Encountered in Behavioral Treatment of Hyperactive Children. In M. Gittelman (ed.), *Strategic Interventions for Hyperactive Children.* Armonk, NY: Sharpe, 1981.
29. Porges, S. W., and Smith, K. M. Defining Hyperactivity: Psychophysiological and Behavioral Strategies. In C. K. Whalen and B. Henker (eds.), *Hyperactive Children: The Social Ecology of Identification and Treatment.* New York: Academic, 1980.
30. Rapoport, J. L. The "Real" and "Ideal" Management of Stimulant Drug Treatment for Hyperactive Children: Recent Findings and a Report from Clinical Practice. In C. K. Whalen and B. Henker (eds.), *Hyperactive Children: The Social Ecology of Identification and Treatment.* New York: Academic, 1980.
31. Reynolds, A. G., and Flagg, P. W. *Cognitive Psychology.* Cambridge, Ma.: Winthrop, 1977.
32. Rosenthal, R. H., and Allen, T. W. An examination of attention and arousal and learning dysfunctions of hyperkinetic children. *Psychol. Bull.* 85:689–715, 1978.
33. Ross, D. M., and Ross, S. A. *Hyperactivity: Research, Theory, and Action.* New York: Wiley, 1976.
34. Safer, D. J., and Allen, R. P. *Hyperactive Children: Diagnosis and Management.* Baltimore: University Park, 1976.
35. Sandoval, J. The measurement of the hyperactive syndrome in children. *Rev. Educ. Res.* 47:293–318, 1977.
36. Schworm, R. W. Hyperkinesis: Myth, mystery, and matter. *J. Spec. Educ.* 16:129–148, 1982.
37. Skinner, B. F. *About Behaviorism.* New York: Vintage, 1976.
38. Spring, C., Blunden, D., Greenberg, L. M. et al. Validity and norms of a hyperactivity rating scale. *J. Spec. Educ.* 11:313–321, 1977.
39. Taylor, E. Food additives, allergy and hyperkinesis. *J. Child Psychol. Psychiatry* 20:357–363, 1979.
40. Walden, E. L., and Thompson, S. A. A review of some alternative approaches to drug management of hyperactivity in children. *J. Learn. Disabil.* 14:213–217, 238, 1981.
41. Weiss, G., and Hechtman, L. The hyperactive child syndrome. *Science* 205:1348–1354, 1979.
42. Wender, P. H. *Minimal Brain Dysfunction in Children.* New York: Wiley, 1971. P. 198, 201.
43. Whalen, C. K, and Henker, B. The Social Ecology of Psychostimulant Treatment: A Model for Conceptual and Empirical Analysis. In C. K. Whalen and B. Henker (eds.), *Hyperactive Children: The Social Ecology of Identification and Treatment.* New York: Academic, 1980.

7 Communication Disorders

Debora D. Kent

Language is a code that enables ideas about the world to be represented through a system of signals for communication [19]. The function of language is to provide symbols that represent relationships observed in the world, objects, and ideas. The components of language are grammar, phonology, and semantics. Grammar consists of morphology and syntax. A *morpheme* is the smallest meaningful unit of language. For example, in the word *reader,* there are two morphemes, read and er. The root word, read, is called a *free morpheme,* which means it has referential meaning and can be used alone. The suffix, -er, does not have referential meaning and cannot be used alone in a sentence; it is a *bound morpheme. Syntax* refers to the order in which the elements of a language can occur, and the relationship between these elements in a sentence; syntax also refers to the rules for forming sentences. Basically, these rules govern the relationship in a sentence between subjects, predicates, and objects that form different sentence types.

Phonology is the sound system of a language that results from the interaction of physical manifestations and their linguistic elements. Physically, utterances consist of continuous movements of the vocal tract. Linguistically, utterances are sequences of morphemes, words, or phrases.

Semantics is the part of language concerned

with the structure of the meanings of speech forms or with contextual meaning. It is the relationship between the symbols and ideas associated with them in the mind of the listener.

LANGUAGE DISORDERS

For a variety of reasons, some children fail to develop or use language normally. They exhibit behaviors that interfere with communication, such as little or no talking, difficulty following directions, unusual use of words or phrases, and grammatical mistakes. There is currently a lack of agreement in defining language problems in children. Commonly used terms include deviant language, language disorder, language disability, and delayed language. The term *language disorder* will be used here to describe any disturbance in the acquisition of a child's native language.

It is estimated that five percent of school-age children have language disorders that are severe enough to interfere with education [96]. Some examples of language disorders are those associated with the hearing impaired or deaf and children who are mentally retarded or autistic who may be slow to develop language. Children with auditory processing deficits or inadequate exposure to language can also exhibit a language disorder.

As part of a language assessment, the speech-language pathologist uses information about the child's cognitive, social, and emotional skills to determine the existence of a language problem. Information about the child's language use is obtained from parents, teachers, and the psychologist to aid in the selection of appropriate test instruments. A variety of assessment tools must be used since no single method is sufficient to provide an adequate description of all areas of language.

Before administering standardized tests, the examiner should observe the child's use of language in an unstructured situation. This setting provides an opportunity to assess the child's pragmatic skills and to observe interaction of language components during actual communi-

cation, which is difficult to obtain during more formal testing.

A transcript of the child's utterances provides information on the mean length of utterance, structural complexity of language, and sentence development [80]. These measures can be compared with normal standards or are used to determine language performance. Examples of standardized tests are the Berr-Talbot Exploratory Test of Grammar [8], Northwestern Syntax Screening Test [52], Peabody Picture Vocabulary Test [27], Vocabulary Comprehension Scale [4], Assessment of Children's Language Comprehension [33], Carrow Test for Auditory Comprehension of Language [21], and Boehm Test of Basic Concepts [16].

Other tests include the Bankson Language Screening Test [5], Illinois Test of Psycholinguistic Abilities [50], Utah Test of Language Development [60], Language Assessment Tasks [47], Basic Concept Inventory [29], Sequenced Inventory of Communication Development [42], Detroit Tests of Learning Aptitude [3], and Token Test for Children [41]. In addition to the language tests, a hearing screening should be given and appropriate referrals made if necessary.

Most speech-language pathologists approach language remediation by using a specific abilities framework that addresses the disabilities associated with the disorder. Others favor a linguistic orientation and focus on specific language behaviors. In either case, the goals selected for the child are dependent on the language behaviors exhibited.

Using a specific abilities approach, a program is designed to deal with perceptual and linguistic processing deficits. Therapy activities involve auditory attention, identification of nonsymbolic stimuli, localization of sounds, auditory figure ground, discrimination of phonemes, sequencing, morphology, and syntactic structure.

If the child has cognitive deficits the program may include methods for improving cognitive processing of semantic units and vocabulary, semantic classification, cognitive processing of

172

semantic relations, and cognition of semantic transformations and implications. Finally, the remediation of language production deficits may use strategies that are directed at improving auditory memory of words, phrases, and sentences, convergent and divergent production of language, and productive control of syntax [91].

A linguistic approach to language disorders focuses on learning and using the language of the community. Goals are selected according to the normal sequence of development and include the development of single word utterance, semantic and syntactic relations, interaction of content and form, and interaction of content, form, and usage [15].

Language learning is most effective during activities that occur in the child's natural environment, with the child as an active participant. Remediation techniques also involve the presentation of correct models of the target behavior, elicitation of the behavior, and reinforcement of the correct behavior or its close approximations. Positive reinforcement can vary from tokens, which can be traded for desired objects, to natural reinforcers, such as activities or objects requested by the child, or simply achievement of successful communication.

LANGUAGE AND READING DISORDERS

Many children experience difficulty in acquiring the complex skill of reading, which requires processing graphic, orthographic, phonologic, semantic, and syntactic information [53, 85]. When difficulty in understanding written language exists with no predisposing factors such as mental retardation, emotional disturbance, visual impairment, or environmental deprivation, it is known as dyslexia [62].

It has been suggested that reading disorders are caused by visuospatial confusion associated with a neurologic deficit [34, 48]. According to this view, therapy should stress training of visual processes as a prerequisite for higher level learning. Other studies suggest reading disorders are a problem with auditory perceptual

processing [49, 55]. This approach in therapy involves the development of sequencing and discriminating isolated sounds or words.

A growing body of knowledge indicates that linguistic performance in semantics, morphology, and syntax is associated with reading ability. For example, poor readers exhibit more errors in the use of morphology than normal readers, and their errors are more idiosyncratic and less predictable than those of normal readers [87, 92].

Vellutino [86] reported that poor readers performed better in copying visual symbols from memory than in naming them, indicating semantic deficits. Because of deficiencies in verbal processing, the child is unable to remember the verbal label associated with its printed symbol. Linguistic awareness and phonetic coding in short-term memory are requirements for skilled reading, and poor readers are found to be deficient in both areas [18, 54].

Readers actively construct the meaning of sentences based on their level of cognition and knowledge of the language [76]. Comprehension of sentences requires competence in decoding the linguistic elements and using appropriate methods for analyzing each sentence. A child's language disorder or immature comprehension strategies may interfere with an accurate interpretation of what is read. Placement of clauses within a sentence may result in a failure to understand the sequence of events described in reading material. Understanding concepts such as comparison, ownership, familial relationships, and spatial and temporal concepts can also be difficult.

The speech-language pathologist can provide teachers with information on the nature of the child's language acquisition problems and work directly with the child to remediate the language disorder. Using the language tests previously mentioned, the speech-language pathologist can assess the child's linguistic skills.

The processing strategies used by the child are also assessed. (Wallach [9] describes methods of assessing the child's ability to integrate, make inferences, and evaluate and interpret information as well as judge synonymy, ambiguity, and grammar. These methods yield information on processing and cognition.) Speech segmentation ability is assessed in order to determine if the child can count the number of words in a sentence, segment words into syllables, and segment syllables into sounds.

Remediation focuses on improving deficient skills. Stark and Wurtzel [78] advocate activities that encourage sentence segmentation, phoneme manipulation, and rearranging words to develop phonetic coding skills. Wallach [88] describes techniques involving actions, gestures, and pictures to assist the child in discerning the meaning of sentences. She uses activities that involve comprehension of cause and effect, integration of ideas, and comprehension strategies.

ARTICULATION DISORDERS

Speech is a process of relating meaning with sound. This sound system is known as the phonological system of a language. American English is composed of approximately 46 sounds or phonemes [7]; other languages have different numbers of sounds. The process of producing and using these sounds is called *articulation*.

The phonemes of a language are described in many ways. One of the most widely used classifications is according to their place and manner of articulation. The place of articulation is determined by the structures used to form the sounds. Bilabial sounds are made with the lips, as in /p/. Labiodental sounds, such as /f/ or /v/, are made with the lower lip and upper teeth. Linguadental sounds are made with the tongue and teeth, for example, /th/, while lingua alveolar sounds are made using the tongue and alveolar ridge located behind the upper teeth. The phoneme /t/ is a lingua alveolar sound. Linguapalatal sounds, such as /sh/, are made with the tongue and palate. Linguavelar sounds, such as /k/, are made with the back of the tongue and soft palate. Labial velar sounds

are made with the lips accompanied by a constriction between the back of the tongue and the velum, as in the initial sound in the word *wheel*. Glottal sounds are made using only the vocal folds, as in /h/.

The manner in which sounds are made is determined by how the breath stream is controlled. Stop sounds are made by blocking off the flow of air completely, then releasing it, as in the sound /p/. Fricatives are made by constricting the mouth opening so that the turbulence of the air passing through creates a noisy sound, as with /f/. Affricates are a combination of stop and fricative sounds. The air is first cut off completely, then released through a small opening, as in /ch/. Sounds made by obstructing the airflow through the mouth and allowing it to escape through the nose are called nasals. The sound /m/ is a nasal. The lateral sound /l/ is made by lingua-alveolar contact at the midline of the tongue but not at the sides, allowing the sound to escape through the sides of the mouth. The rhotic /r/ is produced by turning the tongue tip back or bunching it in the center or near the front of the mouth. Glides, such as the initial sound in *yellow*, are produced by gradually changing the shape of the vocal tract. Vowel sounds are classified as high, mid, or low, and front versus back. For example, the vowel sound in *we* is a high front vowel, while the vowel sound in *ball* is a low back vowel.

Another method of categorizing the sounds of a language is *distinctive feature analysis*, that is, the phonemes of all languages are composed of bundles of features. These features differentiate speech sounds from one another by certain attributes. For example, the sound /k/ is differentiated from /g/ by the feature of voicing. Their other features are the same, but /g/ is voiced while /k/ is unvoiced. Linguists suggest that a child's acquisition of phonology involves the acquisition of phonetic elements that are basic to the phonemes of a language. Each feature is present in several phonemes and serves to distinguish individual phonemes from each other or groups of phonemes from each other. Some

174

of the features of consonants include:

1. Consonantal sounds have a pronounced constriction in the midsagittal area of the vocal tract, distinguishing them from vowels and glides.
2. Vocalic sounds have no marked constriction of the vocal tract and are associated with voicing.
3. Sonorant sounds have a vocal tract configuration that allows the airstream to flow freely.
4. Interrupted sounds have a complete blockage of the airstream.
5. Strident sounds are produced with a great deal of air turbulence.
6. High sounds are made with the tongue above its resting position.
7. Low sounds are made with the tongue lower than its resting position.
8. Back sounds are made with the tongue retracted from its neutral position.
9. Anterior sounds have contact between articulators anterior to the palate.
10. Voiced sounds are produced with vocal fold vibration [2].

When the articulatory productions of an individual deviate sufficiently from normal, the speaker is said to have an *articulation disorder*. The severity of the disorder is judged according to intelligibility, cultural speech standards, vocational goals, cosmetic acceptability, and personal satisfaction.

Traditionally, types of articulation defects have been identified as omissions, substitutions, and distortions. Sound omissions, considered the most severe type of error, are characterized by the deletion of phonemes from words. For example, the sentence "He took my soap" might be articulated as "E tu my o." Sound substitutions are less severe and occur when one phoneme is substituted for another. In the case of a child with a substitution error, the above sentence might be articulated as "He took my toap." Distortions are considered the

least severe type of error and occur when the child produces an approximation of the phoneme but does not produce it acceptably. In the above example, the sentence might be articulated with correct productions of all the sounds except /s/, which might be produced with lateral air emission, resulting in distortion.

Articulation disorders can also include the use of phonologic processes, which are changes in speech that occur regularly for classes of phonemes or sound positions. Hodson and Paden [45] have identified changes in speech that are rarely seen in the speech of normally developing 4-year-olds but occur frequently in the speech of unintelligible children. These changes include noninterrupted sounds replaced with stops; omitted final consonants; consonants involving contact between the back of the tongue and velum produced anteriorly; weak syllables omitted in polysyllabic words; voicing added to prevocalic voiceless consonants; consonants replaced with glottal stops; reduced consonant clusters; omitted strident phonemes; and substituted vowels or glides.

The development of articulation skills is affected by factors that influence phonemic differentiation as well as impair sound production. These factors include sensory problems that affect articulation, such as auditory discrimination skills, or sensation in the oral cavity [72]. Several structural deviations have been found to adversely affect speech production. Missing teeth affect the production of some labial dental, linguapalatal, and linguadental phonemes. Malocclusions, limited lingual movement due to ankyloglossia (restricted lingual frenum), and cleft lip or palate also affect articulation. Other structural deviations that may affect articulation include lip mobility and tongue size.

As part of an articulation evaluation, an audiology screening is performed to determine whether a child has a loss in hearing acuity. It is usually conducted using a pure-tone audiometer that administers the frequencies considered most important for speech. The tones are administered at an intensity level of 20 decibels.

Instruments used to assess the child's auditory discrimination skills include the Wepman Auditory Discrimination Test [90] and the Goldman-Fristoe-Woodcock Test of Auditory Discrimination [37].

An articulation evaluation includes an examination of the speech mechanism. During this evaluation, the facial musculature, tongue, mandible, maxilla, teeth, palate, pharynx, larynx, and muscles of respiration are assessed for adequacy of speech production. A representative sample of speech sounds is made by asking the child to repeat sentences or read a passage aloud to determine the degree of intelligibility of their speech. Available diagnostic tests include the Templin Darley Diagnostic Test of Articulation [81], Fisher-Logemann Test of Articulation Competence [31], Photo Articulation Test [60], Goldman-Fristoe Test of Articulation [36], and McDonald Deep Test of Articulation [58]. These instruments test consonants in the initial, medial, and final positions of words, or in combination with a variety of other sounds. Other tests assess distinctive features, such as the Distinctive Feature Analysis of Misarticulations [59], Compton Hutton Phonological Assessment [25], and Assessment of Phonological Processes [44].

Finally, an analysis of the child's errors is compared with normative data, and articulation skills are judged as adequate or inadequate relative to age. The types of errors (omission, substitution, distortion, or nasal emission) are noted, as well as the position and consistency of errors. The child's ability to produce an error sound correctly following an auditory or visual model is determined. The number of errors and the frequency of occurrence of the error sounds are also noted.

Treatment is made up of three stages: establishment, facilitation of transfer, and maintenance. The purpose of establishment is to enable the child to produce correct utterances of error sounds on request. This determination may be achieved through perceptual or discrimination training, based on the ability to hear the differences between sounds that are believed necessary for correct sound production [7, 82].

Following discrimination training, the target speech behavior is taught by working on the sound in isolation, progressing to syllables, words, and sentences. Five techniques used in establishing production of a target sound are progressive approximation, auditory stimulation, phonetic placement, modification of other sounds already mastered, and use of the key word method. Once a child can produce target sounds on demand, the sounds are said to be established, and the objective of therapy is to facilitate transfer to the appropriate contexts and settings.

The final phase of therapy, maintenance, involves the child's developing the ability to self-monitor articulation. During this phase, reinforcement of the target sounds is retained on an intermittent schedule but is reduced in frequency. Contact with the speech-language pathologist is also reduced.

Articulation disorders can seriously impair communication, particularly if the child has many errors. The prognosis for effective intervention is good if the child is inconsistent in error productions, responsive to error sounds stimulation, motivated to improve, of normal intelligence, can identify errors, and has no other speech or language abnormalities. Other factors which influence the child's progress are the cooperation of the child's parents, teacher, and peers, the emotional and physical health of the child, and the existence of powerful reinforcement for normal speech [28].

CLEFT PALATE

A cleft palate is a slit or opening separating certain parts of the oral structures. Clefts range in severity from openings in the uvula to complete clefts of the hard and soft palates. They can be found alone or in combination with clefts of the lip and alveolar dental arch. The incidence of cleft lip and/or palate varies in different locales,

176

but the condition occurs on the average of 1 in 700 live births [19].

Clefts occur when the facial processes fail to fuse properly during embryologic development. Normally, the bones of the hard palate grow toward the midline and unite with the center partition of the nose, which grows downward from the base of the skull. This growth occurs approximately eight weeks after conception, thus separating the oral cavity from the nasal cavity. When this union fails to take place, clefts of the primary, hard, and soft palate result. Similarly, a cleft lip condition results when the processes that form the lip fail to join during the sixth week after conception.

The existence of a cleft palate may contribute to problems with communication because of direct and indirect influences on hearing, speech, and language development. Feeding problems and dental anomalies often accompany the condition, and the existence of a cleft palate may contribute to psychological problems. Researchers generally agree that there is a higher incidence of middle ear disease and conductive hearing loss among children with cleft palate as a result of drainage and infection of the middle ear due to involvement of the eustachian tube [43].

The speech effects of cleft palate include hypernasality resulting from the failure of the palate to separate the oral and nasal cavities; consonantal distortion due to the nasal escape of air; sound distortions resulting from the use of compensatory adjustments for velopharyngeal incompetence; and weak pressure consonants due to reduced intraoral breath pressure [20]. The most frequent type of misarticulation is omission of a sound altogether. Glottal stops (air blocked by the vocal cords then suddenly released) are generally substituted for plosives (air trapped by the lips before being released). Pharyngeal fricatives (air passed through a constricted area formed by the pharynx and the posterior part of the tongue) are often substituted for oral fricatives (air directed through contact points formed by placing the tongue tip between the upper and lower incisors). Air leakage accompanies both fricatives and plosives. Although characteristic articulatory errors are prevalent, persons with clefts are variable in their errors. Proficiency of speech production varies with the type of cleft and the ability to impound air orally [77].

The relationship of a cleft condition to language development is less clear. In fact, the major differences between the language skills of normal and cleft palate children appear to be decreasing. This decrease may be attributed to early language stimulation in the home, supplemented by the early intervention of a speech-language pathologist. While it is generally agreed that children with clefts are at risk for problems with language development, their skills show great variability and a favorable prognosis.

The personality of the cleft palate individual has received considerable attention. Research has been conducted to find evidence relating cleft palate to maladjustment, to identify behavioral characteristics in individuals with cleft palate, and to determine the effects of cleft palate on the individual's self-image. Although there is some evidence that these children are more dissatisfied with their physical appearance [46], particularly with the parts of their bodies that are directly related to the cleft condition, their self-evaluations were generally found to be high [17]. While the existence of a cleft appears to have subtle effects on an individual's personality, it does not appear to interfere with overall adjustment.

The dental effects of the cleft palate condition are more easily observed. Many persons born with clefts exhibit some type of dental abnormality, such as abnormal size and shape of teeth, malocclusions, missing teeth, and supernumerary teeth. A sizeable number of consonants are produced by the tongue or lips in conjunction with the teeth, and under some conditions dental deviations may affect articulation. Factors that are likely to be important are dental-arch relationships, the presence of open bites, missing central incisors, and any conditions that affect relationships between the tongue and lower incisors.

The multiple problems associated with cleft palate require a team of specialists with a plastic surgeon, orthodontist, and speech-language pathologist as primary members. Other members may include an audiologist, oral surgeon, otologist, and prosthodontist.

Primary physical management should be accomplished before age 3 to allow the development of adequate speech. Some evidence [30] suggests that the best results for speech are obtained when the palate is repaired before 8 months of age. If hypernasality persists following surgery, a speech evaluation is used in conjunction with radiographic, air flow, and breath pressure measures to determine the need for further surgical or prosthetic treatment.

Bloch [10] has identified six areas in which the speech-language pathologist gathers information during an evaluation of a child with cleft palate: (1) adequacy of the velopharyngeal mechanism to determine the need for secondary surgery or the use of a speech appliance, (2) presence of dental-occlusal problems that might affect articulation, (3) adequacy of the child's hearing, (4) etiology of articulation patterns, (5) effects of phonatory habits, and (6) language performance.

Several tests are used to estimate nasal emission, hypernasality, and hyponasality. An index of hypernasality is determined by counting the number of productions in which a perceived change of tone occurs when a patient produces ten words initiated with /b/ and terminated with /t/ while alternately opening and occluding the nostrils. The patient then produces ten words initiated with /m/ and ending with /t/ while alternately opening and occluding the nostrils. The number of words that sound the same under both conditions determines the index. A nasal-emission clinical index is determined by count-

ing the number of productions in which nasal emission is observed when a small paddle wheel is held in front of the nares during production of ten bisyllabic words containing /p/ and /b/ in initial and medial positions [19].

As a result of compensatory movements in the vocal tract, some articulation behaviors of cleft palate children differ from behaviors typically encountered in children without clefts. For this reason, slightly different articulation tests are used. These tests include the Iowa Pressure Articulate Test [61], Bzoch Error Pattern Diagnostic Articulation Test [19], and Receptive-Expressive Emergent Language Scale [20] or Mecham Verbal Language Scale [60].

Various surgical techniques to repair the lip, hard palate, and soft palate have been used for some time, and the prognosis in terms of successful healing and adequate speech is good [26]. To repair a cleft lip, surgery is usually undertaken during the first four months after birth for the main purpose of restoring muscle balance. Recently, more attention has been devoted to correction of nasal deformities at the time of cleft lip repair [2]. The anterior palate may be closed during lip surgery, although it is often left open until the child is older in order to avoid unnecessary scarring. Surgery to repair the soft palate may include closure of the cleft, provision of a functional velum, and secondary operations to improve velopharyngeal closure.

While lip clefts can be closed only with surgery, surgical closure of clefts of the palate may not always be the treatment of choice. Prosthetics may be utilized if there is a wide cleft with a deficient soft palate, wide cleft of the hard palate, neuromuscular deficit of the soft palate and pharynx, need to delay surgery, need to reposition arches before surgery, or need to position teeth in a more favorable alignment.

A prosthetic speech aid must obturate the cleft, provide a surface against which muscles of the pharyngeal wall can squeeze to open and close the nasopharyngeal valve, and be anchored to teeth firmly while being removable for cleaning. Because the presence of a few good teeth is necessary for a speech aid, the arrival of deciduous teeth is usually the minimum age for fitting children with obturators. As growth occurs, speech appliances must be adjusted to the changing dimensions of the nasopharynx and palate.

To be most effective, speech and language stimulation should be provided in early infancy for cleft palate children. Hahn [40] has described a home training program in which the speech-language pathologist meets with the parents shortly after the lip is closed. At this time the structure and function of the normal speech mechanism is explained to the parents, and variations in their child's structure are pointed out. The importance of babbling and vocal play for language development and methods for eliciting them are demonstrated. Subsequent meetings occur when the child is between 7 and 12 months of age, shortly after surgical closure of the palate, and later during the preschool years. The parents are taught language stimulation techniques appropriate to their child's level of development and are given help in explaining to the child the facts concerning physical differences. By the time a child is ready for nursery school or kindergarten, the direct services of a speech-language pathologist are usually required.

Worthley [97] has identified three goals for the speech of individuals with cleft palate:

1. Development of optimal palatopharyngeal sphincter action to produce a breath stream that projects through the front of the mouth rather than the nares, breath pressure for production of consonants requiring varying amounts of pressure, and voice quality so that hypernasality is reduced
2. Development of optimal articulatory proficiency
3. Elimination of facial grimaces, nostril constriction, and gross substitution errors

Therapy involves blowing exercises, activities to increase lip flexibility and to direct breath stream, and articulation training.

STUTTERING

Stuttering is a speech disorder that has long been an enigma to those who seek to understand it. It has been the subject of more investigation than any other disorder of speech, yet answers to the puzzle still elude researchers.

Van Riper [83] defines stuttering as a condition in which the forward flow of speech is interrupted abnormally by repetitions or prolongations of a sound, syllable, or articulatory posture, or by avoidance and struggle behaviors. According to Wingate [93], stuttering involves a disruption in the fluency of verbal expression that is characterized by involuntary, audible or silent, repetitions or prolongations in the utterance of short speech elements, such as sounds, syllables, or words of one syllable. These disruptions are usually frequent or marked in character and not easy to control. Sometimes the disruptions are accompanied by accessory activities involving the speech apparatus that may be related to body structures or stereotyped speech utterances. Also, there may be the presence of an emotional reaction due to excitement, tension, fear, embarrassment, or irritation. The immediate source of stuttering lies in some incoordination expressed in the peripheral speech mechanism, although the ultimate cause is unknown.

Stuttering usually begins before the age of 5 years, and is frequently insidious in onset. It has been found to be associated with the late acquisition of speech. The disorder is significantly more prevalent in males and tends to occur in individuals who have a family history of stuttering. The results of school surveys in the United States indicate the prevalence of stuttering to be approximately 0.8 percent [1].

The severity of stuttering varies among individuals. Bloodstein [11, 12] has identified four phases of the disorder.

I   Children under 6 years of age in which the difficulty is usually episodic. It is characterized by easy repetitions that tend to occur on the initial word of a sentence, or on small units of speech, and is intensified by variable sources of communicative pressure. These children do not regard themselves as stutterers and speak freely in all situations.

II   Children age 6 or 7 years who stutter primarily when speaking rapidly and when they are excited. Stuttering occurs in the major parts of speech. These children view themselves as stutterers yet continue to speak freely in all situations with little or no concern about the stuttering.

III Children who stutter and encounter more difficulty in some situations. Word substitutions, word and sound difficulties, and conscious anticipations develop. Despite the marked stuttering, there is limited fear or embarrassment and essentially no tendency to avoid speaking.

IV   Children who experience vivid anticipation of stuttering. Special difficulty arises in response to various sounds, words, situations, and listeners. Word substitutions are frequent and certain speaking situations are avoided; other evidence of fear and embarrassment is exhibited.

The evaluation of stuttering relies on observation, inquiry, and analysis, utilizing information from both child and parents. The clinician needs to gather data concerning the onset and development of stuttering, nature and results of intervention by the parents, history of stuttering in the family, and parental knowledge of stuttering.

Next, a sample of the child's spontaneous speech is obtained. The number of words stuttered per minute is computed and the types of stuttering behaviors (repetitions, prolongations, struggling), and their severity are noted. During this assessment, the Fluency Interview [32] and

Stuttering Severity Instrument [66] may be used to determine the rate and severity of stuttering. Other measures include the consistency of dysfluencies on the same words during repeated readings of the same passage. Adaptation, the decrease in stuttering that occurs with repeated reading of the same passage, is another measure. Adaptation is viewed by some as having prognostic value, and consistency is thought to indicate how strongly stuttering responses are associated with stimuli or cues to which they have become conditioned. If the child cannot read, repetition of a series of short sentences may be substituted.

Three or four sessions may be necessary to obtain a valid base rate of stuttering behavior. The parents should observe enough of the evaluation to be able to inform the clinician if the child's stuttering behaviors are characteristic of those typically exhibited by the child. The parent also aids in determining the variability of stuttering and identifying situations that seem to precipitate dysfluency as well as situations that increase fluency. The reactions of the child, degree of avoidance of certain words, anticipation of difficulty, and ability to maintain eye contact are noted.

Treatment is provided in a developmental manner including psychological aspects as well as the dysfluency itself. Most clinicians believe that the phase I, or primary stutterer, should not receive direct intervention. For this group, indirect treatment should focus on eliminating the conditions that are thought to precipitate dysfluency. The objective is to prevent the child from developing an awareness of stuttering or fear of speaking, which could cause the disorder to progress.

Intervention for the phase II, or transitional stutterer, continues to focus on preventing the child from viewing talking as stuttering, and also eliminating dysfluency from speech. Controversy exists as to whether direct treatment is indicated. Luper and Mulder [56] state that it is best not to single out a child for therapy if there is doubt about the wisdom of doing so, in which case indirect therapy should be employed. Bloodstein [13] states that when a child's difficulty has become chronic, it is fair to assume that there is an urgent need for some type of symptomatic therapy. The fact that the child already identifies as a stutterer makes it unlikely that a negative reaction will develop from the discovery that someone else also regards the child as a stutterer. Guitar and Peters [39] believe that the choice of direct or indirect treatment should be chosen based on the child's feelings and beliefs about stuttering. They advocate an approach that involves fluency shaping and stuttering modification. They recommend a progression, outlined by Van Riper [83], of desensitization and modification of stuttering. While therapy at this stage may be direct, it generally focuses on speech production with less emphasis on stuttering.

Therapy for the more confirmed stutterers (phases III and IV) must be direct and deal with the child's emotional reactions to stuttering. In addition to providing the child with methods of attaining fluent speech, therapy must eliminate the child's use of avoidance behaviors and associated symptoms. The fluency shaping stuttering modification approaches which are used with adults are used with stutterers in these stages [14, 83].

As many as 80 percent of those who stutter recover from it by the time they are of college age [71]. Many recover without professional help. While recovery can occur at any age, it is a gradual process and is more likely to take place during adolescence [94].

Recovery from stuttering has been found to be related to the severity of stuttering, type of stuttering behaviors, self-image, and time of onset of recovery [56]. A prognosis for complete recovery from stuttering would be expected for someone who exhibits mild or moderate stuttering, has stuttering behaviors consisting of syllable repetitions rather than complete blockings at the onset, does not identify as a stutterer, and begins recovery from stuttering at a young age [38].

Hearing Disorders
Joan M. Izen

The developmental consequences of hearing disorders are most dramatic during the first 3 years of language learning. Early diagnosis and intervention, preferably before 6 months of age, provide the child with maximum opportunity for normal or relatively normal development.

Hearing loss is the most common handicap in the United States today, affecting an estimated 13 million adults and 3 million children. Among those individuals with identified impairments, 40 percent have a mild loss, 20 percent a moderate loss, 20 percent a severe loss, and 20 percent a profound loss [67]. The National Census of the Deaf Population (NCDP) reports that personal earnings were lowest for those born deaf and highest for those deafened after 11 years of age. Additionally, prelingually deaf persons hold fewer professional and technical positions than postlingually deaf persons.

Deaf children of deaf parents perform more successfully on a wide variety of measures including linguistic competence, intelligence, and academic achievement [64]. In addition, this research indicates better social and emotional adjustment with fewer behavioral problems among deaf children who have two deaf parents than among deaf children who have one or no deaf parents.

Children who are either congenitally deaf or become deaf before the acquisition of language will experience greater educational difficulties than their peers who lost their hearing after language had been established.

The degree of hearing loss refers to the loss in sensitivity of hearing that exceeds the normal range of 0 to 20 decibels. As a rule, the greater the degree of hearing loss, the more disabling the developmental effects. The handicapping effects of this type of hearing impairment are associated with the critical role auditory discrimination, that is the ability to understand speech clearly, plays in the language acquisition process. For example, children with conductive losses typically display good to excellent auditory discrimination abilities regardless of the degree of loss. Conversely, the auditory discrimination abilities of children with sensorineural losses may range from good to poor. The distortion of the incoming speech signal, which is a typical feature of sensorineural losses, may be so great as to totally preclude the understanding of the spoken word [57].

At the very least, a mild deficit in auditory abilities may be evidenced in the child's difficulty with speech sound production. At the most complex level, the child with a severe to profound sensorineural impairment will experience difficulties with speech, language, and cognitive, social, and emotional development requiring extensive special services.

Developmental delays attributable to hearing impairment often go undetected during the child's first year of life. Hearing impaired babies may appear to react appropriately to sound and often develop strong compensatory visual abilities that mask their true disabilities. Their early cooing vocalizations, which are purely reflexive in nature, simulate normal development, adding to the difficulty of early diagnosis. At approximately 6 to 7 months of age, the severely impaired child's vocalizations decrease markedly in frequency and fail to change significantly in type. This lack of change, which may serve as the first and most obvious developmental effect, results from the child's severely limited auditory feedback system. In essence, the hearing impaired child exists in a state of sensory deprivation lacking the auditory stimulation so crucial to language development. Without this feedback system the child is unable to connect the speech sounds produced with the oral motor movements used to produce them. As a result the child fails to achieve two major milestones, acquisition of control of speech and conception of speech controls. This leads to difficulty in communication. The child without verbal skills lacks the ability to interact with the environment. The child tends to assume a more passive role in communicative interchange and becomes the receiver of information that is difficult to decode and utilize. This passivity compromises social and emotional development early in the hearing impaired child's life.

In actuality, the effect of hearing impairment on social and emotional development probably began in the first few days of life. The hearing parent and hearing impaired infant may find themselves out of sync, such as the infant not responding appropriately to the parent's soothing auditory stimulation. In addition, the infant's perception of the parent is inextricably tied to the visual presence of the person. Unlike the hearing child who learns to rely on associated sounds to anticipate a parent's presence, the hearing impaired child's parent is present only when seen or felt. These subtle but important disruptions of normal parent-infant interactions can affect the child's ability to develop trusting relationships and object constancy.

The parents face the difficult task of providing positive caregiving to their infant while struggling with the grief they feel as a result of having a hearing impaired child. In many respects, the successful habilitation of the hearing impaired child is dependent on the parents' ability to grieve and cope.

CAUSES OF IMPAIRMENT

Current research has focused on the study of birth defects and their relationship to hearing impairment. Medical specialists have described physical characteristics and functional deficits which have led to the categorization of children who have recurrent patterns of malformations or syndromes [73]. Konigsmark and Gorlin [51] have cataloged more than 150 syndromes with associated hearing loss or deafness. Bergstrom [6] reported that 25 percent of early childhood hearing loss is genetic, 42 percent is nongenetic, and 33 percent is of unknown etiology. He adds that the unknown causes are probably due to recessive genetic etiology or unidentified nongenetic causes.

A genetic, or endogenous, disorder originates as a trait transmitted from parent to child, which is a congenital impairment. Syndromes with associated hearing impairment, such as Waardenburg syndrome, albinism, and Pierre Robin syndrome, fall within this category. The cause of a nongenetic, or exogenous, disorder may be attributed to one or a combination of the following factors: malformation, disease or damage to any part of the auditory system due to prenatal or perinatal factors, middle ear disorders, or environmental factors. Together or individually these factors affect the system's ability to receive and transmit sound stimuli. Examples of prenatal and perinatal factors include rubella (german measles), Rh blood type incompatibility, and premature birth. Problems with middle ear function include eustachian tube dysfunction, inflammation of the middle ear (otitis media), and fluid in the middle ear (serous otitis media). It is of interest to note that research suggests approximately 12 percent of all children suffer from a middle ear infection between the ages of 6 and 24 months. The frequently accompanying mild to moderate conductive hearing loss is thus of nongenetic origin. Environmental factors include childhood diseases such as mumps and meningitis and traumatic injury.

ASSESSMENT

Parents, particularly mothers, are typically the first and most reliable detectors of their child's hearing impairment. Very early in their child's life they may identify a difference, a subjective "gut feeling" that their baby is not reacting normally to sounds. The child may be the "too good to be true" baby who sleeps soundly through household noises, rarely cries or fusses. Based on their suspicions the parents may embark on a period of constant impromptu testing, scrutinizing the child's response to various forms of auditory stimulation. If the child's responses fail to relieve these suspicions, the family physician is usually the first contact with the professional world. The parents bring to this initial meeting all the fears, anxieties, and concerns that have developed since their initial concerns.

Wong and Shah [95] note that all too often the physician rejects the parents' observations in favor of findings on cursory physical examination of the child's ears.

A quick auditory screening is generally performed using uncalibrated sound sources such as toy noisemakers, cowbells, snappers, and whistles. Observations are made of the child's gross responses to these forms of auditory stimulation with specific attention to the palpebral reflex (quick opening and closing movement of the eyelids) and startle responses such as a cessation of movement, a cry, or a head turn in the direction of the sound. Based on the results, child's age, and parents' concern, the need for more extensive testing is determined.

Given the recent advances made in screening techniques, hearing loss can now be identified reliably in the neonatal period, and the degree of deafness can generally be established by 8 to 10 months of age. Early detection offers both an opportunity for early medical intervention, if warranted, and a source of valuable information concerning the etiology of hearing problems. From educational and audiological standpoints, early detection provides the opportunity to initiate auditory habilitation at an age that is most likely to ensure optimum development of hearing function. Newborn screening programs are often limited to high risk infants being cared for in neonatal intensive care units (NICU) [79].

The two most popular diagnostic screening tests used primarily with infants hospitalized in NICUs are the crib-o-gram and the brain stem evoked response audiometry (BSER). The crib-o-gram represents a major technological breakthrough in that the test process is fully automated, enabling increased validity of responses. The infant is placed on a crib mattress that is on top of a motion sensitive transducer. The transducer is sensitive to changes in respiration and almost any motor movement, except eye blinks or disassociated facial grimaces. The test stimulus, a 92 decibel narrow band noise, is presented through a loudspeaker according to a predetermined schedule regulated by an automatic timer. The infant's responses are registered on a stripchart located next to the crib. A positive auditory response is scored if there is a change in the ongoing motion of the mattress within 2.6 seconds of the test sound. Each testing period consists of a 10 second prestimulus recording and a 6 second poststimulus recording of infant activity. This cycle is repeated several times at predetermined intervals to obtain a statistically valid sample of responses for each baby. In this way the sample is likely to be more independent of nursery routines, random responses, and the rapidly changing arousal levels of the newborn. The scoring process takes about 1 minute per baby, and lay persons can be taught scoring techniques in about 1 week.

Brain stem evoked response audiometry is a highly specialized procedure that extracts the brain stem's responses to sound stimuli from ongoing electroencephalographic (EEG) activity. The procedure is most successful when attempted during a sleep or sedated state. Three surface recording electrodes are used. The active electrode is placed on the infant's forehead and the reference and ground electrodes are each placed on an earlobe or a mastoid. The auditory stimuli, referred to as acoustic clicks, are presented through earphones at a rate that varies from 10 per second to 60 per second. Responses are recorded as tracings and interpreted according to their wave formations. Each wave represents an impulse that reaches successively higher levels of the brain stem starting with wave I, which originates in the auditory nerve itself and ends with wave V, located in the brain stem. An absence of one or more wave formations suggests an abnormality in the hearing pathway that leads from the inner ear to the brain. A detectable auditory brain stem response (ABR) indicates that the stimulus presented to the child produced excitation within the peripheral hearing mechanism which in turn stimulated the central auditory pathways. Additional diagnostic information is provided by the length of time between each wave, as this

serves as an indicator of the rate of conduction of the nerve impulse. Thus the professional gains information on the function and integrity of brain stem auditory structures and peripheral hearing status. The use of this procedure is indicated for difficult-to-test children, including infants and very young, hyperkinetic, and multiply handicapped children.

An audiologist specializes in identification and treatment of hearing impairment. This health professional may recommend the use of hearing aids and can assess the impact of hearing loss on speech, language, psychosocial, educational, and vocational development. Otologists, ortolaryngologists, and otorhinolaryngologists are physicians who specialize in diseases of the ear and related structures and provide a much-needed medical perspective.

The goal of the audiologic assessment is to determine the degree and type of impairment and their effect on the child's development. A comprehensive interview, ongoing communication with the parents and associates, and informal observation of the child provide critical information. Specialized testing techniques provide information on type and degree of hearing impairment. The techniques used are determined by the child's age, neurologic maturation, and language capabilities.

Clinical evaluation of an infant's hearing status is indicated if the child (1) is identified as being at risk for hearing loss, (2) fails a screening test, or (3) is suspected of auditory dysfunction. Behavioral observation audiometry (BOA) is the most common procedure used to evaluate infants from birth to 6 months of age. This technique relies primarily on observation of reflexive responses to acoustic stimuli and provides information regarding the extent of impairment.

After 6 months of age a child can be tested using behavioral conditioning techniques. Testing procedures such as conditioned orientation reflex audiometry (COR) and visual reinforcement audiometry (VRA) rely specifically on the child's ability to turn toward and localize the source of a sound stimuli. For example, both a sound and a pleasant visual stimulus are presented simultaneously. After a few such presentations the child will turn in the direction of the visual stimulus every time the sound is emitted. The audiologist then manipulates the testing procedure by presenting the sound without the visual stimulus. If the child turns in the appropriate direction (localizes the visual stimulus), a reward is given. If the child turns in the wrong direction, looks straight ahead, or otherwise responds inappropriately, no reward is given. Using this procedure of stimulus-response reinforcement, the tester employs successively softer sounds of different frequencies until the child stops responding with appropriate localizations. Results of this testing procedure may reveal not only the extent of impairment but also information pertinent to sensitivity in the more responsive ear.

As the child develops speech and language abilities, advanced testing procedures provide more information about overall level of sensitivity. The audiologist capitalizes on these newly developed skills by evaluating the 18- to 30-month-old child's response to various simple questions and commands about clothing items, body parts, and common articles. The intensity level of the tester's vocal presentations can be lowered until it reaches the lowest level at which the child responds.

The most definitive information concerning the type and severity of loss is obtained from the older child, 2 to 6 years of age. The results of pure-tone testing procedures are plotted on an audiogram, which provides a graphic representation of the child's hearing capabilities of intensity and frequency levels. Sounds ranging in intensity from 0 to 110 decibels and frequency from 125 to 8000 Hz are presented. The right and left ears are tested separately to determine whether the loss is unilateral or bilateral. The sounds are first presented through earphones to determine air-conduction hearing levels. Air-

conduction testing assesses the entire auditory system from the pinna (outer ear) to the auditory cortex. The sounds are then presented through a vibrator which is attached to the mastoid bone behind the ear. Theoretically, bone conduction testing assesses only the auditory system from the cochlea (inner ear) to the higher auditory centers. Administration of both tests provides important comparative information needed to determine the type of hearing loss. The results of pure-tone audiometry provide information on the extent, degree, frequency, and type of hearing impairment, and difference in hearing acuity between the two ears.

Speech audiometry provides information on the extent to which a hearing impairment affects the ability to hear, discriminate, and tolerate speech. It serves to verify the pure-tone results and type of hearing loss, and determine appropriate rehabilitative strategies. Speech audiometric procedures are dependent on at least some degree of language development and thus are used with older children.

Impedance audiometry provides an objective evaluation of the integrity of middle ear function. It is used on a wide population, including very young, difficult-to-test children. A plug is placed in the ear canal to create an air tight chamber. Air is then introduced or removed to create a pressure range from -300 to $+200$ mm H_2O. An auditory stimulus is presented and measurements are taken of how the sound bounces off the tympanic membrane (eardrum) at different pressures. This measurement of the eardrum's elasticity is recorded on a tympanogram. A bell-shaped tympanogram is indicative of normal middle ear function. If the eardrum is immobile, as with an acute ear infection, a flat line tracing results. Typically a normal reading will be obtained within a week after the infection clears. A persistent flat line tracing, however, may warrant medical intervention such as a myringotomy. A myringotomy is a minor surgical procedure in which a small tube is inserted into the eardrum, enabling fluid in the middle ear to drain and equalize the pressure between the middle ear and the ear canal.

CLASSIFICATION

The degree or severity of hearing impairment is classified along a continuum that ranges from mild to profound. A child who has a mild hearing impairment cannot hear sounds within the 15 to 40 decibel range. A moderate hearing impairment involves a 45 to 70 decibel loss. A severe loss is between 70 to 90 decibels, and a profound loss is greater than 90 decibels. A severity statement generally correlates with the prognosis for the child's speech and language acquisition. For example, children with mild to moderate losses are expected to develop speech and language abilities that closely approximate the patterns of normal children. The child with a mild impairment may experience difficulty detecting distant noises but is able to participate easily in normal conversation. In contrast, the severe to profoundly impaired child is isolated from normal stimulation, catching only an occasional word, often out of context.

Hearing disorders are also classified according to the location of the damage. There are four types of hearing impairments: conductive, sensorineural, mixed, and central. A conductive hearing loss may result from blockage of the ear canal due to congenital malformation, wax, or foreign objects, or from abnormalities of the middle ear structures resulting from a birth defect, injury, or disease. Sound transmission is obstructed from passing through the ear canal, eardrum, or middle ear resulting in some degree of sensitivity reduction. Auditory discrimination and comprehension capabilities remain unaffected. Otitis media serves as the most frequent cause of conductive losses in young children. Conductive losses often can be treated successfully by medical or surgical intervention.

Sensorineural hearing loss results from damage or malformation of the cochlea or auditory nerve. In young children, it is most often hereditary. Sensorineural loss affects hearing sensitivity (loudness) and auditory discrimination; for example, sounds that are heard may appear to be distorted. While a hearing aid is recommended for children with sensorineural impairment, it is important to note that the aid will only increase loudness levels; it will not serve to increase auditory discrimination abilities.

A mixed hearing loss results from a combination of problems involving the outer, middle, and inner ear. Among young children the most common example is the coexistence of a chronic middle ear infection (conductive component) superimposed on an underlying sensorineural hearing loss.

Central deafness or central auditory impairment results from a lesion in the central nervous system that disrupts the ability to organize and make use of incoming auditory information. Children with central auditory impairment typically demonstrate deficits in the areas of auditory attention, awareness, memory, recognition, association, and comprehension.

EDUCATIONAL ISSUES

Educational programs for hearing impaired children include oralism and manual communication. Oralists believe in the auditory approach to education, that is, a unisensory approach, and acoupedics, in which audition is the focal point. The basis of this approach is that if the hearing impaired child is to be integrated into the hearing world, effective oral communication is essential. Given appropriate amplification and adequate exposure to normal patterns of speech, the hearing impaired child can learn to make proper use of residual hearing to achieve effective oral communication. The method of manual communication commonly recommended is sign language (see Nonvocal Communication Systems).

The total communication approach focuses on all forms of communication, utilizing all types of sensory stimulation as well as sign language. Other methods of training the hearing impaired child include cued speech and the Rochester method.

The enactment of Public Law 94.142, The Education of All Handicapped Children Act of 1975, established a system for individualized, professionally designed educational programs. A typical team might consist of a teacher of the hearing impaired, psychologist, audiologist, speech-language pathologist, resource room teacher, and classroom teacher. Additional services may be required from an occupational therapist or physical therapist depending on the specific needs of the child. Together, in cooperation with the parents, an individualized educational plan (IEP) is developed with the goal of providing the most appropriate educational program for the child. Objectives are submitted by each discipline, accompanied by specified teaching strategies and educational materials. Regular yearly meetings (staffings) are attended by the entire team to reassess the program, discuss the child's progress, and develop new objectives. The IEP details what the child will learn and where the child will learn it, along a continuum of services and settings ranging from partial to full-time regular classroom placements, special classes, or schools.

The impact of public law on the educational programming for hearing impaired children has been significant. Northcott [63] states that the law assumes the classification of children by individual, behavioral, developmental, and educational needs. Classification is based on a difference, rather than a deficit, model of individualized educational programming for all.

NONVOCAL COMMUNICATION SYSTEMS

A large number of children are unable to develop speech that is adequate for communication. This inability may be due to impairment of sensory input, deficiency in integration and mediation function, impairment of behavior-motor

response, deficiency in stimulus analysis-decoding, deficiency in grammatico-semantico-encoding, or impairment of response analysis-feedback [68].

To meet the communication needs of these individuals, a variety of nonvocal communication systems have been used. Nonvocal communication techniques encode and transmit messages without using the articulators and vocal tract. They often are referred to as augmentative communication systems to emphasize that they augment, rather than replace, an individual's existing means of communication.

Nonvocal communication techniques may be classified as aided or unaided. Unaided techniques require no instrumentation and rely on movements of the upper extremities and/or head and neck to decode messages. One of the most widely known unaided techniques is American Sign Language, or Ameslan, which is a manual communication system used by the deaf in the United States. The gestures of Ameslan (signing) may signal letters of the alphabet, words, or phrases, morphologic or syntactic information, or phonemes. Frequently, signing is done simultaneously with speaking, a process known as total communication. This system is quite flexible and can be used to encode messages concerning the past, present, or future. Since signing is not understandable to those who do not use it, an individual can use the system only with those who have had training in its interpretation.

A less frequently used manual communication system using gestures is American Indian Sign Language, or Amerind [75]. This system was originally used by North American Indians for intertribal communication. Its signs are pictographic and ideographic and are fairly easy to interpret without training. This system, however, is less flexible than Ameslan.

Other unaided systems include the use of mime, facial gestures, coded eye blinks, and pointing. These systems require less fine motor coordination than the manual techniques and severely restrict the variety of messages that can be transmitted.

Aided techniques are those that require the use of some type of physical object or device to encode messages. These techniques require a symbol system, method of representing the symbols, and manner to indicate the sequence of elements necessary to encode a message. Visual symbols used for this purpose may include photographs, drawings, Bliss symbols, rebuses, and printed words. Auditory signals include both natural and synthesized speech and sequences of noise.

Photographs and drawings represent the most concrete of the visual symbol systems. They range in complexity from color photographs of familiar objects and people to simple line drawings. They are useful in communicating basic messages, but are less suitable than other symbols for communicating abstract ideas.

Blissymbolics is a writing system that is pictographic and ideographic, and can be read in all languages [9]. In the United States, the English equivalent of a word is printed below its symbol so that a user may communicate with anyone who can read English. The system consists of approximately 100 symbols, which can be modified in a number of ways to change their meanings. The symbols can be used singly or combined in various ways to encode almost any message, creating a very flexible system.

Rebuses are pictographic symbols which may consist of a single drawing, several drawings, or a combination of letters of the alphabet and drawings [23]. The meanings of rebuses are changed by adding appropriate English suffixes. They represent a fairly flexible system and can be easily decoded by untrained interpreters.

Printed words represent the most flexible visual symbol system. They can be used for the transmission of any message, provided both the sender and receiver can spell and read. Most systems include ten digits and some frequently used words and phrases. An English symbol system could consist of as few as 26 symbols.

Visual symbols generally are used in conjunction with one of three types of aided systems. The user can transmit messages by (1) indicating the appropriate sequence of symbols appearing on a communication board, (2) manipulating symbols in an appropriate sequence, or (3) drawing or writing on a piece of paper or other material.

Scanning, encoding, and direct selection [84] may be used for indicating messages on a communication board. Scanning involves the presentation of selections by a person or display and requires the user to select the appropriate symbol by responding only when it is presented. Encoding involves indicating a choice by means of a code of signals that must be memorized or referred to on a chart. Direct selection involves direct indication, through pointing, gesturing, or using motor-driven indicators.

Aided techniques may be automated or nonautomated. An example of an aided, nonautomated, direct selection communication system is a communication board mounted with Bliss symbols that utilizes finger pointing to indicate messages. An aided, automated, indirect selection system would be a communication board equipped with lights that scan selections. The response to this system is made by activating a switch when the desired symbol is lit.

A nonvocal system utilizing the auditory processing capabilities of the user would be machine-generated speech, which may consist of a synthesized voice, natural speech, or Morse code. An example of an aided, automated system with auditory output would be a system that accepts correctly spelled English words and then synthesizes spoken messages.

While the variety of communication aids currently available is extensive, there are still individuals for whom physical limitations impose severe restrictions on communication. An attempt should be made to select the most flexible, efficient, and operative system. Currently, research is being conducted to increase different movements (e.g., eye movement) that can be used with automated communication systems. This research may provide more flexible and efficient communication systems for severely handicapped persons.

The decision to use a nonvocal communication system is based on the child's cognition, oral reflex status, language and speech production, intelligibility, emotional status, chronological age, previous therapy, speech imitative ability, and environment [70]. Once a decision has been made to employ nonvocal communication, an assessment of the child's current functional levels and communication needs is made. The child's prelanguage skills are assessed. These skills include attention, matching, memory, sequencing, and categorization [24]. Vocabulary, grammar, semantics, pragmatics, inner language, speech, writing ability, and physical ability are evaluated as well [74].

Through a task analysis of behaviors the child needs to perform, the appropriate communication system can be developed [24]. The format of the output (e.g., spoken or printed) should be selected with respect to the child's needs and environment. For example, a communication system designed to allow a child to complete school work would be more effective with visual output [35].

The motor function of a child must be assessed to determine the ability to use various communication systems. In general, the more intact the motor function, the wider the variety of choices available. A movement should be identified that is voluntary, reliably controlled, and socially acceptable, while still allowing use of the selected system. Measurements related to the selected movement include activation force, range of motion, resolution of motion, reaction time, and repetition of response [74]. These measurements help to determine the speed, accuracy, and force with which the selected movements can be executed.

The sensory function of the child must be assessed to determine the adequacy of auditory, visual, and tactile-kinesthetic-proprioceptive function for the tasks involved in using various communication systems. Finally, an important area to assess is the child's level of cognitive function [69].

Once a communication system has been selected, the child must be trained in its use. The child and parents may feel uncomfortable with the chosen system, believing that speech development has been sacrificed or that the system will not aid in communication. Thus a primary concern of the team is to help the family and child accept the system.

In order to use the system effectively, the child must be motivated to communicate. A lack of motivation may exist because the child has little need to communicate, particularly if needs are anticipated. The child may not understand the benefits of communication, have few opportunities for interaction, or simply not desire communication. Opportunities must be created for the child to want to communicate so that the communication system will be successfully implemented.

In addition to physically learning how to use the communication system, the child may need to be shown the functions and benefits of communication. Individuals in the child's environment must become familiar with the system for it to be effectively used. They must be instructed in how to interpret messages, and structure situations, such as mealtime, to maximize the child's communication opportunities. Using a nonvocal communication system requires flexibility for everyone involved with the user. The adaptations each person must make when communicating with the user of a nonvocal system may be difficult; the benefits derived from enabling a child to become an effective communicator, however, outweigh any disadvantages involved.

Interested readers may obtain additional information by contacting the following:

The Alexander Graham Bell Association for the Deaf
3417 Volta Place, N.W.
Washington, D.C. 20007

The National Association for Hearing and
Speech Action (NAHSA) (The Consumer
Affiliate of the American Speech-Lan-
guage-Hearing Association)
10801 Rockville Pike
Rockville, Maryland 20852

Both these organizations offer a variety of
printed materials, brochures, pamphlets, and
checklists that address issues specific to hearing
impaired infants and young children. These materials may prove particularly useful for parent
education and community awareness programs.
Examples of brochures available from the Alexander Graham Bell Association include: "Listen!
Hear! For Parents of Hearing Impaired Children," "Hearing Alert!" and "Can Your Baby
Hear?" The NAHSA publishes an informative
pamphlet entitled "Answers and Questions
About Hearing Loss." Also available are two
booklets that are appropriate for parents new to
the problems of a hearing impaired child: *Your
Child's Hearing—A Guide For Parents* and
*About Speech and Hearing Problems—The
ABC's of Speech-Language Pathology and Audiology.* These scriptographic booklets can be
obtained by contacting:

The Channing L. Bete Co., Inc.
South Deerfield, MA 01373

REFERENCES

1. Andrews, G., and Harris, M. *The Syndrome of
Stuttering.* London: Heineman, 1964.
2. Asensio, O. A variation of the rotation-advance-
ment operation for repair of wide unilateral cleft
lips. *Plast. Reconstr. Surg.* 53:167, 1974.
3. Baker, J., and Leland, B. *Detroit Tests of Learning Aptitude.* Indianapolis: Bobbs-Merrill, 1959.
4. Bangs, T. *Vocabulary Comprehension Scale.*
Austin: Learning Concepts, 1975.
5. Bankson, N. *Bankson Language Screening Test.*
Baltimore: University Park Press, 1977.
6. Bergstrom, L. Causes of severe hearing loss in
early childhood. *Pediatr. Ann.* 9:23, 1980.
7. Bernthal, J., and Bankson, N. *Articulation Disorders.* Englewood Cliffs. N.J.: Prentice-Hall,
1981.
8. Berry, M. *Berry-Talbot Exploratory Test of
Grammar.* Rockford, Ill., 1966.
9. Bliss, C. *Semantography (Blissymbolics)* (2nd
ed.). Sydney, Australia: Semantography (Blissymbolics) Publications, 1965.
10. Bloch, P. Clinical evaluation for the cleft palate
team setting. In K. Bzoch (Ed.), *Communicative
Disorders Related to Cleft Palate* (2nd ed.).
Boston: Little, Brown, 1979.
11. Bloodstein, O. The development of stuttering: I.
Changes in nine basic features. *J. Speech Hear.
Disord.* 25:219, 1960.
12. Bloodstein, O. The development of stuttering: II.
Developmental phases. *J. Speech Hear. Disord.*
25:366, 1960.
13. Bloodstein, O. The development of stuttering.
III. Theoretical and clinical implications. *J.
Speech Hear. Disord.* 26:366, 1961.
14. Bloodstein, O. *A Handbook on Stuttering* (2nd
ed.). Chicago: The National Easter Seal Society
for Crippled Children and Adults, 1975.
15. Bloom, L., and Lahey, M. *Language Development and Language Disorders.* New York: Wiley, 1978.
16. Boehm, A. *Boehm Test of Basic Concepts.* New
York: Psychological Corporation, 1969.
17. Brantley, H., and Clifford, E. Cognitive, self-concept, and body image measures of normal, cleft
palate, and obese adolescents. *Cleft Palate J.*
16:177, 1979.
18. Byrne, B., and Shea, P. Semantic and phonetic
memory codes in beginning readers. *Memory
and Cognition* 7:333, 1979.
19. Bzoch, K. (Ed.). *Communicative Disorders Related to Cleft Lip and Palate.* Boston: Little,
Brown, 1979.
20. Bzoch, K., and League, R. *Receptive-Expressive
Emergent Language Scale.* Baltimore: University
Park Press, 1970.
21. Carrow, E. *Test for Auditory Comprehension of
Language.* Austin, Tex.: Urban Research, 1973.
22. Chomsky, N., and Halle, M. *The Sound System
of English.* New York: Harper & Row, 1968.
23. Clark, C., Davies, C., and Woodcock, R. *Standard Rebus Glossary.* Minneapolis: American
Guidance Service, 1974.
24. Coleman, C., Cook, A., and Meyers, L. Assessing nonoral clients for assistive communication
devices. *J. Speech Hear. Disord.* 45:515, 1980.
25. Compton, A., and Hutton, S. *Compton-Hutton
Phonological Assessment.* San Francisco:
Carousel House, 1978.
26. Converse, T. The techniques of cleft palate
surgery. Proceedings of the conference: Com-

municative Problems in Cleft Palate. *ASHA Reports* 1:55, 1965.

27. Dunn, L. *Expanded Manual for the Peabody Picture Vocabulary Test.* Circle Pines, Minn.: American Guidance Service, 1974.

28. Emerick, L., and Hatten, J. *Diagnosis and Evaluation in Speech Pathology.* Englewood Cliffs, N.J.: Prentice-Hall, 1974.

29. Engelman, S. *The Basic Concept Inventory, Teacher's Manual.* Chicago: Follett, 1967.

30. Evans, D., and Renfrew, C. The timing of primary cleft palate repair. *Scand. J. Plast. Reconstr. Surg.* 8:153, 1974.

31. Fisher, H., and Logemann, J. *The Fisher-Logemann Test of Articulation Competence.* Boston: Houghton Mifflin, 1971.

32. *Fluency Interview.* Monterey, Calif.: Monterey Learning Systems, 1976.

33. Foster, R., Giddan, J., and Stark, J. *Assessment of Children's Language Comprehension,* Manual. Palo Alto: Consulting Psychologists, 1973.

34. Frostig, M., and Horne, D. *The Frostig Program for the Development of Visual Perception.* Chicago: Follett, 1964.

35. Gans, B. Physiological and medical considerations in non-vocal communication. Paper presented at Second Annual Course on Pediatric Rehabilitation. Department of Rehabilitation Medicine of Tufts University School of Medicine and New England Medical Center, Boston, 1982.

36. Goldman, R., and Fristoe, M. *The Goldman-Fristoe Test of Articulation.* Circle Pines, Minn.: American Guidance Service, 1969, 1972.

37. Goldman, R., Fristoe, M., and Woodcock, R. *The Goldman-Fristoe-Woodcock Test of Auditory Discrimination.* Circle Pines, Minn.: American Guidance Service, 1970.

38. Guitar, B. Pretreatment factors associated with the outcome of stuttering therapy. *J. Speech Hear. Res.* 19:590, 1976.

39. Guitar, B., and Peters, T. *Stuttering: An Integration of Contemporary Therapies.* Memphis, Tenn.: Speech Foundation of America, 1981. p. 16.

40. Hahn, E. Directed home training program for infants with cleft palate and lip. In K. Bzoch (Ed.), *Communicative Disorders Related to Cleft Lip and Palate* (2nd ed.). Boston: Little, Brown, 1979.

41. Hahn, W., and Weiss, M. Token test: Administration and scoring, unpublished manuscript. Denver: Denver Public Schools Diagnostic Teaching Center, 1973.

42. Hedrick, D., Prather, E., and Tobin, A. *Sequenced Inventory of Communication Development, Examiner's Manual.* Seattle: University of Washington, 1975.

43. Heller, J. Hearing loss in patients with cleft palate. In K. Bzoch (Ed.), *Communicative Disorders Related to Cleft Lip and Palate* (2nd ed.). Boston: Little, Brown, 1979.

44. Hodson, B. *The Assessment of Phonological Processes.* Danville, Ill.: Interstate, 1980.

45. Hodson, B., and Paden, E. Phonological processes which characterize unintelligible and intelligible speech in early childhood. *J. Speech Hear. Disord.* 46:369, 1981.

46. Kapp, K. Self concept of the cleft lip and/or palate child. *Cleft Palate J.* 16:171, 1979.

47. Kellman, M., Flood, C., and Yoder, D. *Language Assessment Tasks.* Madison: Kellman, Flood, Yoder, 1977.

48. Kephart, N. *The Slow Learner in the Classroom.* Columbus: Merril, 1960.

49. Kirk, S., and Kirk, W. *Psycholinguistic Learning Disabilities: Diagnosis and Remediation.* Urbana: University of Illinois Press, 1971.

50. Kirk, S., McCarthy, J., and Kirk, W. *Illinois Test of Psycholinguistic Abilities, Examiner's Manual.* Urbana: University of Illinois Press, 1968.

51. Konigsmark, B. W., and Gorlin, R. J. *Genetic and Metabolic Deafness.* Philadelphia: Saunders, 1976.

52. Lee, L. *Northwestern Syntax Screening Test.* Evanston: Northwestern University, 1971.

53. Levin, H., and Kaplan, E. Listening, reading, and grammatical structure. In D. Horton and J. Perkins (Eds.), *Perception of Language.* Columbus: Merril, 1971.

54. Liberman, I., Shankweiler, D., Fischer, F. et al. Explicit syllable and phoneme segmentation in the young child. *J. Exp. Child Psychol.* 18:201, 1974.

55. Liberman, I., Shankweiler, D., Liberman, A., et al. Phonetic segmentation and recoding in the beginning reader. In A. Reber and D. Scarborough (Eds.), *Reading: Theory and Practice.* Hillsdale: Erlbaum, 1976.

56. Luper, H., and Mulder, R. *Stuttering Therapy for Children.* Englewood Cliffs, N.J.: Prentice-Hall, 1964.

57. Martin, F. N. (Ed.). *Pediatric Audiology.* Englewood Cliffs, N.J.: Prentice-Hall, 1978.

58. McDonald, E. *A Deep Test of Articulation.* Pittsburgh: Stanwix House, 1964.

59. McReynolds, L., and Engemann, D. *The Distinctive Feature Analysis of Misarticulations.* Pitts-

burgh: Stanwix House, 1975.

60. Mecham, M. *Verbal Language Development Scale.* Minneapolis: Educational Test Bureau, 1959.

61. Morris, H. Communication skills of children with cleft lips and palate. *J. Speech Hear. Res.* 5:79, 1962.

62. National Advisory Committee on Handicapped Children: First Annual Report, Subcommittee on Education of the Committee on Labor and Public Welfare, U.S. Senate. Washington, D.C.: U.S. Government Printing Office, 1968.

63. Northcott, W. H. *Implications of Mainstreaming for the Education of Hearing Impaired Children in the 1980's.* Washington, D.C.: The Alexander Graham Bell Association for the Deaf—Information Services Division, 1982.

64. Northern, J. L., and Downs, M. P. *Hearing in Children* (2nd ed.). Baltimore: Wilkins & Wilkins, 1978.

65. Pendergast, K., Dickey, S., Selmar, J. et al. *The Photo Articulation Test* (2nd ed.). Danville, Ill.: Interstate, 1969.

66. Riley, G. A stuttering severity instrument for children and adults. *J. Speech Hear. Disord.* 37:314, 1972.

67. Schein, J. D., and Delk, M. T. *The Deaf Population of the United States.* Silver Spring, Md.: National Association of the Deaf, 1974.

68. Schiefelbusch, R., and Hollis, J. A general system for nonspeech language. In R. Schiefelbusch (Ed.), *Nonspeech Language and Communication.* Baltimore: University Park, 1980.

69. Shane, H. An overview of augmentative communication. In N. Lass, L. McReynolds, J. Northern et al. (Eds.), *Speech Language and Hearing Volume. II. Pathologies of Speech and Language.* Philadelphia: Saunders, 1982.

70. Shane, H., and Bashir, A. Election criteria for the adoption of an augmentative communication system: Preliminary considerations. *J. Speech Hear. Disord.* 45:408, 1980.

71. Sheehan, G. Stuttering and its disappearance. *J. Speech Hear. Res.* 13:279, 1970.

72. Shelton, R., Johnson, A., and Arndt, W. Delayed judgement, speech-sound discrimination, and /r/ or /s/ articulation status and improvement. *J. Speech Hear. Res.* 20:704, 1977.

73. Siegel-Sadewitz, V., and Shprintzen, R. J. The relationship of communication disorders to syndrome identification. *J. Speech Hear. Disord.* 47:338, 1982.

74. Silverman, F. *Communication for the Speechless.* Englewood Cliffs, N.J.: Prentice-Hall, 1980.

75. Skelly, N., Schinskey, L., Smith, R. et al. Ameri-can Indian sign: A gestural communication system for the speechless. *Arch. Phys. Med. Rehab.* 56:156, 1975.

76. Snyder, L., and Johnston, J. P. Cognition and reading in normal and language/learning disabled children. Paper presented at ASHA Convention, Detroit, 1980.

77. Spiestersbach, D. The effects of orofacial anomalies on the speech process. Proceedings of the conference: Communicative problems in cleft palate. *ASHA Reports* 1:111, 1965.

78. Stark, J., and Wurtzel, S. Reading: Why do educators need the speech/language pathologist? Paper presented at the ASHA Convention, Detroit, 1980.

79. Stewart, I. F. Newborn infant hearing screening—a 5 year pilot project. *J. Otolaryngol.* 6:477, 1977.

80. Templin, M. Certain language skills in children: Their development and interrelationships. Child Welfare Monographs, 26. Minneapolis: University of Minnesota Press, 1957.

81. Templin, M., and Darley, F. *The Templin Darley Tests of Articulation.* Iowa City: University of Iowa, 1969.

82. Van Riper, C. *Speech Correction: Principles and Methods* (6th ed.). Englewood Cliffs, N.J.: Prentice-Hall, 1978.

83. Van Riper, C. *The Treatment of Stuttering.* Englewood Cliffs, N.J.: Prentice-Hall, 1973.

84. Vanderheiden, G. Providing the child with a means to indicate. In G. Vanderheiden and K. Grilley (Eds.), *Non-vocal Communication Techniques and Aids for the Severely Physically Handicapped.* Baltimore: University Park, 1976.

85. Vellutino, F. Toward an understanding of dyslexia: Psychological factors in specific reading disability. In A. Benton and D. Pearl (Eds.), *Dyslexia: An Appraisal of Current Knowledge.* New York: Oxford University Press, 1978.

86. Vellutino, F., Steger, J., and Kandel, G. Reading disability: An investigation of the perceptual deficit hypothesis. *Cortex* 8:106, 1972.

87. Vogel, S. Syntactic abilities in normal and dyslexic children. *J. Learn. Disabil.* 7:103, 1974.

88. Wallach, G. Language processing and reading deficiencies: Assessment and remediation of children with special learning problems. In N. Lass, L. McReynolds, J. Northern et al. (Eds.), *Speech, Language, and Hearing, Volume II: Pathologies of Speech and Language.* Philadelphia: Saunders, 1982.

89. Wallach, G., and Goldsmith, S. Language-based learning disabilities. Reading is language too! *J. Learn. Disabil.* 10:178, 1977.

90. Wepman, J. *Auditory Discrimination Test.* Los Angeles: Western Psychological, 1973.
91. Wiig, E., and Semel, E. *Language Disabilities in Children and Adolescents.* Columbus: Merril, 1976.
92. Wiig, E., Semel, E., and Crouse, M. The use of morphology by high risk and learning disabled children. *J. Learn. Disabil.* 6:457, 1973.
93. Wingate, M. A standard definition of stuttering. *J. Speech Hear. Disord.* 29:484, 1964.
94. Wingate, M. Recovery from stuttering. *J. Speech Hear. Disord.* 29:312, 1964.
95. Wong, D., and Shah, C. P. Identification of impaired hearing in early childhood. *CMA* 121:529, 1979.
96. Wood, N. *Verbal Learning, Dimensions in Early Learning Series.* San Rafael: Dimensions Publishing, 1969.
97. Worthley, W. *Sourcebook of Articulation Learning Activities.* Boston: Little, Brown, 1981.

SUGGESTED READING

HEARING DISORDERS

Bess, F. H., and McConnell, F. E. *Audiology, Education and the Hearing Impaired Child.* St. Louis: Mosby, 1981.
Boothroyd, A. *Hearing Impairments in Young Children.* Englewood Cliffs, N.J.: Prentice-Hall, 1982.
Downs, M. P., and Sterritt, G. M. A guide to newborn and infant screening programs. *Arch. Otolaryngol.* 85:15, 1967.
Fine, P. J. *Deafness in Infancy and Early Childhood.* New York: Medcom, 1974.
Fulton, R. T., Gorzycki, P. A., and Hull, W. L. Hearing assessment with young children. *J. Speech Hear. Disord.* 40:397, 1975.
Hodgson, W. R. Testing Infants and Young Children. In J. Katz (Ed.), *Handbook of Clinical Audiology* (2nd ed.). Baltimore: Williams & Wilkins, 1978.
Jaffe, B. F. (Ed.). *Hearing Loss in Children.* Baltimore: University Park Press, 1977.
Moses, K. L., and Van Hecke-Wulatin, M. The socio-emotional impact of infant deafness: A counseling model. In S. E. Gerber, and G. T. Mencher (Eds.), *Early Diagnosis of Hearing Loss.* New York: Grune & Stratton, 1978.
Protti, E., and Evans, J. E. Neuroaudiology: A challenge for the future. *Hearing Aid J.* 35:19, 1982.
Rubin, M. Meeting the needs of hearing impaired infants. *Pediatric Annals* 9:46, 1980.
Salamy, A., Somerville, G., and Patterson, D. The infant hearing assessment program. *Hearing Aid J.* 35:10, 1982.
Simmons, F. B. Diagnosis and rehabilitation of deaf newborns: Part II. *ASHA* 22:475, 1980.
Weber, B. A. Auditory brain-stem response audiometry in children. *Clinical Pediatrics* 18:746, 1979.

Juvenile Rheumatoid Arthritis

Diane M. Erlandson

THE DISEASE PROCESS

Juvenile rheumatoid arthritis (JRA) is the most common of the childhood connective tissue diseases. It is a chronic condition that occurs before the age of 16 and is one of the leading causes of childhood disability. Diagnostic criteria developed by the American Rheumatism Association indicate that arthritis must be present and persistent in one or more joints for a minimum of 6 weeks and all other disease possibilities must have been ruled out in order for JRA to be diagnosed [11]. Even with strict guidelines, JRA can still be difficult to diagnose. It is currently divided into three subsets based on the signs and symptoms manifested during the first 6 months of the disease. These include pauciarticular JRA (four or fewer joints affected), polyarticular JRA (five or more joints affected), and systemic onset JRA (Still's disease). In general, outcome is favorable, but early diagnosis, careful treatment, and close follow-up are essential to minimize long-term impairment [12].

The use of the term *rheumatoid* is somewhat misleading since those unfamiliar with JRA, especially newly diagnosed families, tend to associate it with the adult form of rheumatoid arthritis (RA). Even though both types of arthritis mean that there is chronic inflammation in the joints, there are crucial differences to keep in mind during treatment as described by

Cassidy [13]. Children will often present with large joint involvement especially in the pauciarticular group whereas adults more typically present with small joint disease. While approximately two thirds of children may expect to achieve permanent remission, the majority of adults with RA develop progressive joint changes. Blood tests also vary. The rheumatoid factor is present in only about 20 percent of children with JRA in comparison to 80 percent of adults with RA. Systemic features such as uveitis, pericarditis, hepatitis, rash, and fever are far more common in children. Cervical spine disease may be present in both children and adults; however, children more characteristically have inflammation and ankylosis of the epiphysial joints. Also, atlantoaxial subluxation is a risk factor in both groups. For indeterminate reasons children appear to have less joint pain than adults. Lastly, the type of joint deformities also varies. Children very often develop radial drift at the metacarpophalangeal (MCP) joints whereas adults develop an ulnar drift. Valgus deformities of the elbows and flexion contractures of the wrists are more commonly seen in children.

There is one exception to these differences between JRA and RA. Older children, usually in the adolescent age group and female, who have a positive rheumatoid factor and rheumatoid nodules, tend to develop the same joint problems as an adult with RA would. The long-term prognosis for these children is generally worse in terms of severity of disability. They often require multiple replacements as adults and have significant mobility and self-care impairment.

EPIDEMIOLOGY
Approximately 150,000 to 250,000 children in the United States have JRA. It is 2 to 3 times more common in females, but this varies in each subset. In general, polyarticular JRA is more common in females. Systemic-onset JRA occurs with almost an equal frequency in both males and females. Pauciarticular JRA is more commonly seen in females. Another type of pauciarticular arthritis is seen in boys over the age of 5 who are HLA-B27 positive, which probably represents a mode of onset of juvenile ankylosing spondylitis. Traditionally these boys have been included in discussions of JRA.

The incidence of JRA is equivalent among the races. It is rarely seen in more than one family member or in first-degree relatives with other connective tissue diseases [40].

ETIOLOGY
The cause of JRA is unknown. Possible etiologies include infection, autoimmunity, trauma, and genetic predisposition. The relationship of stress to the onset of disease is not certain. Clearly there is some triggering event that initiates the inflammatory process and alters the body's defense mechanism. Current research is investigating the relationship of JRA with viruses, bacteria, immunodeficiency, stress, trauma, and HLA typing [13].

INFLAMMATORY PROCESS IN JRA
The term *arthritis* means that the synovium of a joint becomes inflamed. Since synovium is present in all diarthrodial joints, arthritis could potentially occur in any of them. The synovium lining the tendon sheaths and bursae may become inflamed in the presence of JRA. The joint is also made up of the articular cartilage and is held in alignment by the joint capsule, ligaments, and muscles. The synovium is a very thin piece of tissue about the width of a piece of cellophane. It produces synovial fluid for the purpose of lubrication and cartilage nourishment since cartilage does not have its own direct blood supply. Joint movements assist in the process.

When inflammation is present in a child's joint, the volume of synovial fluid usually increases, which causes a rise in joint pressure. The fluid and the inflammation lead to swelling. The joint loses its normal contour, which may only be noticed when compared to a normal joint. This swelling should not be confused with the swelling associated with bony overgrowth that is the result of the hyperemia of the inflammatory process.

Joint pressure may be further increased by forced flexion. For this reason this motion should be avoided in activities of daily living and in therapy. Even though not a common occurrence in JRA, flexion of inflamed knee joints while weight bearing (squatting, bending, kneeling) can cause rupture of a Baker cyst, tracking synovial fluid from the joint capsule down into the calf.

Stretching of the joint capsule usually results in pain. In order to reduce the stretching of the capsule and relieve the pain, children tend to flex the joint into a position of comfort very often with the use of pillows, which can lead to flexion contractures. Flexion contractures also occur because of the increase in bulk of the synovium and the effort of the joint cavity to accommodate it [49]. As the disease progresses, flexion contractures may also occur as a direct result of destructive enzymes damaging ligaments, tendons, and muscles.

Tenosynovitis in the flexor tendons of the hands is relatively common in children with polyarticular JRA. Bursitis is far less common but may be seen in such joints as the shoulders and the first metatarsophalangeal (MTP) joint of children with polyarticular involvement.

COURSE OF THE DISEASE

JRA is a chronic disease characterized by remissions and exacerbations. The frequency and duration of remissions and exacerbations is variable from child to child. They may last weeks, months, or years. Remissions may be drug induced or may occur as part of the natural course of the disease. Exacerbations may also occur as part of the natural course of the disease but may also occur after trauma or with infection as well.

Chronic disease implies lifelong disease usually with progressive physical changes and very often some degree of disability or impairment. Since the majority of children with JRA usually recover, the term takes on a slightly different connotation. It is possible for any child with JRA to have ongoing disease that will last a lifetime. This would be seen more commonly in adolescents with seropositive nodular disease. It is also possible for a child to go into remission during childhood and again suffer exacerbation in adulthood.

These children who remit permanently may, nonetheless, be affected chronically with the repercussions of the disease that was active during childhood. Lifelong problems can result from flexion contractures, growth retardation, limb discrepancies, bone deformities, and visual impairment [17].

If parents are uninformed regarding some of these problems, they may go undetected. Leg-length discrepancies, scoliosis, and uveitis associated with JRA have chronic implications and should be carefully observed for so that appropriate remedial action can be taken. For the most part, resulting gait abnormalities, spinal deformities, and blindness are preventable if treated early and correctly. The observation and prevention of chronic problems of JRA are major parental responsibilities especially since children usually do not understand the concept of chronicity until the age of 12 or 13.

Acute situations associated with JRA are relatively uncommon. High spiking fevers to 105°F may be typical for some children. However, if the temperature is unresponsive to medication and cooling baths, then emergency medical assistance may be necessary. Immediate medical attention would also be required in the presence of uveitis, pericarditis, and pleuritis. Even though uncommon, a sudden neurologic deficit may be suggestive of atlantoaxial subluxation. Vasculitis of the bowel, which is rare, may cause sudden and severe abdominal pain.

A side effect from drugs may also cause acute problems. The most likely acute situation would be created by a gastrointestinal bleed. Of greater concern would be the suppression of bone marrow resulting in a drop in blood counts.

CLINICAL MANIFESTATIONS OF JRA

The signs and symptoms of JRA may occur at any time up until the age of 16. Even though it is uncommon, there have been case reports of disease present at birth. The systemic type of JRA may be seen in adult years and is known as adult Still's disease. In general, the signs and symptoms in children at onset can vary from one child to the next. For example, toddlers may first show signs of disease by not walking in the morning whereas another child may present with fever of unknown origin. The most common signs, however, are morning stiffness, fatigue, pain, loss of appetite, irritability, limping, and fever. Eliciting symptoms from the child can be quite difficult when the child is very young. If there is no initial joint swelling in the lower extremity, for instance, it may be difficult to determine why the toddler is not walking. Symptoms of stiffness such as limping can be intermittent and improve with mobility. This can become confusing to parents and health professionals because it may appear that something is wrong initially and then the symptoms resolve unexpectantly. Since pain may not be present in all children with JRA, some children may lose considerable range of motion before a problem is even noticed.

The *pauciarticular disease,* also known as oligoarticular disease, is seen in 40 to 50 percent of children with the disease. Four or fewer joints are involved with no systemic features. It is usually asymmetrical and very commonly occurs in the lower extremities, especially the knees. Other commonly affected joints include ankles, hips, elbows, and singular finger joints. It is relatively rare in the temperomandibular joints, cervical spine, or the shoulders.

The pauciarticular variety of JRA can be further subdivided [44]. Young girls 2 to 3 years of age with positive antinuclear antibodies (ANAs) very frequently develop uveitis. Because the uveitis is asymptomatic, it can easily go undetected. Since the inflammation could ultimately lead to visual impairment and even blindness, slit-lamp examinations by an ophthalmologist are essential at frequent intervals usually every 3 to 4 months. Young boys with pauciarticular arthritis usually around the age of 9 or 10 at onset have a 90 percent chance of being HLA-B27 positive [27]. These boys are also likely to develop sacroiliitis, and as they get older they may develop ankylosing spondylitis. In both subgroups rheumatoid factor is almost always negative. In general the prognosis is favorable for these subgroups with an average of disease duration of $2\frac{1}{2}$ to $7\frac{1}{2}$ years [44].

Functional limitations with pauciarticular JRA are usually attributed to joint stiffness, deformity, and loss of range of motion. Frequently, children will participate in their usual play and recreational activities while holding the joint or limb affected in extension. Boys with positive HLA B27 may show greater signs of discomfort during recreation especially with knee synovitis, tendonitis, and sacroiliitis. Because of these complaints participation in sports often is erratic depending how the child feels on any given day.

The *polyarticular type* of JRA affects 5 or more joints. About 30 percent of children with JRA fall into this category. The most commonly involved joints are the small joints of the fingers and feet as well as knees, ankles, wrists, elbows, shoulders, temporomandibular joints, and cervical spine. Systemic signs of disease may also occur. These include a low-grade fever, hepatomegaly, splenomegaly, lymphadenopathy, and mild anemia. Pericarditis is relatively rare in this group, and chronic uveitis tends to occur in less than 5 percent of the cases [23].

In general, polyarticular JRA occurs far more frequently in girls than in boys. Most children have a negative rheumatoid factor. However, this test creates a further distinction in this particular type of JRA. Those who are rheumatoid factor negative usually develop their disease between the ages of 2 to 5 and have a fairly good prognosis in the long term. Children who are rheumatoid factor positive tend to develop their disease a little later in childhood, usually after the age of 11 [44]. The arthritis in these children tends to look more like that in adult RA than that in a seronegative polyarticular group, with regard to course of disease and prognosis. These children very often develop subcutaneous nodules, and significant erosive disease may develop. They also very often progress to total joint replacements as adults.

Some children with polyarticular disease may also have what is termed *dry arthritis*. These children tend to have little in the way of joint effusions but have major problems with joint contractures and stiffness.

Functionally children with polyarticular disease are limited for a number of reasons. Fatigue can be very limiting especially in the school situation. The pain and stiffness usually affects mobility and, therefore, the ability to take part in self care, activities of daily living, socialization, and recreation.

The systemic variety of JRA also known as *Still's disease* occurs in about 20 percent of children with the disease. The sex ratio is virtually equivalent. It can occur at any age during childhood with no true peak incidence. It is characterized by daily high spiking fevers and arthritis in one or more joints. The fever usually occurs as a single daily spike peaking in late afternoon and evening and going back to normal by the morning. It is possible for the fever of Still's disease to precede any signs of arthritis by months. These children very often are categorized with fever of unknown origin until further symptoms manifest themselves. They very often complain of fatigue and myalgia and can be noticeably irritable. Systemic features of the disease also include a rash, hepatomegaly, splenomegaly, lymphadenopathy, pleuritis, pericarditis, and occasionally abdominal pain. Laboratory tests very often reveal leukocytosis, thrombocytosis, and anemia. The rheumatoid factor is usually negative.

The most characteristic feature of this type of JRA is a rash. It is usually a salmon pink color and is most pronounced during the spiking fevers. Lesions are usually macular, about 2 to 5mm in diameter and surrounded by erythema.

Larger lesions tend to be clear in the center. The rash is most commonly seen over the trunk and proximal extremities and over the affected joints. It may also occur over the face, palms, and soles of the feet. Usually transient in nature from one to a few hours in duration, it is possible for the rash to occur on a daily basis. It may even sometimes be reproduced by scratching and pressure (Koebner's phenomenon) or after a hot bath. It is rarely itchy [23].

The arthritis seen in Still's disease can be variable, ranging from one to many joints. However, many children do develop a polyarticular type of disease and shed the systemic features of the disease as they get older. These children can progress to severe polyarticular disease with erosions and deformities. Functional limitations may be due to the systemic features of the disease, the arthritis, or both. In the presence of fever most children feel rather ill and retire to bed. Fatigue and general malaise can be quite severe. Fevers that occur in the afternoon and evening can, therefore, be completely disabling and, thus, affect school activities, ability to do homework, play, and recreation. The functional limitations of children with polyarticular involvement in Still's disease are similar to those discussed with polyarticular disease.

LABORATORY TESTS AND PROCEDURES
No specific blood test or diagnostic procedure can make the diagnosis of JRA conclusively. For the most part, the diagnosis is based on clinical findings. Laboratory tests and radiographs may then provide support to the diagnosis only. It is not uncommon, therefore, for the diagnosis to be misjudged or go undetermined for long periods of time if the practitioner is inexperienced.

Blood tests provide a certain amount of information related to the JRA. The rheumatoid factor is only positive in less than 20 percent of children. Again, these children are usually female and older. The antinuclear antibody (ANA) is positive in many children, especially those with pauciarticular disease and is helpful in identifying those children at risk for iridocyclitis. The HLA B27 can be helpful in identifying those children, especially boys, with pauciarticular disease, who are at greater risk for developing sacroiliitis and ankylosing spondylitis as they get older.

Some blood tests are helpful in monitoring the disease as well as treatment progress or side effects. The erythrocyte sedimentation rate (ESR) is very often elevated with JRA. Platelets may also be elevated as part of the acute phase reaction. Similarly, hypergammaglobulinemia may also be present. Elevated white blood counts are more frequently elevated in the children with the Still's variety of JRA during a flare of inflammatory activity. Anemia may also be present, characteristic of the anemia of chronic disease. It is usually present in those children with polyarticular JRA or those with Still's disease. Occasionally one may see a minor rise in the serum glutamic-oxaloacetic transaminase (SGOT) and serum glutamic-pyruvic transaminase (SGPT) in children with low-grade hepatitis related to the JRA. However, elevation in liver enzymes may also be seen with the use of salicylates and less commonly with the other nonsteroidal anti-inflammatory drugs. The urinalysis should be normal. Proteinuria may be the first indication of ankyloidosis affecting the kidney, even though it is very rare.

Children who are on salicylates require periodic monitoring of their salicylate level in an effort to maintain a therapeutic level in the blood. Generally, this range is considered to be 20 to 30 dl in most labs. However, the standard may be different from one laboratory to the next, and this would need to be determined from the laboratory being used.

The synovial fluid is usually inflammatory in nature; however, it is possible to obtain very low white blood counts in the joints of children with chronic synovitis. There also may be exceptionally high white blood counts in the synovial fluid, making one suspect infection when in fact no infection is present [13]. Ordinarily, synovial fluid aspirations are done infrequently

in children due to the emotional trauma involved and the limited information obtained.

Radiographs may be ordered initially but are usually unhelpful. Soft-tissue swelling may be the only finding. Later findings include widening of the joint space as well as periarticular osteoporosis. More aggressive synovitis results in erosions and narrowing of the joint space. Other abnormalities include premature epiphysial effusion, overgrowth of the joint, and subluxation. X rays are often helpful in determining bone age. Scanograms may also be ordered to provide a more precise measurement of limb-length discrepancies.

Other laboratory tests for the most part depend on the systemic features of the illness. Laboratory tests such as electrocardiograms, chest x rays, and echocardiograms may be required.

PHYSICAL IMPACT OF JRA

GROWTH ABNORMALITIES

Because JRA occurs in a growing child, a number of significant problems may ensue. The inflammation itself, which causes localized hyperemia can result in overgrowth of the bone, thus creating obvious bony enlargement of the joint, or a longer limb or digit. However, if the epiphysial plate itself is involved, then the growth in fact is retarded [23]. General stature of the child may also be reduced permanently. This is more commonly seen in children with severe polyarticular disease, especially with the onset in early childhood, as well as those with the systemic variety of JRA. Children who require daily steroids for control of disease are also at risk for growth retardation. The growth of the mandible may also be retarded, resulting in micrognathia, which gives the child a chipmunklike appearance. This not only causes cosmetic problems but significant dental problems as well. The child may develop an abnormal bite, crowding of teeth, and an abnormal location of tooth eruption [1]. The child's height may also be affected by cervical spine disease.

200

Usually the inflammation occurs in the apophyseal joints, resulting in eventual effusion of the posterior spine. The subsequent loss of motion can cause the growth of the intervertebral disks and vertebral bodies to be stunted [7]. Significant scoliosis as well as vertebral collapse on the basis of steroid therapy may also reduce the child's stature. When the child's growth has been affected by active disease, it is possible for the height to return to normal within a 2 to 3-year period if remission occurs, only if premature fusion of the epiphysis has not occurred [3].

JOINT DEFORMITIES

The most common joint deformity in children with JRA is flexion contracture. Joint deformities, however, do depend on the joints affected, the aggression of the synovitis, and the degree of tendon and ligament involvement. Common problems seen in the hands of children with JRA as outlined by Athreya include lack of extension of the wrist, ulnar deviation of the wrist, proximal interphalangeal (PIP) swelling, and possibly distal interphangeal (DIP) swelling, swan neck, or boutonnière deformities, unequal growth and MCP subluxation of the thumb [4]. Palmar subluxation and radial or ulnar deviation of the MCPs may also occur. Hand involvement has a significant impact on self-care activities, grip, dexterity, and endurance.

Flexion contractures of the elbows can range from very mild to severe and debilitating. As the disease persists, valgus may eventually occur. Loss of supination may go undetected since many children will compensate for this by moving the entire arm for motion. Major problems with flexion contractures in the elbows are that the child and parent may not notice them or they may occur relatively quickly. These deformities can cause significant problems with feeding, grooming, brushing teeth, and putting the hand out to receive an object, especially if there is also wrist synovitis or deformity.

Significant shoulder abnormalities are usually seen in children with polyarticular disease. Range of motion is usually reduced, especially in rotation and extension. Muscle atrophy may also be present. Activities affected include combing and washing of the hair, buttoning or zipping clothing in the back, personal hygiene, toileting, and lifting.

Cervical spine disease creates loss of motion mostly from the epiphysial involvement. Extension, rotation, and lateral flexion can be significantly limited. The loss of extension can be so severe that the child's actual line of vision is slanted downward. The most severe problem from cervical spine disease is atlantoaxial subluxation even though a neurologic deficit may not be present [13]. Children undergoing surgery requiring general anesthesia must have cervical spine films beforehand due to the risk of interruption of the spinal cord during intubation. Torticollis is relatively uncommon. Children are most bothered by cervical spine involvement if participating in sports that require neck motion as well as driving a car in the teen years. As the child progresses into adulthood, cervical spine abnormalities create greater functional limitations. An interesting functional limitation seen in mothers with JRA caring for infants is that fusion of the cervical spine would prevent the mother from seeing the child well while feeding when the child is held close to her chest.

Temporomandibular joint abnormalities (previously discussed) can create a difficulty with chewing and less so with talking. Hip synovitis can reduce the range in all planes. Flexion contractures are relatively common, creating problems with standing, walking, and posture. A lordotic curve may be accentuated. Limited rotation, abduction, and adduction may also occur. Functional limitations include ambulation, bike riding, horseback riding, and participating in active sports. In the adult years, women may have some difficulty with sexual relations, which they generally adapt to. Also, women at childbirth may not be able to keep the hips flexed in abduction and may deliver the infant more easily in a side-lying position.

Flexion contractures in affected knees are relatively common. Genuvalgum may also occur, especially in the longer limb. A child's activities are not only affected by the flexion contracture of the knee but also by the degree of muscle atrophy and ligamentous laxity. Activities that may be affected include rising from the floor, ambulation, stair climbing, running, jumping, active sports and recreation, and sitting cross-legged. Disease in the feet can create a number of problems depending on the actual joints involved. Ankle range may be significantly impaired, resulting in a very stiff walk. The forefoot may become quite splayed, and the toes may develop cocked-up deformities. Some children may also develop hallux valgus. Foot abnormalities are very often created by hip and knee deformities as a compensatory mechanism. A valgus knee may very well cause a varus ankle. Simple walking and fitting into standard shoes may become major problems.

GAIT DISTURBANCE

The gait of a child with JRA is dependent on the presence of joint synovitis and deformities, growth discrepancies, and muscle strength. Synovitis of the knee may cause pain, a flexion contracture, quadriceps weakness due to stretching, decreased use, and instability. The opposite leg, therefore, becomes the longer leg, and the stress shifts to the longer limb. Hip flexion contractures also cause the affected limb to shorten. Children with a hip that is ankylosed very often compensate with a greater lordosis of the lumbar spine as well as increased movement in the opposite hip [19]. Hip synovitis and contracture may also cause hip flexor weakness, which creates a backward thrust of the trunk and pelvis in an effort to lift the leg [19]. Hip disease may result in an antalgic gait, which is characterized by a shortened stance phase on the affected side, thus limiting weight-bearing time on the painful hip. Foot involvement can affect both the stance phase and swing phase of gait usually because of significant stiffness or pain.

POSTURE

The posture of a child with JRA is altered for a number of reasons. These might include cervical spine involvement with a torticollis or forward flexion. Equal hanging of the upper extremities is a function of the structure of the limbs as well as the trunk. Inequalities may be seen, therefore, with tilting of the shoulders and hips, spinal deformities, flexion contractures of the elbows, or limb growth discrepancy [48]. Scoliosis, and lordosis are fairly common problems of the spine in children with JRA. Flexion contractures in the hips and knees, leg-length discrepancies, joint deformities, or pain will all contribute to an abnormal posture.

IATROGENIC EFFECTS

Iatrogenic effects of drugs may also cause physical abnormalities in children with JRA. The greatest offenders are steroids. Children on daily steroids may suffer from major body-image changes. The face may become very bloated and puffy. Weight gain and redistribution of adipose tissue can also grossly affect the child's usual appearance. A thoracic kyphosis with a noticeable "hump" on a side view may cause concern to both children and parents. Steroids may also cause vertebral collapse resulting in loss of height. As mentioned earlier, the growth of the child may also be retarded, causing the child to be much shorter than his or her peers. Acne may also result from the use of corticosteroids in adolescence, which will improve or abate after the drugs are discontinued.

Other drugs such as gold or nonsteroidal anti-inflammatory drugs have the potential of causing skin rash. This is more commonly seen with the use of gold injections. The rash usually recedes following withdrawal of the drug, but this may be a slow process. Rashes due to the nonsteroidal anti-inflammatory drugs are usually mild and resolve quickly once the offending drug is stopped.

IMPACT OF JRA ON THE CHILD AND FAMILY

PSYCHOSOCIAL RESPONSE

The child's response to having a chronic illness such as JRA can be a rather complex one [41]. Apparently the response is also not always consistent with the degree of disability [31, 37]. Unlike adults who tend to go through a cycle of grieving before acceptance of the disease, children tend to have a more individualized response largely because of the differences in developmental stages, level of understanding, and environmental support. Regardless of the age of the child, the child inevitably develops some perceptions of what is happening [20]. Perceptions about illness are largely based on the child's knowledge base, experience, and response of others [16]. Perceptions about health and illness in general change in conjunction with cognitive development [25]. Therefore, to simply tell a 5-year-old child that he or she has juvenile rheumatoid arthritis would have very little personal value for that child. Therefore, a meaningful response may be nonexistent. On the other hand, if the child has heard the word *arthritis* before and associates this with a neighbor in a wheelchair, he or she then has a different perception that may be very frightening. Because children are often unable to verbalize a response to their illness or treatment, this should not be ignored.

In a child's mind having an illness may be one problem but having a chronic illness is an entirely different matter [22]. Children under the age of 12 do not understand "part healthy" and "part unhealthy" [36]. Hence it is difficult for children to understand the unpredictability of JRA as well as remissions and exacerbations. It is not until a child reaches the age of 12 or 13 that the concept of chronic disease can be understood.

By the time a child reaches school age and has more interactions with children of the same age, he or she then begins to take note of differences between him- or herself and other children. These differences are usually related to ambulation and speed. Between the ages of 7 and 11 children with arthritis are very often exposed to unkind comments from other children about their disease, disability, or appearance [32]. This is not only upsetting to children but can actually result in depression.

From early childhood through adolescence, acquiring skills to become independent, to problem solve, to develop relationships, and to develop positive self-esteem are additive and ongoing. Because of the nature of the disease as well as the implicit problems with mobilization and, therefore, interraction and socialization, opportunities to improve on these skills are at risk [34]. Therefore, by the time the child reaches adolescence, significant psychological problems may be present. Adolescence alone is a very critical stage of development because of the many changes that occur physically and emotionally but also because it immediately precedes adulthood. Therefore, there is a certain amount of pressure on an adolescent to resolve certain issues in an effort to function well as an adult.

There is clearly a difference in the psychological response in adolescents who have had JRA in early childhood as opposed to those who acquire it later in childhood. Those who develop it early in life tend to view the presence of the disease as "their normal." Very often, too, early dependent relationships on parents, especially the mother, are continuous and progressive to the point of being pathologic. This then creates other problems that relate to the development and nurturance of other relationships as well as positive self-esteem. When JRA develops in older childhood and adolescence, the child may become quite fearful of what will happen to him or her. This is especially true in those children who understand the term *chronic*. Rapid growth and body changes as well as a fluctuation in emotions place adolescents in a very stressful situation. More bodily changes due to the disease as well as compromised performance or participation very often lead to a feeling of worthlessness and depression. At times, these feelings can create a psychological immobility that requires psychiatric interventions.

Small children are sensitive to the reactions not only of their peers but more importantly their parents, their siblings, and other family members. Children very often form their opinions about their disease and themselves based on parental influence. Those parents, therefore, who convey a "disabled" attitude on the child are placing the child in jeopardy of internalizing the same attitude. Children may resent their siblings because they themselves have an illness and the siblings do not. Siblings in fact very often have strong feelings toward the child with JRA because of the time spent by parents with the child as well as a number of fears that may surface regarding getting the illness or causing the illness. Children at times may even use their disease to manipulate their environment when reasonably assured that they will get the expected or hoped for response.

Noncompliance with medical treatment is a common response to illness in adolescents. Frequently, they will attempt to alter their medications or stop taking them. More commonly, however, they will cease all prescribed physical and occupational therapy. The issue of noncompliance is also very complex in origin [8]. The adolescent needs a very careful assessment to determine not only perceptions but attitudes, understanding, expectations, and environmental influences.

Hospitalization and the performance of frightening or invasive procedures create other psychological responses consistent with the developmental stage of the child [39]. Toddlers, for instance, have great difficulty in separating fantasy from reality. They also have a great fear of separation. Therefore, fear and anxiety are very common in this age group during hospitalization as well as with certain treatment. Simple things such as goniometers, tape measures, and splints may become sources of fear.

Preschoolers have very magical thoughts.

They are also literal in their interpretation of events. Their greatest fear tends to be that of mutilation to their body. As a result, misunderstanding and misperceptions also result in significant fear and anxiety. School-age children are very concerned about their peers. It is the time for developing identity and promoting self-esteem. Hospitalization and procedures can be threatening because of separation as well as the fear of losing control.

The adolescent is also very much concerned with control, independence, and appearance. Hospitalization may impose barriers to keeping one's appearance up. Washing hair and applying makeup may be a low priority to the hospital staff but a major priority to the adolescent. Temporarily becoming dependent due to immobility procedures such as bed rest, traction, or casting not only can create anxiety but can be devastating.

FAMILY RESPONSE TO JRA

When parents are first told that their child has juvenile rheumatoid arthritis, many emotions emerge. As with children, these emotions are influenced by the parents' understanding of the disease, prior experience, and the response of others. Often parents have never known a child with JRA and, unfortunately, expect that their child will appear to have adult RA. Most parents, if not all, enter into the grieving cycle. The grief largely stems from their loss of a "normal" child and, therefore, their dreams and expectations for the future. Initially, the parents may suffer from disbelief, guilt, and anger. Later, anxiety and depression occur. The grieving cycle differs in severity not only from family to family but also among family members. The child with JRA as well as the siblings may enter into the cycle. This can create major family disruption primarily because family members are not usually at the same stage in a cycle at the same time. In other words, one parent may have completed the cycle and come to the point of acceptance of disease while the other is in a state of denial. This makes communication and follow-up care difficult. The cycle is also dependent on the child's physical and emotional status. For instance, parents of children who are in remission may be in a state of acceptance of disease once again. A flare of disease may then interrupt this acceptance and trigger the whole grieving cycle over again.

Guilt is frequently a major problem within a couple's relationship. One spouse may feel that the other spouse is at fault for the child developing the disease even if told that the disease is not hereditary per se. This can create marital tension and at times even separation. Home treatment is also a major source of couple conflict. More often, mothers are responsible for the child's care at home. The mother may then become resentful of the father who does not have to spend the time or the anguish of caring for the child.

When a family of a child with JRA is also trying to contend with other family issues, the psychological equilibrium within the family is at stake. Health problems, behavioral problems, social problems, and financial burdens are especially overwhelming in anyone's life. Any one of these in conjunction with coping with a chronic childhood disease can be psychologically immobilizing.

FUNCTION OF A DEVELOPING CHILD

The function of a child with JRA is affected by the number and location of the joints involved. Those developmental tasks at risk in the presence of JRA also affect general function if not successfully achieved (Table 8-1). The pain, immobility, instability, and muscle weakness associated with JRA all can also influence normal childhood function. Each of these has an impact not only on the activities of daily living and self-care practices of a child but more importantly on the accomplishment of the expected developmental tasks. Children may in fact complete certain tasks but may do so in a modified way. Parents of an only child who has JRA may be inexperienced and may not realize that some of these approaches are deviant. Children who develop JRA in infancy or as toddlers seem to be at greatest risk for disrupting their normal development. The reason for this is that many of the developmental tasks are additive in nature. For instance, if a child cannot stand, then he or she will not be able to walk. Also, a child who cannot turn the faucets on will not be able to wash when alone.

Accomplishing developmental tasks also plays a major role in the child's development of independence, positive self-esteem, and a sense of identity. Thus, the professional team may be more concerned about these issues rather than the actual carrying out of certain tasks since children very often adapt physically in some way to the alteration from the norm. The child will eventually learn how to button and how to put on shoes but may not in fact do these things because of an abnormal dependency on the parent. Children who are allowed to function below their capacity tend to do so unless redirected. However, a major problem that results from not performing activities of daily living and self care can be that the child loses this ability mostly due to the loss of range of motion. Even though these tasks are additive as the child gets older, the health professional cannot assume that the child can still perform any one activity. Therefore, if a child learned to dress by the age of 4, the health care provider cannot assume that at the age of 8, the child is still doing this.

One of the most common reasons for parental interference with a child's performance is that the child "takes too much time" and it would be "faster to do it myself." Many children have lost their ability to dress themselves completely because of this attitude.

Infancy is the time when the child is developing cognitively from sensorimotor input. Because of this it is vital for the child to interact with the environment, which would imply the need to be very mobile. The inability to do simple things such as reaching out for an object, kicking the legs, and crawling could greatly impair a child's opportunity to experience the environment. Toddlers are busy with play, explo-

TABLE 8-1. Developmental tasks at risk in children with JRA

INFANTS 1–6 MONTHS
Upper extremities
   Raises head when prone
   Reaches up with arm
   Head erect when sitting
   Spreads fingers to grasp
   Picks up with one hand
   Uses both hands in coordination
   Roles over
   Picks up small objects
Lower extremities
   Kicks legs when flexed
   Roles over
   Locks knees to stand
   Bears weight
INFANTS 7–14 MONTHS
Upper extremities
   Holds own bottle
   Pulls self up
   Holds cup with both hands
   Cooperates with dressing
   Opens and shuts small doors
Lower extremities
   Stands holding on
   Sits without support
   Stoops
   Crawls
   Creeps
   Walks
   Cooperates with dressing
TODDLERS 15 MO–2½ YEARS
Upper extremities
   Climbs up and down furniture
   Carries large objects
   Turns pages
   Turns door knobs
   Undresses
   Unbuttons
   Can screw on bottle cap
   Drinks with small glass with one hand
   Feeds self with spoon
   Holds pencil and crayon properly
   Throws ball overhand
Lower extremities
   Kneels
   Squats
   Walks on tippy toes

   Walks well
   Climbs up and down furniture
   Jumps
   Walks up stairs
   Slides down stairs feet first
   Runs
   Tricycles
   Sits with legs straight
   Kicks ball
   Puts on shoes
   Gets out of bed or crib
Social
   Plays in company of children
PRESCHOOLERS 2½–5 YEARS
Upper extremities
   Climbs jungle gym
   Uses scissors to cut
   Laces shoes
   Dresses completely
   Buttons
   Uses small tools
   Brushes teeth
   Does own toileting
   Turns faucets
   Opens and closes doors
Lower extremities
   Sits on heels
   Hops on one foot
   Stands on one foot
   Climbs
   Laces shoes
   Dresses completely
   May skate
   Skips
   Does own toileting
   Stairs one after the other
   Heel to toe walk
Social
   Plays with other children
SCHOOL AGE 6–12 YEARS
Upper extremities
   Swims
   Plays sports
   Uses tools well
   Washes own hair
   Bathes self
   Cuts own food

206

TABLE 8-1 (CONTINUED)

Pours from a container	Applies makeup
Opens car door	Hygiene after toileting
Opens new jar or can	Drives
Writes/draws/paints	Performs vocational tasks
Does crafts	Types
Lower extremities	Hobbies
Runs well	Sews
Bicycles	Plays instruments
Swims	Does housework
Skates	Employment
Plays sports	Lower extremities
Social	Dances
Plays with friends	Employment
ADOLESCENTS 12–20 YEARS	Social
(Functional level comparable to adult)	Socializes in groups
Upper extremities	
Shaves	

ration, and learning new activities. It is a time during which they learn about themselves and their surroundings. They gain a sense of autonomy and confidence from doing so. These successes are dependent, however, on their ability to interact with their environment and to receive positive reinforcement for their achievements. Preschoolers start to see themselves in relation to those around them. They begin to understand and participate in social roles and self-care habits. They also are beginning to learn a sense of their own identity. In order to accomplish these tasks the preschooler must, therefore, be able to play and practice self-care activities. Mastering of certain tasks also needs strong encouragement and reinforcement. The school-age child tries to become adept at physical skills including sports. Peer contacts and socialization help to promote self-concept development. Independence also seems to make great strides during this time and is enhanced by being able to carry out new tasks by themselves. Absence from school, inability to participate in recreational activities, and physical immobility would impair the child from learning these new tasks. By the time a child enters adolescence it is hoped that he or she will have become independent, self-accepting, and at ease with his or her appearance, that personal identity will become clearer in society, and that he or she will be making appropriate plans for adulthood. If in fact the child has been delayed developmentally up to this point by lack of opportunities for achievement of developmental tasks, then this becomes a problem not only for the child but the family as well. Very often it is apparent that the adolescent has never had the chance to socialize with other children of the same age. They also are very inexperienced in social situations and have great difficulty with personal interactions. A healthy identity also suffers because the child may visualize him- or herself as "abnormal" and find it difficult to fit into a normal world. Emancipating from the parents if independence was never fostered is, therefore, impossible at this time. Personal skills and good emotional development help to make independence easier and more desirable. Two common but unfortunate problems seen in some older adolescents can occur due to delays in previous accomplishments of tasks. The first problem is that adolescents 18 and 19 years of age, for instance, have the emotional development of 13- or 14-year olds. When they try to transfer into a college or job situation, they have enormous difficulty trying to relate to others, especially those of the opposite sex. They also have very little idea how to make their own decisions. The second problem is found primarily in those children who have had JRA most of their lives. When it comes time for these adolescents to make plans to leave the home, they are literally incapable because of their lack of experience and gross dependency on the family. Parents often are surprised that the child is not making plans and have little insight as to why this is not possible. It is a rude awakening and a sad situation when a mother comes to realize that she herself will not be given her long-awaited freedom from caring for a disabled child.

One of the greatest influences of childhood development is school participation. It provides a medium for children to learn about themselves and others and to learn and test out new skills. Through the interactions with other children and teachers in the school environment, the child learns to communicate, to speak out independently, and to share and work with others. The school environment also serves as a medium for being exposed to new situations and learning how to handle them. They learn to become self-disciplined and to experience the consequences of their decisions. School usually provides many opportunities for the child to gain a sense of self-accomplishment, which assists in the development of self-esteem.

Children with JRA suffer from problems that can impinge on all of these things. The most significant problems affecting school attendance and participation in the usual activities include pain, fatigue, stiffness, immobility, and limited endurance. School-related activities that are affected by these problems are listed in Table 8-2.

Because JRA is so unpredictable, attendance at school can be erratic. Children may be out for 1 or 2 days at a time, which can cause serious difficulty in keeping up with the school

TABLE 8-2. School problems in children with JRA

Writing
Holding a pen or pencil
Typing
Working with hands creatively
Learning to play an instrument
Attention span when uncomfortable
Carrying books
Doing homework
Writing on the blackboard
Staying at school for a full day
Going to school every day
Writing long reports
Walking to classes
Getting to class on time
Sitting, standing, or walking for long periods
Participating in gym
Climbing stairs
Going on field trips
Using the bathroom independently
Carrying a tray at lunch
Finishing lunch on time
Taking medication
Doing exercises
Using walking aids
Wearing splints

work if the child is not tutored each time. Some children are also not well enough to attend school all day and may in fact only be required to do the scholastic work but miss out on the socialization and recreation. Gym and physical education are usually compromised because of the illness. Even though the child may not be able to do all of what is required during that time interval, he or she may be able to participate in some other way.

Schoolmates may not be aware of the arthritis but may notice some differences in the child. Usually schoolmates will ask questions that the child may not be able to answer. Many children are embarrassed by their condition and tell their playmates that they fractured a bone. Adolescents may operate under the assumption that their peers do not even notice their arthritis and refuse to discuss it. Teachers' responses vary depending on their knowledge about the condition. Many parents seem to think that it is not necessary to tell the teacher. This in fact usually causes many unfortunate repercussions. The teacher may think that the child is lazy or simply does not care. Some teachers find it very hard to believe that a child can feel so unwell on one day and perfectly fine the next. In addition to this, most children do look rather healthy with JRA and this may give not only the teacher but the schoolmates the impression that the child is "putting it on." On the opposite end of this spectrum, some teachers may go overboard in being solicitous to the child. This calls a lot of attention to the child, usually in an embarrassing way. Many teachers, however, are very understanding of the implications a chronic disease can have on the development of a child and try to, therefore, integrate the child into the normal school environment as much as possible.

Since the institution of Public Law 94-142, children with JRA are allowed the opportunity to have a core evaluation by a team of professionals in an effort to develop an individual education plan (IEP). The goal of this plan is to allow the child to get the best possible education while working with the illness or disability. There are many benefits to having an IEP, which include getting physical and occupational therapy during the school day. Therefore, if the health professional feels that the child requires regular therapy, it can be written right into the plan. An IEP can also help the child get a tutor more quickly since many schools insist that a tutor cannot be provided until the child is absent for 2 weeks. This of course is impractical for children with JRA since they may only be out for a few days at a time. It is possible to incorporate the need for a tutor into the IEP as early as day 1 or day 2 of being absent. Other things such as grades may also be addressed in the IEP. Since many children are so fatigued and are required to carry out a home exercise program at the end of the day, it may not be possible for them to do a large amount of homework. The health professional may request that the child, therefore, only be graded on the work that he or she is able to do rather than be penalized for the work that cannot physically be accomplished. IEPs should also address the physical setting of the school system. Location of bathrooms, stairs, distances, and transportation all need careful consideration.

EVALUATION

The child with JRA must be evaluated on three levels prior to the initiation of any therapeutic program. The extent of the evaluation may vary from one child to the next depending on the child's status. No professional should assume that all therapeutic programs are standard for these children. Instead, the program should be individualized, taking into consideration all facets of the child's and family's life-style. Due to time constraints, the health professional may need to use a series of screening questions that will give a fairly good sense of the child and family. The health professional should first determine who lives with the child and what the living arrangements are. If parents are out working, participation in a therapeutic program may be difficult. If transportation or finances are a problem, attending clinic or getting rehabilitation services may be close to impossible. The level of adjustment to disease within the family is essential for the health professional to be aware of. Educating parents about a home program may be futile during times of anxiety and depression. The professional, therefore, must assess where the parents are in the grieving cycle in order to integrate them into the treatment program (Table 8-3).

The health professional should seek out the child's and family's perceptions, attitudes, and motivations since they all have an impact on the treatment program's success. Screening questions to help elicit information in these areas are as follows [16]:

TABLE 8-3. Relationship of grieving cycle to instruction on home program

Stage of grieving cycle	Parent reaction	Health professional's role
Anxiety/denial	May be forgetful, may not want to "hear," may try to control the treatment program, may be noncompliant with the treatment program.	Support productive behaviors; start with a full assessment; keep home program very simple and only include what is absolutely necessary; incorporate other "helpers" until the parent is able to be more involved
Depression	Withdrawal; emotional; immobility; sadness, grief, and anger; beginning stage of awareness of the situation and its implications	Be supportive; provide information and involve parent at a slow rate depending on tolerance; provide repetition and clear explanations; involve others to relieve the parent
Reorganization	Starting to adjust and make changes in life that will help, participates in child's care, becomes more open with health professionals	Provide information and involve more in treatment; reinforce new behaviors and successes thus
Resolution	Starts to seek out or becomes involved with others in similar situations. May become more articulate privately and publicly about JRA, feels comfortable with day-to-day living and treatment program	Reinforce program as necessary; evaluate parent's involvement in the program periodically; may wish to seek out the parent's services in helping another parent; promote the child's independence in therapy especially as child gets older

1. What is the child's and family's previous experience with illness, especially with arthritis, and what was the outcome?
2. What does the child/family think caused the arthritis?
3. What do they think the child will be like in 10 years?
4. How has the arthritis affected the family routine?
5. What does the child/family think treatment (medication, exercises, splinting) will accomplish?
6. What has the child/family been told by the health team about the arthritis?
7. How threatening is the arthritis to the family structure?
8. Does the child/family feel that they have any decision-making power in the treatment?
9. How much hope do they have?
10. What are the cultural attitudes and beliefs of the family that would affect treatment?
11. Does the family usually participate and comply with treatment programs?

The child's function should be evaluated in the home, at school, and outdoors. It may be done by interview, by observation, or through questionnaires. Standardized testing for function in children with musculoskeletal deficits is limited. MacBain and Hills Functional Assessment Tool was developed for children with JRA [28]. It measures timed walking, running, stair climbing, donning socks and a vest, as well as grip strength. Other instruments appropriate for adolescents may be used (Fig. 8-1).

In general, the evaluation should probably include both objective and subjective data. It is

Name: _____ Functional Class: _____

Rate each task from 1–5 based on the following:

1. Can perform without help; performs as usual *before* onset of JRA
2. Since onset of JRA performs activity differently; needs help from another part of body, e.g., uses 2 hands, must sit, etc.
3. Performs with assistive device, e.g., jar opener, cane, raised toilet seat, etc.
4. Accomplishes full activity only with someone's help
5. Unable to do even with help
6. Pain. *P* should be placed next to each number if child has pain when performing activity

Activity	Date	Date		Activity	Date	Date
1. In and out of bed without holding on				27. Go to school 1-daily all day 2-absent 1–2 x/mo 3-part of each day 4-absent 4 or more x/mo 5-cannot attend		
2. Bra on and off						
3. Tee shirt/pull over on and off						
4. Slacks/panty hose on and off				28. Carry school books		
5. Socks				29. Write		
6. Shoes on and off				30. Participate in gym 1-always 3-sometimes 5-never		
7. Tie laces						
8. Pull up zipper in back						
9. Snap clothing				31. Carry lunch tray		
10. Button				32. Crafts		
11. Wash hair				33. Socializes with friend(s) away from home and school at least once a week 1-always 3-sometimes 5-never		
12. Comb hair front and back						
13. Brush teeth						
14. Shave						
15. In and out of tub						
16. In and out of shower				34. Ride bicycle		
17. On and off toilet				35. Dance		
18. Perineal care (after elimination, with menses)				36. Walk around house		
				37. Walk at least 2 blocks		
19. Cut serving of meat				38. Drive		
20. Open new jar				39. Get in and out of car		
21. Lift pan or kettle from stove with one hand				40. Use public transportation or take school bus		
22. Lift glass or cup to mouth with one hand				41. Turn key		
23. Wash dishes				42. Open car door		
24. Do laundry				43. Turn door knob		
25. Make up fresh bed				Subtotal		
26. Go up and down one flight of stairs without holding on				Total		

Score = number answered divided by total score

Function score rating: 90–100 Excellent • 70–89 Good • 60–69 Fair • less than 60 Poor

FIG. 8-1. Functional inventory for children with juvenile rheumatoid arthritis.

not enough to simply ask a child and family if the child is able to do certain things, especially self-care tasks since many may be able to do them but in fact do not because a family member wishes to help. Therefore, in addition to the usual questions related to "Are you able to . . ." the health professional should also ask if the child does these things on a regular basis.

A child should also be evaluated for the accomplishment of the expected developmental task for his or her particular age. The play activities of the younger child should be elicited and evaluated. Special emphasis is placed on play because it specifically aids in the development of the child's biophysical, cognitive, affective, and social development in the long run [45]. The health professional should be aware of the type of play the child enjoys as well as what the child is capable of doing. By observing the child in play, the professional can gain an understanding of the child's personality and then incorporate the most suitable play activities in the treatment program. Because of the overall impact play has on development, the health professional may alter treatment in such a way that the child sees the treatment as play.

The child's physical environment should be questioned in detail. The health professional should ask the family about physical layout of the house and school, architectural barriers, assistive devices, mobility and transportation problems, and the availability of others to assist the child.

The child's usual rest and activity patterns may be determined by asking the parents or child to describe an average 24-hour period. It is even more effective to have the child or parent keep a journal of all activities for two weekdays and one day on the weekend. This provides important information regarding how feasible it will be to add a therapeutic program into the family's usual routine. It also gives a fairly good picture of the child's fatigue and endurance levels. When keeping the journal the child may indicate those times during the day

there was pain, stiffness, or fatigue, and what was done to relieve these symptoms. Understanding the pain, stiffness, and fatigue cycle of a child will enlighten the health professional as to how much emphasis needs to be placed on these areas. It also provides key information as to when and how to interrupt this cycle with treatment strategies.

PHYSICAL EVALUATION

The physical evaluation should begin with very careful inspection of the child, preferably with as little clothing on as possible but with respect for the child's privacy. The child's posture, gait, and general mobility should be observed [47]. Height and weight should be measured and compared to normal growth patterns. Deformities, growth discrepancies, muscle atrophy, and favoring of body parts should be recorded. The health professional should also appreciate how visible the general condition really is and compare this to the child's perception. Speed, hesitancy, and endurance can be determined by watching the child ambulate and move from one position to another. If possible, it may also be helpful to observe the child undress and redress.

The type of footwear and its efficacy should be assessed. Watching the child walk with shoes on as well as off will assist in this process. In order to determine the necessity for any change in treatment, the child should demonstrate the use of any aids, especially walking aids, as well as the home exercise program and the use of splints.

A full musculoskeletal examination is required. Each joint should be observed for swelling, bony enlargement, effusion, range of motion, stability, and deformity. Further distinction should be made in those joints that are swollen as to whether there is an active synovitis or chronic synovial thickening. The range of motion must be evaluated actively and passively. Tenosynovitis and tendon nodules should be sought since they may prevent the smooth movement of tendons. Measurement of muscle bulk and strength is essential in those groups surrounding the affected joints.

The health professional must seek out whether systemic features of the disease are present. Fever and fatigue especially can grossly interfere with any treatment program. The health professional should also be aware of the child's current medications and instructions provided by the physician. This information will be helpful in determining the content of an educational plan and how to integrate all parts of the treatment program into the child's daily life.

TREATMENT PROGRAM

The treatment program for all children with JRA, even though highly individualized, has goals that can be applied universally. The most important goals are to alleviate the inflammation and to prevent physical and emotional abnormalities and disabilities. Other long-term goals related to these are for the child to (1) master each developmental stage, (2) adjust to the many disease implications of JRA successfully, (3) make rational and intelligent decisions about behaviors affecting health and disease, (4) participate in self-care responsibly, and (5) progress to a normal and fulfilling adulthood.

The physical and emotional problems related to JRA dictate the necessity for a team approach [2]. The team of professionals usually consists of a pediatric rheumatologist, nurse, physical therapist, occupational therapist, social worker, opthalmologist, and orthopedist. A physiatrist, psychiatrist, and nutritionist are commonly consulted. The team is usually directed by the pediatric rheumatologist and coordinated by the nurse. The coordinator also acts as the liaison between the health team, the family, the school system, and other professional referrals. Team meetings on a regular basis to update all members on the child's status are helpful in making the necessary adjustments to the treatment program. It is generally agreed that the management of the child should be conserva-

tive in nature, using careful thought and discretion with any addition or change in the program.

DRUG THERAPY

There is no medication that will cure the disease. Instead, the focus of drug treatment is to suppress the inflammation as much as possible. Aspirin continues to be the drug of choice because of its efficacy in reducing inflammation and its relative safety. The dose is based on the child's weight usually from 75 to 100 mg/kg/day in four divided doses. The side effects include stomach upset, constipation, bleeding, tinnitus, lethargy, hyperactivity, and hepatitis. The aspirin should always be taken with food in an effort to prevent gastric irritation. Brushing the teeth after chewing baby aspirin may be helpful in reducing dental caries.

The only other nonsteroidal anti-inflammatory drug that is approved for children of all ages is Tolectin 25 to 30 mg/kg day in three to four divided doses with food. If aspirin or Tolectin proves ineffective or causes toxicity, naproxen, ibuprofen, and sulindac are sometimes used. It should be emphasized that these drugs have not been subjected to trials in children and are not approved for use in children by the Food and Drug Administration.

Some children require the added assistance of slow-acting anti-inflammatory agents. The two most commonly used to suppress disease activity are gold salts and hydroxychloroquine. Each is used in the presence of aspirin or another nonsteroidal anti-inflammatory drug. The gold is given intramuscularly on a weekly basis for 20 weeks. If at that point the child is doing well, then it may be extended to every 2 to 3 weeks. Side effects include rash, mouth sores, dry skin, proteinuria, and bone marrow suppression. This form of treatment requires additional family time simply to have blood tests drawn routinely as well as going for a weekly injection. Injections at the pediatrician's office may not be covered by health insurance and add to the expense of the treatment.

Hydroxychloroquine (Plaquenil), usually used in the older child, is given orally on a daily basis. Like gold, it may take several weeks before its efficacy is evident. The main concern with using hydroxychloroquine is the potential for causing retinopathy. Even though this is not common, it may impose the risk of serious visual problems.

D-penicillamine, which is commonly used in the treatment of adult RA, is not approved for use in children. Some physicians have chosen to use D-penicillamine nonetheless, especially if the child has very aggressive unrelenting disease in spite of the standard drug therapy.

Steroids are used as infrequently as possible because of the severity of side effects, especially disturbance in growth. It may be necessary to use steroids in the event of a life-threatening situation such as pericarditis or myocarditis. They also may be required in the presence of uveitis. Ordinarily, the eye is treated with steroid drops, but in some cases, oral steroids may need to be added. The administration of intrarticular steroids is relatively uncommon in children. However, if the child is unresponsive to the standard oral medications, and a single joint is very active, the physician may choose this method. Children also do not seem to benefit from the same degree of relief as adults with this form of treatment.

Steroids taken on a daily basis orally have a number of serious side effects. They include weight gain, redistribution of adipose tissue, osteoporosis, hypertension, Cushing's syndrome, major body-image changes, cataracts, glaucoma, increased susceptibility to infections, and reduced healing ability. High doses of steroids may also cause the child to become quite depressed or hyperactive. Most side effects are reduced when the steroids are taken on an alternate-day basis.

EYE CARE

Because of the seriousness of uveitis in children with JRA, it is the responsibility of all team members to remind the parent and child of eye follow-up care. Preferably, a flow sheet should be kept in the child's chart to record ophthalmologic exams. Parents and children tend to forget about these examinations because of the lack of symptoms associated with the inflammation. The physical therapist is usually the team member seen by the family most frequently and is in an excellent position to provide close follow-up of these appointments.

PHYSICAL THERAPY

The physical therapist is involved with improving the child's motion and strength, preserving the best possible function, preventing musculoskeletal abnormalities, and promoting childhood development [15]. The physical therapist also acts as a health educator. Both parents and children require instruction from the therapist about what is expected of them in the home and school situation. However, the therapist must make the child as independent as possible in the treatment program. Almost all children with JRA require a physical therapy program at some time during the course of their disease. Most exercises should be performed at least once a day but preferably twice a day depending on the home and family assessment. Even joints that are acutely inflamed need physical therapy. Acute synovitis requires gentle passive range of motion by the child, parent, or appropriate delegate. During a period of active synovitis, one of the worst motions a child can endure is a forced flexion of the affected joint. This can be especially harmful to the finger joints, wrists, hips, and knees. As an example, children who flare a knee joint may not have been told to discontinue their more aggressive flexion program. This may not come to the health provider's attention until it becomes evident that the synovitis is not improving. Frequently, once the forced flexion is discontinued, the knee joint will begin to settle down.

All the joints of children with JRA must go through range of motion daily. No one should assume that participating in the usual activities of daily living will suffice. If the joints are not moved through their entire range on a regular basis, usually daily, the joint will slowly lose its full range. Both parents and children find this very difficult to understand when the child is physically active. During acute flares passive range of motion is initiated. As the flare decreases, active assisted exercises are added. Most children, especially in the younger age groups, require an active assisted program especially since they are not able to gauge their own range and progress or lack of progress. Active range of motion programs may be the ideal but are usually not practical for just these reasons. Range of motion may be assisted with the use of overhead pulleys as well as daily prone lying, especially while watching television. The therapist cannot assume that because the child is capable of doing an active program that he or she in fact is disciplined enough or interested enough to do so. Children expect an immediate response to any of their actions. Exercises do not provide this and, as explained earlier, children cannot appreciate the long-term benefits or problems related to their behaviors. This, therefore, places much of the burden of the program on the parent. Because of the risk of promoting dependency as a result of this, the therapist may wish to suggest another adult to monitor the child's program.

If the child is especially stiff during the day in between exercises, the physical therapist might suggest simple movements, especially in the classroom that would go unnoticed but would allow the child to range the joint and limber up. For instance, the child may slide the feet back and forth under the chair and desk, open and close the hands, or place the hands behind the head and stretch the elbows back.

A common complaint of families and adolescents is that they do not have time to exercise. The therapist should try to work around these concerns and make suggestions for performing exercises during other activities. Younger children may be able to carry out range of motion

exercises while at play such as throwing balls, sitting on the floor with the legs apart and swinging them in, and reaching activities. Bath time is important for carrying out exercises also because of the beneficial effects of the warmth and bouyancy of the water. The parent can include exercise play activities while in the tub and pretend that they are simply playing. Adolescents may wish to do exercises while in the shower. Cervical spine range and upper extremity ranges can be done quite easily and effectively with the assistance of the heat of the water to promote relaxation. The adolescent can actually walk the hands up the wall of the tub to stretch out the shoulder joints while the water is directed at the shoulder. Children who are stiff in the morning are significantly helped by taking their medication 30 to 60 minutes before arising with a glass of water and some crackers and then doing as many of the range of motion and isometric exercises in bed before arising as possible. The warmth of an electric blanket or down comforter can also be helpful in loosening up in the morning.

Isometric exercises are essential in most children with arthritis. Isometrics in the presence of knee synovitis not only provide strength to the quadriceps muscle but often alleviate the stiffness when going from a sitting to a standing position. After sitting for a while at a desk at school or at the movies, the child may wish to extend the knee and tighten up the quadriceps muscle slowly 10 times before arising. This also helps to reduce limping when present. Isometric exercises should be taught from firm surfaces; thus, soft mattresses should be avoided. Parents may be taught to provide resistance to certain muscle groups to improve on the muscle strength.

Some children may also require postural exercises. Even if the child does not have to carry out a specific program, the child should be aware of how he or she is standing and walking and ways to improve on these. Special attention should be paid to the child's sleeping habits. Firm mattresses as a rule are more supportive to the musculoskeletal system. Flat pillows and cervical pillows are helpful in promoting extension of the cervical spine. The role of waterbeds in children with JRA is uncertain even though children may feel more comfortable in the morning and more mobile when they awaken. It is unclear as to how this type of bed, which conforms to the shape of the body, affects posture, joint contractures, and deformities.

Hydrotherapy should be incorporated into the treatment program for as many children as possible. This may be done in the form of simple tub baths. Many children also benefit from the use of the whirlpool, hubbard tank, or large hydrotherapy pool. Children should be encouraged to swim as much as possible, preferably twice a week. It is noteworthy that the range of motion is actually seasonal because they are only able to swim during the summer months. Group games and exercises in a pool for children with JRA are helpful not only in assisting the range of motion but also in promoting socialization and a sense of accomplishment. Games with balls and hoops are often enjoyed by all children and help with upper extremity mobility and strength.

The physical therapist may be involved with gait analysis as well as splinting or casting of the lower extremities. Gait analysis is more commonly being used in children with JRA and requires observation and analysis by trained experts.

Splints are often used in the lower extremities to rest a greatly inflamed joint. Splints may also help in preventing or reducing deformity. They are usually made of plastic or plaster. Bivalve casts are relatively common for children with knee synovitis and flexion contractures. They are worn when in bed and are removed in the morning. As the flexion contracture improves, the splint will either be altered to meet the changes or a new one will be fabricated. Some physicians also prefer serial casting. This has not been well studied in JRA. Serial casting for some can mean keeping a cast on for 7 to 10 days at a time or bivalving a cast and using the same one for 7 to 10 days but allowing the joint

to go through its range of motion twice a day. The fear with keeping a cast on for several days is that the joint will stiffen. With any form of splinting it is essential to pay careful attention to the surrounding muscles, making certain that their strength is maintained.

Most children adapt well to the use of splints in bed. If, however, they find bilateral splints cumbersome, the family may wish to alternate the splints from one night to the next. In an effort to promote independence, the physical therapist should encourage even the younger children to assist with the application and removal of splints.

Physical therapists usually participate in the decision regarding the use of walking aids. In general, children with lower-extremity involvement do not require the assistance of walking aids over the long term. However, some children do require periodic assistance with their mobility. Other children who have severe disease will require the use of crutches until they are able to have joint replacements. Children with upper-extremity disease often find it difficult to use axillary or forearm crutches. Instead, platform crutches or a platform walker are used. Children who have severe disease and require such walking aids often need even more assistance when trying to ambulate even greater distances. For this reason, some children may require the use of large strollers and wheelchairs in order to be mobile on a temporary basis. Generally, pediatric rheumatology teams are against these modes of transportation. They appear to contradict the philosophy of the child's care. However, there are certain circumstances whereby the use of wheelchairs and strollers may in fact assist the child's function and independence. In any case, the decision to use these measures should be carefully and critically thought out.

OCCUPATIONAL THERAPY
The goals of the occupational therapist are similar to those outlined under the section on physical therapy. However, the occupational thera-

pist should place greater emphasis on the child's development in relation to function. For this reason, the occupational therapist is concerned with those children who have upper-extremity involvement. The same principles relating to exercise, hydrotherapy, and splinting outlined for the physical therapist also apply. The most commonly used splints in the upper extremities are for the wrists. Wrist splints are usually custom made with the wrist joint placed in a neutral position, approximately 10 to 15 degrees of dorsiflexion. Like other splints, wrist splints are used to help reduce inflammation and prevent deformity. They are also used to help maintain the motion of the wrist, especially extension. Many children with wrist involvement tend to adapt to a flexed position and use their hands in this position for much of the day. A common posture in these children who are concerned about the appearance of their hands is to stand with their arms crossed and their hands located in the opposite axillae. This position only encourages flexion. Because of the continuous assumption of a flexed position, many children may also require the use of functional splints. A functional splint may be quite helpful in assisting the child with writing at school or even playing certain games. Most children do not like to wear splints during the day because they are noticeable. The splints should therefore be fabricated to be as inconspicuous as possible.

Lightweight plastics are usually the most practical materials for splints in children because they can be modified as the child grows and cleaned easily. Corrective or dynamic splinting in children is relatively uncommon. Its efficacy has never been determined and it is rather cumbersome for a child to become accustomed to. There are occasions, especially after hand surgery, that the surgeon may request dynamic splinting. Finger splints may be helpful in resting PIP joints when a single joint is involved.

The principles of joint protection and energy conservation are major parts of the home program for an adult with RA. These principles, even though important in the long run, probably do not need the same emphasis in a child. It is not clear whether these principles have any impact on the preservation of the joint. An average home program often consists of medication 4 times a day, exercises twice a day, splints at bedtime, lying prone, and hydrotherapy. This means that the child is asked to do nine specific activities on a daily basis that not only affect him or her but the family as well. To add a regimented program for joint protection and energy conservation in light of the uncertainty of its success or failure may be completely overwhelming. Instead, as the child gets older and learns new tasks, the therapist may wish to include joint protection gradually. There are obvious situations, however, in which it would probably be counterproductive for a joint not to be protected. As a rule most children and parents can be advised against repetitive and aggressive motion of an involved joint. An example of this would be jumping, running, or playing basketball on a swollen knee. Since the goal of the team is to promote the child's normal development, it is essential to encourage a healthy attitude about life rather than living life around an illness.

A child's independence may be enhanced by the institution of assistive devices [6]. These might include a long-handled sponge, a long-handled brush, self-help clothing, and elasticized shoe laces. Again, assistive devices should be implemented with discretion to prevent the child from developing the attitude of being disabled.

The occupational therapist plays a key role in promoting the developmental tasks of the child. He or she may wish to identify activities that would be fun for the child but would assist with range of motion, function, and accomplishment of the expected developmental task [29]. Suggested activities would depend on the areas the therapist wishes to improve on. Table 8-4 outlines suggestions for fun activities that would assist with range of motion and development.

Children will frequently limit their own activi-

TABLE 8-4. Fun activities to promote range of motion and development

TODDLERS	SCHOOL-AGE CHILD
Finger painting	Swim
Stack blocks	Ride bicycle
Play with Play Doh	Cut and fold paper
Pattycake	Play with clay
Place stickers in books and on paper	Do card tricks
Pick up small objects with fingers and place them in containers	Play instruments
Button play clothes	Play with marbles
Make hand impressions on paper with paint	Dance
Roll a ball on the floor with legs spread	Play with Nerf or rubber ball
Turn pages	Skate
Ride a tricycle	Knit or crewel
Run hands through sand	Type
PRESCHOOLERS	Finger puppets
	Twirl baton
Play Simon Says	Play charades
Make hand impressions in Play Doh	TEENAGERS
Lie on floor and pretend to make angels	
Lie prone on floor while playing	Hairdos
Cut with scissors	Cook
Tie shoes and make bows	Sweep
Play with toy tools	Paint
Make bubbles in water with hands	Sculpt
Paste	Play instrument
Throw ball overhead	Swim
Paint	Pingpong
Ride a tricycle	Apply makeup
Roll Play Doh to make balls and snakes	Do light housework
Write on a blackboard	Sew, knit, crewel, and macrame
Paste picture high on a wall	Dance
Play in pool	Play cards
	Play ball
	Badminton

ties depending on how they feel. However, some children do not use good judgment because they wish to participate with their friends. The child should be encouraged to discuss what he or she wishes to do with the team when in doubt. Most health teams are in tune with the child's needs and desires and try to place as few restrictions on the child as possible. However, usually contact sports should be avoided.

RELIEVING PAIN
Some children with JRA never experience pain in any of their joints. This is most commonly seen in children who have pauciarticular disease. Other children with polyarticular disease have chronic pain. Pain-relieving strategies are not used as frequently in children as they are in adults. Many of these strategies have not been well tested in children and therefore are not proved to be safe. Also, many need close supervision as well as cooperation from the child.

Medications are sometimes helpful. Acetaminophen, while it does not reduce inflammation, may relieve some of the discomfort and can be taken in conjunction with the nonsteroidal anti-inflammatory drug. Taking nonsteroidal anti-inflammatory drugs 30 to 60 minutes prior to the exercise program may facilitate movement and comfort.

Heat is probably the most commonly used pain reliever in children. Temporary relief may be provided with the use of hydrocollator packs, heating pads, warm water, or paraffin. The child should be supervised with all of these methods for delivering heat. Diathermy modalities appear to be inappropriate for children even though they are widely used in adults. Children may not communicate discomfort during this procedure and may suffer from internal burns.

Cold therapy is sometimes helpful in reducing pain and muscle spasm. It may be provided in the form of ice, ice water mixtures, commercial chemical cold packs, and ethyl chloride spray [5]. In children with JRA it is more common for cold to be delivered in the form of ice cubes in a plastic bag or from frozen vegetables in plastic bags, especially peas and corn. The cold is usually applied until numbness occurs and then is discontinued.

The choice of heat or cold to relieve pain is essentially an individual decision. It is a matter of preference and convenience.

Massaging of muscles may also provide significant although temporary relief. The use of relaxation techniques and visual imagery can be very effective in children over the age of 9. By distracting the child with an image that the child decides beforehand, the child is assisted into a state of relaxation by the health provider, and then the visual image is repeated for the child using all of the senses. This method for relieving pain requires a fair amount of concentration and therefore discipline on the child's part. It is effective in assisting children with coping with intra-articular injections and blood tests.

OTHER INTERVENTIONS
Children with JRA affecting the lower extremities, especially the feet, should wear well-fitting and comfortable footwear. Proper footwear may serve more to relieve discomfort rather than to correct or prevent deformity. Time-lapse studies of children reveal that the efficacy of shoe corrections is probably minimized because the greater proportion of the child's time is spent sitting, kneeling, and lying down [24]. Many children are also very self-conscious of their footwear. Fortunately, children with JRA have benefitted from research in jogging sneakers. Children enjoy wearing these sneakers, which are usually well made and provide the proper support. For children with foot involvement of the polyarticular type, the jogging sneaker should provide a wide forefoot with adequate depth. A high arch with weight slightly off the metatarsal heads makes the sneaker even more comfortable. Occasionally wedges are inserted within the shoe to help reduce deformity. Some authorities use medial heel wedges to aid in correcting forefoot valgus deformity [24]. Occasionally, in the older child, custom-made orthoses may be ordered to accommodate or cushion the forefoot. These are usually made from plaster foot molds rather than from tracings of the foot [50]. The health professional should evaluate the shoes and orthoses to ensure that common childhood deformities such as calcaneal valgus and equinovarus deformities are being treated. Adolescent females may find it uncomfortable to wear flat shoes due to a slow loss of dorsiflexion of the ankle. The adolescent may wish to wear shoes with heels, which further promotes the problem; stretching exercises may be helpful. The child's foot should be examined both with shoes on and off.

Children with limb-length discrepancies may also require the use of a lift on the shorter side. The lift should be slightly less than the discrepancy. The lift should be applied to all of the child's shoes on that side.

Cervical collars are used relatively infrequently in children with cervical spine involvement. Soft collars may be used for partial immobilization. They also may be used to prevent further flexion deformities. The child may be asked to wear the cervical collar while reading or doing homework, both being activities that would cause forward flexion of the cervical spine. Children with subluxation of the spine may require the use of a more rigid neck collar. This type of collar is very often prescribed for use while riding in an automobile because of the risk involved with a sudden unpredictable force to the neck [13].

Many parents ask about the role of diet in their child's treatment. Thus far there is no scientific evidence that diet affects the onset or course of the disease. It is usually recommended that the child eat a well-balanced diet to promote normal growth and that children maintain their weight within a range consistent with their height. Some children, mostly in the adolescent years and primarily females, may become obsessed about their weight. In our clinic population we have only observed this in females who have had polyarticular disease for many years. It has been assumed that much of this behavior is on the basis of having very little control in their lives. Eating and choices of food appear to be the only areas of control that they have. We have never seen this progress to severe anorexia nervosa.

ROLE OF SURGERY IN JRA
The most frequently performed surgery in the patient with JRA is the epiphysiodesis, synovectomy, and arthroplasty of the hip and knee. Arthrodesis (fusion of a joint) and soft tissue release usually of the hip are performed relatively infrequently [26].

The epiphysiodesis is performed to prevent growth of the epiphysis in the presence of a leg-length discrepancy. This is ordinarily done by a stapling procedure that is reversible if necessary. Isometric exercises are required postoperatively.

Synovectomy, the excision of synovial membrane or sheath, is usually indicated if there is a persistent synovitis in spite of adequate medical treatment and in the presence of a near normal joint space [18]. The fear for any health team when one joint continues to be active and aggressive in spite of all methods of conservative treatment is destruction and deformity in the joint. The joint most commonly requiring a syn-

ovectomy is the knee. Synovectomy of the MCPs and wrists may also be performed. Results of large-joint synovectomies are good in about two thirds of the joints with regard to reduction in synovitis [21]. Those children with "boggy" synovitis show far better results than those who have "dry" joints. Postoperative care for synovectomies of the knees requires intense training for the quadriceps muscle. Isometric exercises should be instituted immediately if synovitis occurs in the knees. Very often though as the synovium becomes more boggy, isometrics become more difficult to perform. Children should be encouraged to do their isometrics as close to the surgery as they are able so that they will need as little retraining as possible postoperatively. Prevention of postsurgical contractures are of the utmost importance. Resistance exercises and crutch walking should be gradually added as the child progresses. Synovectomy through the arthroscope is now being done in some children, especially in the knee joint. It is still too early to compare these results with those done through arthrotomy. A major advantage of the synovectomy through the arthroscope is that the recovery period is much shorter.

Reconstructive surgery (arthroplasty) now offers a great deal of hope for many children with severe JRA. It is primarily done to improve the young adult's function. Most orthopedic surgeons feel that it is best to wait for bones to stop growing before this type of surgery is performed. Therefore, most of the joint replacements are done between 17 and 30 years of age. Hand surgery is the most common type of reconstructive surgery in this population. Total hip and knee replacements are done less frequently. Those patients with severe polyarticular disease usually require multiple surgical procedures [46].

Children with severe deformity and functional limitation may benefit from reconstructive surgery. Multiple joint involvement creates problems for the rehabilitation process. Ambulation after hip and knee surgery requiring the use of walking aids can be hampered due to upper-extremity disability. Adolescents and even young adults with JRA anticipating reconstructive surgery very often perceive the rehabilitation and the results in a somewhat distorted way. The child's expectations as well as those of the parents should be clarified prior to the surgery. The orthopedic surgeon as well as the other health professionals on the team should also discuss the surgery and its potential risks and benefits realistically. Physical therapy and occupational therapy in children postoperatively are consistent with those provided to adults with total joint replacements. Special concerns, however, exist in this population regardless of age. When reconstructive surgery is done to joints in the lower extremities, upper-extremity range and strength should be monitored. A careful evaluation of function, disease activity, joint measurements, stability, and muscle strength should be followed. Some young adults develop an attitude that the joint replacement is the cure for their disease, and that therapeutic exercises can be cut back. It is also very difficult to request young adults to increase their therapy programs when they have been doing exercises for many years for their arthritis. Some feel that the exercises never helped them and that is why they require joint surgery. Ambulation postoperatively after lower-extremity reconstructive surgery can be difficult if there is upper-extremity deformity or active disease. Patients usually require the assistance of platform walkers or crutches to redistribute the weight over the upper body. It is hard to convey that exercises postoperatively will be beneficial. Preoperative assessment of attitude, motivation, and expectations will help the therapist to determine reasonable goals and outcomes for the patient.

PSYCHOSOCIAL SUPPORT
Medical or surgical treatments for the child with JRA may be in vain if there is no psychosocial support. It is the responsibility of the health team to evaluate this support system as previously described and to intervene appropriately. Support from health team members is usually greatly appreciated by the family. However, the family members may need some professional assistance in helping themselves and one another. Parents may need assistance with learning better communication skills with their children, especially adolescents. Professional counselling may be required to help with anger, guilt, and depression [30]. Children who are usually silent about their feelings must not be ignored simply because they cannot express themselves well. The health professional should assume the child has feelings about the illness and limitations. Play therapy is an effective means for helping children to express themselves [43]. It is usually successful up until the age of 9. It can take on many forms such as the use of dolls, puppets, and doll houses. School children may be helped with play acting and role playing. Therapy groups for adolescents can be quite successful in helping them vent their feelings and frustrations [38]. Integrating role playing is also beneficial by using other adolescents in the role playing. Since all children with JRA at any age suffer from a feeling of powerlessness at one point or another, a tremendous amount of support can be provided to the child by giving back some of this control. The members of the health team can do this simply by allowing the child to make choices even for simple things. Questions such as "Would you like to do your exercises now or in ten minutes?" or "Would you like to take your pills with crackers or cookies?" allow the child to make the decision and to feel that he or she has some power over the situation. Participating in the decision making also assists with the promotion of independence and self-esteem. Independence can be fostered even further by directing the questions and treatment program to the child rather than to the parents. This can be done in the younger children starting at the age of 7. Parents also learn from this that the health team is placing the responsibility on the child rather than just on them [14]. As the child gets

older, usually after the age of 12, the health team should encourage the child rather than the parent to call if there are problems. This may need to be done with parent's guidance, but the child should learn to be at least partly responsible.

Feeling independent and confident about decision making in turn helps to develop good self-esteem. Children with JRA are at a disadvantage because of their disease and limitations. It is up to the health team to highlight and promote the child's assets and guide the child in positive behaviors. Children who are comfortable with themselves are better equipped to form meaningful relationships. Children should be allowed to have interactions with children their own age and not just with an adult population. Children who become too dependent on their parents often have little exposure to children of their own age. Helping the child and parent to separate even at the time of visits when the child is older can be quite helpful in promoting other interactions. Adolescents should be interviewed and examined privately. Parents may also be interviewed separately, and then the plan can be outlined with both the child and parents present.

Forming relationships at school provides experience for the child for later years. Learning to play with peers, to respond to their questions especially about their illness, and to care for oneself away from home are invaluable experiences. The health team shares the responsibility for the child's school attendance. Since school is so important in the development of independence, self-esteem, communication skills, and relationships, the child's exposure to the school environment on a regular basis is essential. If the accomplishment of school work or attendance is in jeopardy, then an IEP should be adopted for the child with input from the health team members. In some circumstances one of the health team members may be present at the core evaluation especially to reflect the philosophy of the team and act as an advocate for the child and family. When possible, the physical

therapy and occupational therapy program may be integrated into the child's school day. This is not a standard procedure but careful consideration is required before instituting this type of program. Therapy at school may call too much attention to the child and make the child feel too different. This would make the program counterproductive. If on the other hand the therapist is trying to help the parents promote the child's independence, then it may be more beneficial for the child to have therapy at school. Suggestions for IEPs that would integrate the treatment program into the child's environment as well as promote independence, self-esteem, socialization, and relationships are outlined in Table 8-5.

Many of the services provided by the health team are preventative and preparatory in nature. The team focuses on the child's physical and psychosocial status, trying to prevent problems in both and improve on deficits and assets. The long-term goal of "normal adulthood"

TABLE 8-5. Team suggestions for individual education plan

Keep set of books at school and another set at home
Have backpack or frontpack for carrying books
Have tape recorder for notes and homework
Use widegrip or built-up pens and pencils
Keep classes on same floor
Use elevator
Allow extra time to get to classes
With irregular school attendance supplement tutor
Make sure child gets seat on bus daily
Take medications on own (9 yr and over)
Keep physician's prescription in child's school file with directions
Allow child to move around the classroom when stiff
Allow child to choose a classmate to assist with lunch activities
Use electric typewriter
Promote art and music
Plan ahead for fire safety and field trips
Institute tutor after the second day of absence from school

should be a prime mover in the philosophy of the team. When the child has a chronic disease, this needs to be considered earlier than in other children. Issues commonly discussed in the high school years may have to be addressed in elementary school. These children may not be able to rely on their physical skills for employment and therefore must focus on their intellectual skills. Vocational counseling in the high school years is especially helpful. Good vocational counselors who are knowledgeable about chronic diseases can help direct the child and family for future planning. Testing of intellectual abilities and personal preferences can give additional information and direction. Assessment by the occupational therapist should be performed prior to the evaluation by the vocational counselor. This would guide the counselor in determining realistic employment goals. The rheumatologist should also indicate whether future reconstructive surgery would be necessary that would interfere with employment. The counselor should also be informed as to the individual's decision-making skills, attitude, and motivation.

Children who continue to have active disease in the adult years may also have continued problems with variations in health status on a day-to-day basis. Thus, the counselor develops a plan with the patient based on the physical status, psychosocial status, rehabilitation potential, educational background, possible physical and psychological stresses of employment, environmental factors, and the patient's personal long-term goals [42].

EDUCATING THE CHILD AND PARENT

One of the most important aspects of the treatment program for the child with JRA is the educational process [9]. The team can develop the greatest plan in the world for the child, but if the child and the parents do not understand it, then the efforts would be in vain. Members of the health team, often the nurse, should assess the child's and parents' impression about the illness, their knowledge base, experience, re-

sponses of significant others, and general expectations [37]. Learning the information about JRA is not simple and is influenced by many personal variables that include age, developmental stage, intelligence, physical and emotional status, environment, support, attitudes, motivation, personal concern, moral development, previous experience, and observational skills [16]. The educational plan must address not only pertinent factual information about the disease and treatment but also how to cope, make decisions, and enhance the child's and family's development and adaptation. The parents' status, especially in the grieving cycle, influences their ability to absorb and retain information that is discussed with them.

In all age groups one of the most important responsibilities of the health team prior to educating the child is to determine the child's perceptions. Children at the preoperational level

TABLE 8-6. Audiovisual aids for teaching parents and children

Preschool	School age	Adolescents and adults
Dolls	Pictures	Blackboard
Puppets	Stories	Overhead
Games	Posters	transparencies
Storybooks	Models	Slides
Hospital equipment (age appropriate)	Coloring and painting	Films
Coloring	Television	VCRs
Painting	Photographs	Magazines
Imitating	Drawings	Pamphlets
Cartoons	Records	Actual objects
Television	Games	Other patients
	Books	Flip chart
	Flannel boards	Pictures
	Hospital equipment (age appropriate)	Posters
	Play acting	Television
	Imitating	Computers
		Photographs
		Drawing
		Games
		Hospital equipment
		Role playing

TABLE 8-7. Incorporating developmental needs into treatment plan

INFANTS 24 MONTHS

Focus education on parents' and child's needs

Stress the importance of allowing child to experience environment through movement even if child has JRA

TODDLERS 2–4 YEARS

Allow child to have some control in plan

Elicit child's understanding and meaning of terms

Determine child's fantasies and fears

Spend ample time with parents possibly one at a time while the other holds the child

Use simple and concrete explanations with the child

Do not use child's favorite object in the demonstration

Reassure the child that he or she is not being punished

Use toys to distract child and make situation less threatening

Allow child to be held and comforted as much as possible by the parent

Use puppets, dolls, etc., especially to get child to imitate a behavior

Use stories related to situation that is being taught

Be honest; do not tell child something will not hurt if it will

PRESCHOOLERS 4–7 YEARS

Determine child's perception and understanding of situation through play (dolls, games, play acting)

Respect child's ritual in the drug program

Allow child to have some control; use positive reinforcers for new behaviors

Do not expose child to unnecessary frightening situations or objects

Be honest with child

Explain simply and sequentially

Discuss separately from parents

Play act situations

Use dolls, puppets, and toys to demonstrate

Model behaviors and have child imitate

Use three-dimensional experiences; pictures may give a distorted perception

Allow child to handle objects related to what is being taught

Reinforce positive behaviors

Play out experience whenever possible

SCHOOL AGE 7–11 YEARS

Remember to continue to promote child's independence

Plan with child's input

Present information factually in a simple and logical sequence

Be clear on child's perception of the situation

"Play therapy" (with dolls, etc.; no longer used after age of 9)

Acting out the situation is very helpful

May use pictures, models, and diagrams

May need to role play ways of relating illness to peers

May need to provide teaching for peers and siblings

Reinforce learned skills

Promote the child's active participation

Do not discuss JRA in terms of concepts (chronic disease, possible disabilities, unpredictability) unless child is advanced in concept development

After educating child have child respond in own way (verbally, acting, storytelling)

TABLE 8-7 (CONTINUED)

ADOLESCENTS 12–20 YEARS

Educational techniques include role modeling, board games, and group interaction
Have adolescent actively participate
Respect privacy
Teach adolescent one on one in clinic and parent separately
Have adolescent repeat or demonstrate what was taught
Next explain disease and medications with associated concepts (chronicity, unpredictability, etc.)
Use appropriate terminology with explanations and definitions
Teach with the goal of adolescent assuming responsibility and practicing self care
Incorporate adolescent in teaching by problem solving and decision-making skills
Teach in groups as much as possible
Encourage questions
When appropriate, use hypothetical situations to determine if adolescent can apply what was taught

should not be asked questions or provided information that would require abstract thinking. The health provider should instead identify the child's perception and provide the child with information through play such as using pictures, dolls, puppets, and games. As the child gets older, he or she will be able to understand more concrete thoughts but still will not be able to understand the concepts related to information. Adolescents are capable of thinking conceptually and forming conclusions from the information that is presented to them.

All educational experiences with the parents and child should take into consideration not only the psychosocial status but also the physical status, the learning style, the timing, and the setting [35].

The teaching strategies are age dependent. A minimum of three are considered to be adequate. One of these should always include audiovisual aids (Table 8-6).

All of the health team members should be concerned about incorporating developmental needs into the treatment plan itself. This can be accomplished through certain approaches, techniques, and educational strategies consistent with the child's stage of development (Table 8-7).

SUMMARY

Care of the child with JRA is complex. Not only does it take into consideration the needs of the child but those of the parents and family members as well. The medical and surgical management is individualized and requires the efforts of the child, family, and a full team of dedicated professionals. The psychological and social needs of the family require special consideration in the treatment plan. Educating the child, parents, and family is an ongoing process starting with making the diagnosis. All members on the team have a certain responsibility to provide relevant information to the family as each member works with them on the treatment program. The long-term outcome of these children is not only a function of the physical management of the child but also the successful attainment of developmental goals, psychological and social reinforcement, and the development of independence, self-esteem, and sound communication skills.

REFERENCES

1. Alepa, F. P. Juvenile Rheumatoid Arthritis. In G. K. Riggs and E. P. Gall (ed.), *Rheumatic Diseases: Rehabilitation and Management*. Boston: Butterworths 1984.

2. Allen, K., Holm V., and Schiefelbusch, R. *Early Intervention—A Team Approach*. Baltimore: University Park, 1978.
3. Ansell, B. Rheumatic Disorders in Childhood. In B. Kiernander (ed.), *Physical Medicine in Paediatrics*. London: Butterworths, 1965.
4. Arthreya, B. The Hand in Juvenile Rheumatoid Arthritis. *Arthritis Rheum.* 20:573, 1977.
5. Banwell, B. F. Therapeutic Heat and Cold. In G. K. Riggs and E. P. Gall (eds.), *Rheumatic Diseases: Rehabilitation and Management*. Boston: Butterworths, 1984.
6. Bare, C., Boettke, E., and Waggoner, N. *Self-Help Clothing for Handicapped Children*. Chicago: The National Society for Crippled Children and Adults, Inc., 1962.
7. Barry, P., and Stillman, J. S. Characteristics of juvenile rheumatoid arthritis. *Orthop. Clin. North Am.* 6:641, 1975.
8. Becker, M., and Maiman, L. Sociobehavioral determinants of compliance with health and medical care recommendations. *Med Care* 13:10, 1975.
9. Boutaugh, M., Amundson, S., Falco, J., et al. Learning Needs of Parents of Children with JRA: Perceptions of Parents and their Health Care Team. *Arthritis Rheum.* 28:S150, 1985.
10. Brewer, E. J. *Juvenile Rheumatoid Arthritis*. Philadelphia: Saunders, 1970.
11. Brewer, E. J., Bass, J., Baum, J., et al. Current proposed revision of JRA criteria. *Arthritis Rheum.* 20:195, 1977.
12. Brewer, E. J., Blattner, R. J., and Wing, H. Treatment of rheumatoid arthritis in children. *Pediatr. Clin. North Am.* 10:207, 1963.
13. Cassidy, J. *Textbook of Pediatric Rheumatology*. New York: Wiley, 1982.
14. Clark, N., Feldman, C., Freudenberg, N., et al. Developing education for children with asthma through study of self-management behavior. *Health Educ. Q.* 7:278, 1980.
15. Donovan, W. Physical measures in the treatment of juvenile rheumatoid arthritis. *Arthritis Rheum.* 20:553, 1977.
16. Erlandson, D. The Disease Process of JRA. In *Understanding Juvenile Rheumatoid Arthritis: A Health Professional's Guide to Teaching Children and Parents*. Atlanta: Arthritis Foundation, 1987.
17. Erlandson, D. The Teaching-Learning Process. In *Understanding Juvenile Rheumatoid Arthritis: A Health Professional's Guide to Teaching Children and Parents*. Atlanta: Arthritis Foundation, 1987.
18. Fink, C., Baum, G., Paradies, L. et al. Synovectomy in juvenile rheumatoid arthritis. *Ann. Rheum. Dis.* 28:612, 1969.
19. Gerber, L. Rehabilitation of Patients with Rheumatic Diseases. In W. Kelley, E. Harris, S. Ruddy, et al. (eds.), *Textbook of Rheumatology* (2nd ed.). Philadelphia: Saunders, 1985.
20. Gochman, D. Some correlates of children's health beliefs and potential health behavior. *J. Health Soc. Behav.* 12:148, 1971.
21. Granberry, W. M., and Brewer, E. Results of synovectomy in children with rheumatoid arthritis. *Clin. Orthop.* 101:120, 1974.
22. Howell, S. E. Psychiatric aspects of habilitation. *Pediatr. Clin. North Am.* 20:203, 1973.
23. Jacobs, J. *Pediatric Rheumatology For the Practitioner*. New York: Springer-Verlag, 1982.
24. Jahss, M. Shoes and Shoe Modifications. In American Academy of Orthopedic Surgeons. *Atlas of Orthotics*. St. Louis: Mosby, 1975.
25. Kalnins, I., and Love, R. Children's concepts of health and illness and implications for health education: An overview. *Health Educ. Q.* 9:104, 1982.
26. Kelley, W., Harris, E., Ruddy, S., et al. *Textbook of Rheumatology* (2nd ed.). Philadelphia: Saunders, 1985.
27. Levinson, J., and Brewer, E. *Juvenile Rheumatoid Arthritis: Diagnosis and Management* (monograph). Fort Washington, Pa.: McNeilab, 1978.
28. MacBain, K. P., and Hill, R. A functional assessment for juvenile rheumatoid arthritis. *Am. J. Occup. Ther.* 26:326, 1973.
29. MacDonald, E. M. (ed.). *Occupational Therapy in Rehabilitation*. London: Bailliere, Tindall & Cox, 1960.
30. Mattsson, A. Long-term physical illness in childhood: A challenge to psychosocial adaptation. *Pediatrics* 50:801, 1972.
31. McAnarney, E., Pless, B., Satterwhite, B. et al. Psychological problems of children with chronic juvenile arthritis. *Pediatrics* 53:523, 1974.
32. McCollum, A. *The Chronically Ill Child*. New Haven: Yale University Press, 1981.
33. McCormick, R. D., and Gilson-Parkevich, T. *Patient and Family Education*. New York: Wiley, 1979.
34. Miller, J., Spitz, P., Simpson, U., et al. The social function of young adults who had arthritis in childhood. *J. Pediatr.* 100:378, 1982.
35. Narrow, B. *Patient Teaching in Nursing Practice*. New York: Wiley, 1979.
36. Natapoff, J. N. Children's views of health: A de-

velopmental study. *Am. J. Public Health* 68:995, 1978.

37. Neill, K. Behavioral aspects of chronic physical disease. *Nurs. Clin. North Am.* 14:443, 1979.

38. Okamoto, G., and Phillips, T. *Physical Medicine and Rehabilitation.* Philadelphia: Saunders, 1984.

39. Petrillo, M., and Sanger, S. *Emotional Care of Hospitalized Children.* Philadelphia: Lippincott, 1972.

40. Petty, R. Epidemiology and Genetics of the Rheumatic Diseases in Childhood. In J. Cassidy (ed.), *Textbook of Pediatric Rheumatology.* New York: Wiley, 1982.

41. Rose, M. Coping behavior of physically handicapped children. *Nurs. Clin. North Am.* 10:329, 1975.

42. Sales, A. P. The Role of the Vocational Counselor. In G. K. Riggs and E. P. Gall (eds.), *Rheumatic Diseases: Rehabilitation and Management.* Boston: Butterworths, 1984.

43. Schaefer, C. (ed.). *The Therapeutic Use of Child's Play.* New York: Aronson, 1976.

44. Schaller, J. Juvenile rheumatoid arthritis: Series 1. *Arthritis Rheum.* 20:165, 1977.

45. Schuster, C. Play During Childhood. In C. Schuster and S. Ashburn (eds.), *The Process of Human Development.* Boston: Little, Brown, 1980.

46. Scott, R., and Sledge, C. The Surgery of Juvenile Rheumatoid Arthritis. In W. Kelley, E. Harris, S. Ruddy (eds.), *Textbook of Rheumatology* (2nd ed.). Philadelphia: Saunders, 1985.

47. Scrutton, D., and Gilbertson, M. *Physiotherapy in Paediatric Practice.* Boston: Butterworths, 1975.

48. Swezey, R. *Arthritis: Rational Therapy and Rehabilitation.* Philadelphia: Saunders, 1978.

49. Wallace R., Heiss, M., and Bautch, J. *Staff Manual for Teaching Patients About Rheumatoid Arthritis.* Chicago: American Hospital Association, 1979.

50. Wood, B. The Painful Foot. In W. Kelley, E. Harris, S. Ruddy (eds.), *Textbook of Rheumatology* (2nd ed.). Philadelphia: Saunders, 1985.

9 Physical Disorders

Martha K. Logigian

Birth Defects

There are numerous genetic and birth defect syndromes, skeletal dysplasias, and chromosomal abnormalities. Some can be detected prenatally through amniocentesis, fetoscopy, and radiographic visualization. These diagnostic tools assist the physician in establishing a definitive diagnosis, which enables accurate genetic counseling. Once a diagnosis is made, the genetic counselor can discuss the prognosis, availability, and value of possible treatment [16].

Table 9-1 presents some of the more common musculoskeletal abnormalities seen in rehabilitation programs. (For an in-depth discussion of these disorders, see the primary references cited in the table.)

CONGENITAL LIMB DEFORMITIES

Most limb abnormalities develop during the third to eighth week of embryonic growth. Teratogenic factors inhibit the orderly differentiation of the developing part, resulting in deformity determined by the stage in limb development and location of the destructive process. Causes of limb anomalies include genetic and environmental factors. Environmental agents, which account for approximately 10 percent of the defects include industrial chemicals and pollutants, caffeine, aspirin, nicotine,

TABLE 9-1. Musculoskeletal abnormalities commonly seen in rehabilitation programs

Syndrome	Clinical findings	Associated problems	Treatment	Reference
Achondroplasia	Short-limbed dwarfism (<50 in.), macrocephaly, hydrocephalus, prominent forehead, broad nasal bridge, short upturned nose, crowded teeth	Autosomal dominant, 80% new mutations, 1 in 10,000, otitis media	Orthopedic management, emotional support, genetic counseling	[8, 12, 20]
Arthrogryposis multiplex congenita	Intrauterine immobility due to neuromuscular disorders; fibrous ankylosis, deformed postures: elbow extension, club hand, hip dislocation, knee extension, club foot	Scoliosis	ROM exercises, splinting, postural supports, orthopedic surgery	[1, 6, 9]
Brachial plexus palsy	Often following traumatic delivery: shoulder internal rotation, adduction; scapulohumeral winging; elbow extension, pronation; if C7 spared: finger, wrist flexion; C7, C8, T1 involved: flaccid hand with autonomic dysfunction, loss of sensation	Fractured clavicle, humerus, cervical spine; torticollis; Horner's syndrome	Positioning; ROM exercises; later bilateral hand activities, strengthening, postural exercises; orthopedic surgery	[7, 10]
Diastrophic dysplasia	Severe dwarfism, short limbed, ear deformity, cleft palate, flaring nostrils, mouth abnormalities, hyperelastic skin	Progressive hearing loss, facial paralysis, optic atrophy	Hearing aids, genetic counseling	[8]
Legg-Calvé-Perthes disease	Avascular necrosis of femoral head/neck	Short stature, lower birth weight, delayed bone age, 7 in 1000	Infant: traction, active/assistive ROM exercise; once full ROM, ambulation with containment orthosis. Older children: orthopedic surgery (femoral osteotomy)	[17]
Marfan's syndrome	Tall, thin stature; hyperextensible joint; arachnodactyly; dislocation of lens and optic anomalies; aortic aneurysm and cardiac abnormalities	Scoliosis, 1 in 16,000, autosomal dominant	Orthopedic surgery/therapy, ophthalmologic management, cardiac surgery	[8, 16]
Noonan's syndrome	Short stature, variable manifestations: craniofacial, cardiac, genitourinary, skin, skeletal	Mental retardation (MR) may be present, 1 in 1000	Management of congenital anomalies, special schooling for MR, genetic counseling	[4, 8]
Osteogenesis imperfecta (OI)	Four forms: OI congenita (OIC), OI tarda (OIT) most common; OIC more severe; varying degrees of short stature; fractures with resulting deformities; craniofacial en-	Hearing loss; blue sclera (OIT) bruise easily. OIT usually autosomal dormant, OIC usually auto-	Orthopedic surgery, dental care, improve hearing function, postural supports, environmental	[8, 14]

	largement; teeth discolored, break easily	somal recessive, 1:20–60,000	controls, emotional support, genetic counseling	[8]
Phenylketonuria	Microcephaly, skin problems, neuromuscular abnormalities, blond hair	Mental retardation, hyperactivity; 1 in 15,000, autosomal recessive	Dietary restrictions, special schooling, genetic counseling	[3, 8]
Prader-Willi syndrome	Short stature, craniofacial and genitourinary abnormalities	Diabetes, obesity, mental retardation, scoliosis, small hands/feet, hypotonia, poor coordination, seizures, lack of emotional control	Dietary restrictions, behavior modification, special schooling, genetic counseling	
Rubinstein-Taybi syndrome (broad thumb–broad toe syndrome)	Short stature with skeletal, craniofacial, skin, cardiac, and renal abnormalities, including broad fingers/toes; large, beaked nose	Mental retardation, seizures, 1 in 600 in MR clinics	Medical/surgical management of abnormalities, special school, genetic counseling	[8, 18]
Stickler syndrome (arthroophthalmopathy, Wagner-Stickler syndrome)	Craniofacial abnormalities with cleft palate, deafness and blindness; joint enlargement; stiffness and limitation	Spondyloepiphyseal dysplasia and other skeletal problems (scoliosis, hip subluxation)	Early treatment of eye and joint abnormalities, repair of cleft palate; genetic counseling	[8, 11]
Torticollis (congenital)	Infant (2–3 weeks of age): head tilt with facial asymmetry, narrowing of palpebral fissure, flattening of occiput on contralateral side, fibrosis of affected sternocleidomastoid muscle	Limited ROM cervical spine affects chin rotation to affected side, lateral flexion to opposite side; long C-curve of spine; possible ipsilateral hip dislocation	ROM exercises, neck collar, surgical tenotomy followed by stretching exercises positioning of mobiles and crib	[5, 6]
Thrombocytopenia with absent radius (TAR syndrome)	Bilateral absence of radius and limb abnormalities, thrombocytopenia	Craniofacial changes, may have heart disease and mental retardation	Orthopedic management; platelet transfusions	[8]
Treacher Collins syndrome (mandibulofacial dysostosis)	Craniofacial abnormalities with hearing loss	Facial skeletal abnormalities	Hearing aids, reconstructive facial surgery, genetic counseling	[8]
Tuberous sclerosis (Bourneville's syndrome, epiloia)	Café au lait spots, acnelike lesions, congestive heart failure, cystic areas in phalanges, calcium deposits in brain	Mental retardation, seizures	Anticonvulsants, surgical removal of tumors, special schooling, genetic counseling	[13]

TABLE 9-1 (CONTINUED)

Syndrome	Clinical findings	Associated problems	Treatment	Reference
Turner's syndrome (XO syndrome)	Short stature, lack of secondary sexual characteristics, webbed neck, heart disease	Ptosis, craniofacial changes, skeletal changes of metacarpal and metatarsal sterility	Surgical intervention where necessary, estrogen therapy, psychotherapy for adjustment, genetic counseling	[8, 15]
Vater anomaly	Growth deficiency: vertebral defects; cleft palate; heart, skeletal, and ear abnormalities; radial dysplasia, scoliosis, lower limb defects	Anal atresia, esophageal stricture, tracheoesophageal connection, kidney anomalies	Treatment of skeletal, gastrointestinal, and cardiac defects; genetic counseling	[19]
XXY syndrome (Klinefelter's syndrome)	Long limbs, thin appearance, small penis/testes, sterility	Low-normal intelligence, behavior problems, seizures, clinodactyly of 5th fingers	Testosterone replacement therapy, special schooling, genetic counseling	[2]
XYY syndrome	Tall stature, asymmetry of face and large ears/teeth	Mild mental retardation, aggressive behavior, ECG changes	Psychotherapy for behavior problems, special schooling, genetic counseling	[8]

1. Arthrogryposis Association, Inc., 106 Herkimer St, North Bellmore, NY 11710.
2. Caldwell, P. D., and Smith, D. W. The XXY syndrome in childhood: Detection and treatment. *J. Pediatr.* 80:250, 1972.
3. Clarren, S. K., and Smith, D. W. Prader-Willi syndrome: Variable severity and recurrence risk. *Am. J. Dis. Child.* 131:1977–1978.
4. Collins, E., and Turner, G. The Noonan syndrome—A review of clinical and genetic features in 27 cases. *J. Pediatr.* 83:941, 1973.
5. Eng, G. D. Congenital torticollis. *Clinical Proceedings, Children's Hospital National Medical Center* 24:75, 1968.
6. Eng, G. D. *Musculoskeletal Disorders.* Boston: Tufts Research and Training Center, 1981.
7. Eng, G. D., Koch, B., and Smokvina, M. D. Brachial plexus palsy in neonates and children. *Arch. Phys. Med. Rehabil.* 59:378, 1978.
8. Feingold, M., and Pashayan, H. *Genetics and Birth Defects in Clinical Practice.* Boston: Little, Brown, 1983.
9. Fisher, R. L., et al. Arthrogryposis multiplex congenita: A clinical investigation. *J. Pediatr.* 76:255, 1970.
10. Johnson, E. W., Alexander, M. A., and Koenig, W. C. Infantile Erb's palsy (Smellie's palsy). *Arch. Phys. Med. Rehabil.* 58:198, 1977.
11. Liberfarb, R. M., Hirose, T., and Holmes, L. B. The Wagner-Stickler syndrome: A study of 22 families. *J. Pediatr.* 99:394, 1981.
12. Little People of America, Box 126, Owatonna, MI 55060.
13. Monaghan, H. P., et al. Tuberous sclerosis complex in children. *Am. J. Dis. Child.* 135:912, 1981.
14. Osteogenesis Imperfecta, Inc., 1231 May Court, Burlington, NC 27215.
15. Palmer, C. G., and Reichmann, A. Chromosomal and clinical findings in 110 females with Turner syndrome. *Hum. Genet.* 35:35, 1976.
16. Pyeritz, R. E., and McKusick, V. A. The Marfan syndrome: Diagnosis and management. *N. Engl. J. Med.* 300:772, 1979.
17. Saturen, P. Skeletal Disorders in Children. In G. E. Molnar (ed.), *Pediatric Rehabilitation.* Baltimore: Williams & Wilkins, 1985.
18. Simpson, N. E., and Brissendes, J. E. The Rubinstein-Taybi syndrome. *J. Genet. Hum.* 25:225, 1973.
19. Temtamy, S. A., and Miller, J. D. Extending the scope of the Vater association: Definition of the Vater syndrome. *J. Pediatr.* 85:343, 1974.
20. The Human Growth Foundation, Maryland Academy of Science Bldg., 601 Light St, Baltimore, MD 21230.

hormones, irradiation, and some viral infections [57].

Congenital limb defects are classified by Swanson [57] into seven major categories. Table 9-2 presents a summation of these categories and rehabilitation highlights. Many general birth defect syndromes, particularly the skeletal dysplasia syndromes, have associated limb abnormalities. (For a more complete review of these syndromes, see Feingold [16] and Molnar [42].)

Rehabilitation management of the juvenile amputee addresses the child's growth potential and muscle coordination and development. There needs to be an early replication of function for both upper- and lower-limb deficient children, including a training program that recognizes that children's activities are different from adults'. Team members must make an effort to decrease demands on the parents, including controlling costs of equipment. The parents' acceptance and that by other children and school personnel is critical to the successful rehabilitation of the juvenile amputee. The overall goals of the rehabilitation program are to improve function and cosmesis.

UPPER-EXTREMITY TRAINING

In general, children are fit with a passive prosthesis by the age of 5 months and a prosthesis with a cable by the age of 2. During the fitting period, the therapist completes a developmental evaluation of the child and introduces the family to the prosthesis. This includes the function, components, and maintenance of the prosthesis and care of the stump. The limb remnant is exposed to different textures and shapes to encourage environmental exploration and develop tactile awareness. The constant use of the passive prosthesis enables the child to continue to develop normal motor milestones such as trunk control, equilibrium reactions, balance, and sitting.

The initial prosthetic period focuses on parental instruction. The parents must encourage the child in age-appropriate activities. They need to feel comfortable with donning and removing the prosthesis so that they can encourage the child to do the same at the appropriate time. Wearing patterns and expectations should be carefully discussed. Operation and positioning of the terminal device are also explained so that parents can carry over all activities at home. Operation of the terminal device is usually initiated by the age of 2 1/2 (Fig. 9-1).

The below-elbow amputee is fitted with a standard upper-limb prosthesis that consists of a socket fitted to the residual limb and terminal device. It is held in place by a harness of canvas webbing and a cable that connects to the terminal device. Relaxation allows closure via elastic bands on the terminal device [9]. Parents are taught these principles, and progress is monitored through clinic visits [23].

The above-elbow amputee has a prosthesis fitted with an elbow joint. This is activated by a second cable that uses humeral flexion and extension to initiate elbow flexion and extension (i.e., unlocking the elbow). Shoulder depression locks the elbow in flexion. Wrist and elbow rotation is completed passively by the uninvolved hand [9]. Parents and child are taught how to lock and unlock the elbow, position the elbow, and operate the terminal device. As appropriate, the child is trained in one-handed techniques. Activities may also be adapted to the child's ability.

For the child with a shoulder disarticulation, one-handed methods are used early in the rehabilitation program. Myoelectrically controlled prosthetic components are particularly useful in high-level amputees [58].

In the event of a bilateral amputation, the training for the below-elbow amputee is the same as for the unilateral amputee. However, for the above-elbow and shoulder disarticulation amputee, the child should be allowed to develop foot skills. A variety of adaptive equipment is made available and age-appropriate skills are encouraged in this manner by the family and therapist.

TABLE 9-2. Congenital limb defects

Category	Rehabilitation plan
I. Failure of formation of parts	
A. Transverse: All congenital amputation-type conditions, classified by the level at which the existing portion of the limb terminates. All elements distal to that level are absent	
1. Phalangeal deficiency (aphalangia): one or more digits, any level of digit	1. Mild: no treatment; severe (function impaired): cosmetic prosthesis or surgical reconstruction (bone lengthening, digit transposition, or transplant); if foot, need shoe correction
2. Transmetacarpal amputation: usually unilateral and with D. Hand short, wide, with skin nubbins	2. Opposition palmar-pad prosthesis
3. Transcarpal amputation: total absence of phalanges and metacarpals; may have five skin nubbins and fusion of carpal bones	3. Opposition palmar-pad prosthesis
4. Transtarsal amputation: absence of phalanges, metatarsals, cuneiform and cuboid bones (forefoot). Triceps surae is underdeveloped, knee hyperextends	4. High shoe with reinforced steel shank and felt or foam shoe filler allows normal push-off in gait
5. Wrist disarticulation	5. a. Forearm dorsopalmar socket with terminal device activated by contralateral scapular abduction
a. Unilateral: long stump, skin nubbins, no skeletal elements distal to radius and ulna	b. Krukenberg forceps (Swanson) on dominant extremity and artificial limb on assisting, opposite extremity
b. Bilateral	
6. Forearm amputation: below-elbow defect	6. Below-elbow prosthesis[a] with prehensile hook and flexible elbow hinge
7. Elbow disarticulation: absence of bony elements distal to distal humeral epiphysis	7. Elbow prosthesis[a] with prehensile hook and flexible elbow hinge
8. Above-elbow amputation: absence of distal epiphysis	8. Above-elbow prosthesis[a] with prehensile hook, elbow lock, and turntable
9. Shoulder disarticulation: complete absence of upper limb	9. a. Shoulder disarticulation prosthesis with prehensile hook, elbow lock, turntable, shoulder cap
a. Unilateral	b. Compensatory skills with feet; externally powered prosthesis
b. Bilateral	
10. Ankle disarticulation: ankle and foot bones absent; distal tibial and fibula epiphyses present	10. Below-knee socket[b] with solid ankle-cushioned heel (SACH) foot
11. Below-knee amputation proximal tibia present, fibula slightly shorter—both taper distally; stump may be in varus	11. Below-knee prosthesis[b] with plastic socket, condylar cuff and SACH foot

12. Knee disarticulation: as K. with symmetrical stump without distal tapering
13. Above-knee amputation
14. Hip disarticulation: femur absent, no acetabular development

B. Longitudinal: all nonformation of limbs other than transverse
  1. Radial deficiency (preaxial deformity): radius and thumb, radius only, thumb only (radial clubhand)
  2. Tibial deficiency:
    a. Complete: leg short, varus foot, great toe absent, knee unstable, tibia absent, fibula bowed
    b. Incomplete: partial tibia, fibula present, yet may be positioned abnormally
  3. Ulnar deficiency: often seen with radial defects and shoulder girdle/proximal humerus defects; anomalies of elbow, wrist, hand, and digits
  4. Fibular deficiency:
    a. Total: bilateral (25%) and unilateral with leg-length discrepancy as tibia short, leg bows anteriorly, valgus foot, 3/4 digits; fibula absent, minimal distal tibial epiphysis
    b. Partial: minimal shortening of tibia and fibula
  5. Central ray deficiency (carpal or digital, or both): affecting 2nd–4th rays (lobster claw or cleft hand)
  6. Phocomelia: proximodistal failure of limb development
    a. Upper limbs: complete, proximal, distal
    b. Lower limbs: complete, proximal, distal

II. Failure of differentiation of parts
  A. Shoulder defects
    1. Sprengel's deformity: shoulder undescended
    2. Poland's syndrome: absence of pectoral muscles
  B. Elbow defects
    1. Dislocation
    2. Synostosis: proximal radioulnar joint
  C. Hand defects
    1. Symphalangism: intermediary digit joint missing, usually PIP, bilaterally
    2. Syndactyly: webbing of fingers, usually at 3rd and 4th digits
    3. Congenital flexion deformities

---

12. Knee disarticulation prosthesis[b] with SACH foot
13. as 12
14. Hip disarticulation[b]

1. Casting, surgery, e. g., osteotomy
2. a. Knee disarticulation amputation and prothesis
   b. Below-knee amputation and prosthesis
3. Above-elbow prosthesis with fenestration for residual digit
4. a. Ankle disarticulation amputation and prosthesis
   b. Shoe lift
5. Surgical reconstruction to improve function/cosmesis
6. a. Complete: use lower extremities for function, shoulder disarticulation prosthesis/myoelectric arm. proximal/distal: may need reconstructive surgery
   b. Complete: hip disarticular prosthesis proximal: electric wheelchair. distal: prosthesis

A. 1 + 2 may require surgical correction and therapy

B. 1. May require surgery and therapy
   2. Surgical correction and therapy

C. 1. Arthroplasty or osteotomy and therapy
   2. Surgical repair
   3. Splinting and range of motion exercises, early. May require surgery.

TABLE 9-2 (CONTINUED)

    4. Camptodactyly: congenital flexion contracture of PIP, 5th digit   4. Same as 3

    5. Clinodactyly

  D. Arthrogryposis (see Table 9-1)

III. Duplication

  A. Polydactyly: duplication of digit

    1. Duplication of thumb   1. Surgical correction

IV. Overgrowth (gigantism)

  A. Macrodactyly: digital enlargement

    1. All elements of digit enlarged   1. and 2. Surgical correction

    2. Excess tissue, along with neurofibromas, lymphangiomas,

       hemangiomas

V. Undergrowth (hypoplasia)

  A. Brachydactyly: digital shortening   A. Surgical correction not indicated

VI. Congenital constriction band syndrome (focal necrosis at the limb

    during fetal development)

  A. Constriction band, usually at distal extremities   A. and C. Surgical correction and therapy

  B. Amputation

  C. Acrosyndactyly: annular grooves, transverse amputations of distal

    parts, web space between fused digits

VII. Generalized skeletal abnormalities

  A. Dyschondroplasia (see Table 9-1 and reference [19])

  B. Marfan's syndrome (see Table 9-1)

  C. Diastrophic dwarfism (see Table 9-1)

[a] Upper extremity: Children fit with prosthesis when 5 mo. Children fit with cable when 2 yr.
[b] Lower extremity: Children fit with prosthesis when standing.

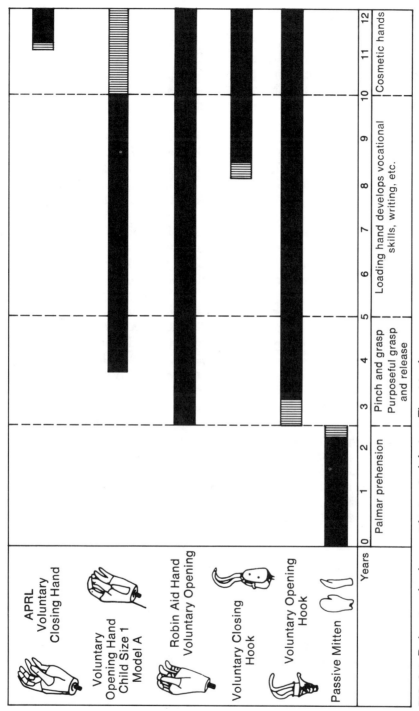

FIG. 9-1. Prehension development for terminal devices. The striped bar indicates use of device is in flux. (Adapted from the Area Child Amputee Program, Michigan Crippled Children Commission.)

237

Children are fit with a prosthesis by the time they are standing. As scoliosis is associated with a unilateral limb deficiency, postural training is important to begin early as well as strengthening of the residual and intact limb. Once the child is standing, weight-shifting and balance activities begin, progressing to ambulation and gait training on a variety of surfaces. Climbing and more complex skills are encouraged as motor control increases [9].

Challenor [9] suggests that for a proximal-limb deficiency, a lightweight extension limb should be in use by age 6 months, with weight bearing by 9 to 10 months. For the above-knee amputee, the initial prosthesis may not have a joint; however, by the age of 3, a lockable knee is used. As the child is able, activities are encouraged using the knee joint in an unlocked position.

Prostheses are fitted with a solid ankle cushion heel or SACH foot, which is available in a variety of pediatric sizes. Below-knee amputees are fitted with a modified patellar tendon weight-bearing socket. Auxiliary means of suspension are recommended for the early years to allow for normal childhood activities. Frequently this is a lateral knee joint with a thigh corset added to a patellar tendon-bearing socket. Depending on the type of prosthesis (involving hip, knee, or ankle articulations), suspension may be slip on (patellar tendon socket, suction, harness, or pelvic belt). Size and weight of the child and prosthesis are general considerations in fitting the prosthesis.

Muscular Dystrophy

Of the inherited neuromuscular disorders, perhaps the best known are the muscular dystrophies [1, 43]. These are hereditary, degenerative disorders of muscle characterized by progressive weakness and atrophy:

Becker (benign): X-linked

Duchenne (severe)
Resembling Duchenne (rapidly progressive)
Limb girdle (benign)
Fascioscapulohumeral
Distal
Ocular
Oculomotor
Dystrophia myotonica: floppy baby

The most common form of this disease is Duchenne's muscular dystrophy (DMD), with an incidence of 1 in 100,000. This is an X-linked, recessive disease causing progressive muscle weakness in boys. It is noticeable at about age 4 and leads to death at about age 20, usually of respiratory complications. Although muscle fiber degeneration begins soon after birth, for a number of years regeneration keeps up with degeneration. Eventually the muscles are replaced by fat and fibrous tissue [7]. Typically, there is a history of late motor milestones (e.g., the child learns to walk late, falls frequently, and has difficulty with stairs and rising from the floor). A waddling gait with increased lordosis and toe walking is common [15]. Gower's maneuver is exhibited, which involves pushing up when rising from the floor using the arms rather than the legs to push off to stand. Eventually, with great weakness, the child must climb up the legs with the hands to get to a standing position [28, 29]. By age 11 to 14 the adolescent loses the ability to walk due to instability of the trunk and requires the use of a wheelchair. Once in the wheelchair, a scoliosis may develop toward the dominant extremity. Muscles of the shoulder girdle are affected later. Psuedohyertrophy of the gastrocnemius is a distinctive characteristic of DMD [22].

There is an association of mental retardation with the disease due to inadequate formation of the cortex in utero, that is, amentia rather than dementia. There is also a progressive degeneration of the myocardium, leading to cardiomyopathy [7].

Genetic counseling is required as sisters of an

affected male will have a 50 percent chance of being carriers of the abnormal gene. Muscle biopsy is necessary to establish the diagnosis of DMD. An elevated creatinine kinase (CK) is important in early diagnosis and identifies carriers. The disease is believed to be due to membrane abnormalities in the muscle fibers (sarcolemma) allowing calcium to leak into the cell, poisoning mitochondria and inducing muscle fiber degeneration (fiber dies) [7].

As there is no effective drug therapy available, management of the patient focuses on the quality of life, no matter how shortened that life may be. Therapy is aimed at reducing side effects, such as contractures, and ensuring availability of adaptive equipment and psychological support. Frequent reassessments of the child's abilities are required to identify specific treatment strategies relative to the stage of the disease. For example, swimming is advocated for mobility, range of motion, and conditioning and can continue when the child can no longer walk [15].

Early in the disease, the child and parents should learn range of motion and stretching exercises, particularly of the flexors, to maintain posture and alignment. Strengthening of unaffected muscles is also indicated. As the child becomes weaker, lightweight night splints may be considered.

The child should be prepared for the use of a wheelchair, which includes adaptations for appropriate positioning and head support. An electric wheelchair can be useful as the disease progresses as well as electronic controls on the bed. Other necessary equipment can include commodes, hydraulic lifts, and accessibility devices designed to enable wheelchair independence.

Children should be encouraged to continue in regular school for as long as possible. Educational programs are directed away from career planning, toward the enhancement of the quality of daily life. Emphasis on short-term goals and avocational and functional activities can be useful and supportive [32]. Helping the child

and family cope with a degenerative disease is the major task of the health care team.

Neuromuscular Diseases

SPINAL MUSCLE ATROPHIES

There is an estimated incidence of spinal muscle atrophies (SMAs) of 1 in 25,000 births. They are a group of neuromuscular disorders that include the following disorders:

1. Infantile SMA (Werdnig-Hoffmann disease) develops before the age of 5 months, and death occurs usually by 2 years of age. Infants may be referred to as floppy babies with diffuse muscle weakness. There is an acute and chronic form of the disease; a scoliosis may be seen in the latter.
2. Benign infantile SMA usually develops after 6 months of age with survival into childhood or adolescence, but with severe disability due to weakness of skeletal muscles.
3. Juvenile and early adult SMA (Kugelberg-Welander disease) affects children between 5 and 15 years of age. It frequently simulates a muscular dystrophy with proximal muscle weakness and wasting. Myopathic changes are frequent [7].

All of these diseases are characterized by progressive degeneration of the alphamotor neurons in the spinal cord and brain stem causing denervation of skeletal muscles. They are usually inherited in an autosomal recessive manner, which makes genetic counseling critical. This is particularly important in the infantile forms, as there is a 1 in 4 risk of recurrence in subsequent children, if one child has the disease. If by the age of 5 there is no disease, the child is unlikely to develop it [7].

These diseases are of unknown etiology, with no accepted method for identifying carriers and no effective drug therapy for treatment. Supportive care is necessary and can include careful feeding with suctioning and postural drainage, positioning, and passive range of motion. If the infant survives into childhood or adolescence, assistive devices can be useful such as ambulation devices and electronic aids. A school program is important as well as emotional support for the child and parents.

CONGENITAL MYOPATHIES

These are a heterogeneous group of diseases characterized by muscle weakness and wasting from birth. The etiology is not clearly understood, and there is no effective drug therapy [7]. However, the more favorable outcome for those affected allows a more aggressive physical therapeutic intervention. Rehabilitation management would be similar to that of a child with a muscular dystrophy [15].

PERONEAL MUSCLE ATROPHY

Peroneal muscle atrophy (Charcot-Marie-Tooth disease [CMT]) includes a number of different diseases considered inherited neuropathies. All present with distal muscle wasting and weakness, beginning in the legs and later involving the hands. Most are diseases of early adulthood and do not limit life. Bradley [7] identifies three main categories:

I. CMT hypertrophic neuropathy: segmental demyelination of the peripheral nerves
   A. Dominant: adult onset
   B. Recessive (Dejerine-Sottas disease): childhood onset
II. CMT neurosensory motor type: degeneration of the neurons of the motor and sensory nerves
   A. Dominant: usually adult onset
   B. Recessive: usually adult onset
III. CMT spinal muscle atrophy type: degeneration of the anterior horn cells. Usually recessive: may have childhood onset

Detection of a patient with a preclinical form of the disease is possible to enable genetic counseling. The etiology is unknown, and there is no drug therapy. Exercise is important to prevent contractures and muscle imbalance. Orthotic and ambulation devices are useful. Adaptive devices are helpful particularly when there is weakness of the hand muscles [15].

NEUROFIBROMATOSIS

Neurofibromatosis (von Recklinghausen's disease) occurs in 1 in 20,000 live births. Inheritance is autosomal dominant with varied expressivity [16]. It is a chronic, progressive disease manifested in multiple organ systems. It first appears in infancy or childhood and is characterized by café au lait spots or tumors [17]. The most frequent pathologic changes are in the musculoskeletal and nervous systems, including scoliosis, unilateral limb enlargement, craniofacial defects, seizures, mental retardation, and optic nerve involvement. Treatment includes surgical removal of cutaneous tumors, medical/surgical treatment of malignant tumors, orthopedic management of musculoskeletal abnormalities, and anticonvulsants for seizures. Genetic counseling is indicated, and special schooling is needed if mental retardation is present.

POLIO

Poliomyelitis (polio, infantile paralysis) is a viral disease of the central nervous system characterized by destruction of motor neurons (anterior horn cells, brainstem nuclei). Before the introduction of the Salk vaccine (1953), 10,000 to 25,000 cases were seen annually [36]. Now, 50 to 60 cases are seen annually, occurring among unvaccinated young children, often of lower socioeconomic groups. Clinical signs include an incubation period of 5 to 35 days. The disease peaks in August and September. In the acute stages of viral infection of motor neurons, there may be tremor, fasciculations and twitching of muscles, and resistance to passive movement. Back and leg pain are common. Fever and signs of meningeal inflammation are usually present. Later, the patient may exhibit flaccid asymmetric motor paralysis and areflexia of cranial and spinal musculature. In most cases, however, the disease looks like aseptic meningitis, which usually has a benign course. It is usually more severe in adults than children [36]. Medical management of the acute illness is essential. Rehabilitation management addresses residual motoric involvement.

SPINA BIFIDA

Spina bifida, described by Tulp [47] in 1652, is a syndrome of multisystem anomalies due to abnormal embryonic development of the neural tube and its surrounding structures. Failure of the laminae to close can be seen at any spinal level, with or without spinal cord involvement. However, it is most common in the lumbosacral area. It occurs in 1 to 6 in 1000 births. As 5 percent of these malformations occur in families with one affected member, genetic counseling is suggested. Amniocentesis has a 99.2 percent accuracy with open neural tube defects [10].

The degree of impairment depends on the site and size of the defect, whether it is open or closed or infected. The mildest form is spina bifida occulta in which external signs are minimal. Internally there may be a bony malformation or congenital neoplasm but no neurologic involvement.

Spina bifida with meningocele indicates that through the defect in the vertebrae, the meninges are displaced, forming a spinal fluid-filled sac under the skin. The spinal cord is not involved. A meningomyelocele, which is the most severe form of spina bifida, involves displacement of the meninges and spinal cord. The lesion may be covered by skin but requires immediate surgical attention. Due to the neurologic involvement, this defect results in paraplegia and is often complicated by hydrocephalus (90%). Hydrocephalus usually requires a shunt to relieve ventricular pressure. Other complications seen in this condition include anomalies of the kidneys, neurogenic bladder, respiratory problems associated with vocal cord paralysis (Arnold-Chiari syndrome), and musculoskeletal deficits such as scoliosis or dislocated hips [4, 10].

Current treatment for urologic problems involves the use of clean intermittent catheterization with and without surgery [1]. Orthopedic intervention must consider the child's potential for ambulation. A potential ambulator needs plantar grade feet and hips and knees that fully extend and flex to 90 degrees [10]. If the child is nonambulatory, standing in a parapodium is necessary to maintain joint alignment. However, the child needs early instruction in wheeled mobility [10, 24].

Although ambulation [18] is of prime importance, rehabilitation management addresses the needs of the whole child with the goal of maximum functional independence [53]. Functional activities include self care, ambulation, mobility, socialization, communication, sexuality, education, and vocation. Psychological support for the child and family is important throughout the rehabilitation process.

Visual Disorders
Judith Falconer

Each of our senses provides us with unique information about the world. The reception, interpretation, and integration of information from multiple senses help us to develop purposeful behaviors and skills and to function within the physical and social environments. One sense cannot replace the information provided by another sense, nor do the other senses increase in acuity when one is absent or impaired.

The blind child, therefore, cannot substitute vision with hearing or touch, nor does auditory and tactile acuity increase because vision is absent. Blind children may learn to use the other senses more efficiently than the sighted child, but this alone does not explain why some blind children successfully develop motor, cognitive, perceptual, personal, social, and language abilities. Perhaps the blind child has the mental capacity to reorganize the world in a manner consistent with his or her sensory experience of it, that is, to interpret and integrate sensory experiences differently from a sighted child, but in a meaningful, organized, and functional fashion [13]. Alternatively, perhaps blindness alters the pattern and the rate of development, but not the level of achievement possible.

Despite the potential for successful development, blind children are at significant risk for both delayed development (significant age-related lags in performance) and deviant development (abnormal movements or behaviors). Because vision, like all the senses, is intricately bound with other functions, it is easy to illustrate how the absence of vision could compromise development. For example, visual stimuli promote motor skill development; seeing an object motivates the child to reach and grasp or lift the head when lying prone. Visual feedback provides cues to successful problem-solving behavior, an essential part of cognitive development. Vision provides information about size, shape, distance, position, and color from which some perceptual abilities emerge. A child's ability to maintain visual contact with the parent helps to decrease separation anxiety, which facilitates healthy personality growth [19]. The child learns acceptable social mannerisms and postures by imitating the behaviors he or she has seen in other children and adults. Through vision, the child associates objects and experiences with words, which is necessary for vocabulary growth.

In each example, vision provides sensory information about, and mediates the child's interactions with, the physical and social environments. When these normal child-environmental interactions are restricted or altered through a loss of vision, changes from expected developmental patterns may occur; conversely, if the child experiences appropriate physical and social interactions, abnormal development is preventable or correctable. In short, the child's basic needs and potential may not differ significantly from that of a sighted child, but when vision is absent or impaired, the child's environment and learning experiences must be retooled to circumvent the functions of the visual sensory processes.

The fate of a blind child depends on factors other than the degree of visual loss. Like the sighted child, the blind child who has security, freedom to explore, and an enriched sensory and social environment successfully reaches adulthood [45]. Identification and implementation of appropriate nonvisual sensory and social environmental conditions are the primary tasks of parents and professionals who care for the blind and the visually impaired child.

PREVALENCE, CAUSES, AND TYPES OF BLINDNESS

There are many definitions of blindness, all of which refer to vision with the best possible correction. The most common definition is the legal definition, which is important because it is often used as the eligibility criterion for financial assistance and services. Legal blindness is defined as visual acuity in the better eye with correction of not more than 20/200 or a defect in the visual field so that the widest diameter of vision subtends an angle no greater than 20 degrees [44]. This means one cannot see the same detail at 20 feet even with correction that a normal sighted person can see at 200 feet, or that the visual field, the area within which objects are seen by the eyes in a fixed position, is very narrow. Most children who meet legal or other criteria for blindness in fact do have some vision. Only one third of all visually impaired children have no useful vision, and greater than one half have vision of 5/200 or better [25].

Clinicians and educators are less concerned with the specific visual acuity than they are with functional visual efficiency—how well the child uses residual vision. Therapists and teachers can help partially sighted children improve their functional visual efficiency through training and identification of the conditions under which residual vision is maximally used. Functional visual efficiency is a more important concept than visual acuity in therapeutic and educational settings because it focuses on the aspect of visual function, which can be trained and improved. However, because functional visual efficiency is difficult to quantify, it is less commonly reported.

Blindness, fortunately, is a low-incidence impairment. Precise estimates of the number of visually impaired children is not known because of methodologic problems in the defining, measuring, and reporting of visual impairment. The number of legally blind school-age children in the United States based on school enrollment figures is in the neighborhood of 30,000; the number of visually impaired school-age children based on household sample surveys is higher [31]. Worldwide prevalence of visual impairments is considerably higher because of poor sanitation, nutrition, and medical care. Blindness also is more common in multiply impaired children. As many as 70 percent of all visually impaired children may have additional problems such as mental retardation, cerebral palsy, and hearing loss [30].

Approximately 76 percent of visually impaired children are born with the impairment or lose sight before age 1 year (congenitally impaired) [25]. Congenital blindness is genetically or prenatally determined. In the United States prenatally acquired visual disorders are caused by maternal infections including syphilis, gonorrhea, toxoplasmosis, and rubella, or by fetal exposure to toxic physical agents such as drugs, radiation, alcohol, and excessive oxygen administered to premature infants (retinopathy of prematurity). However, in many cases the cause of congenital blindness remains unknown. Children who lose sight later in life (adventitiously impaired) are at an advantage because they had vision during early phases of development, but they may experience adjustment difficulties that are unusual among the congenitally impaired. Acquired visual deficits result from infections, vascular disease, neoplasms, trauma, and exposure to toxic agents.

Visual diseases and anomalies common to children under age 20 are cataracts, albinism, glaucoma, macular and retinal degeneration, aniridia (incomplete iris formation), retinitis pigmentosa, anophthalmos (absence of eyes), microphthalmos (small eyes), coloboma of uveal tract, dislocated lens, retinoblastoma, retinopathy of prematurity (retrolental fibroplasia), other damage along the nerve path (retina, optic nerve, optic chiasm, optic tract, optic radiations, visual cortex); and various types of nystagmus, a rhythmical horizontal, rotary, or vertical oscillation of the eyes, which has many causes.

Common refractive errors such as myopia, hyperopia, and astigmatism produce blurred vision but are usually correctable with lenses. Elongation of the eye (myopia, or nearsightedness) causes the light image to fall in front of the retina. If the eye is too short, as in hyperopia or farsightedness, the light image falls behind the retina. Astigmatism occurs when the cornea or lens is misshaped and different portions have different focal points. Misalignment of the eyes, or strabismus, prevents the eyes from focusing in a coordinated movement on the same image. The most common types of strabismus are esotropia (crossed eyes) and exotropia (walled eyes). Esotropia and exotropia may result in double vision or diplopia. To avoid diplopia and confusion, the visual cortex suppresses one of the images that produces strabismic amblyopia, a condition characterized by a visual loss from the weaker eye. Therapy for strabismus can include eye patching, lenses, eye muscle exercises, and surgical correction.

GOALS OF REHABILITATION

Blind children and their families need help. The nature and the intensity of their needs varies significantly from child to child. Some families require only routine medical assistance and information about special educational services and materials. Others need close contact and multidisciplinary services. The circumstances of each child are unique and require an individual assessment.

The first purpose of rehabilitation is to periodically monitor the child's total development. This is a part of routine medical and pediatric care and involves some standard developmental assessment. Monitoring also implies some form of parental interview to determine if further services are warranted or requested. Routine monitoring helps ensure that problems are detected and corrected early.

The second purpose of rehabilitation is to create the conditions favorable for normal development of the blind child. This broad goal captures the complexity of the task. It may include parental training about normal child development, parental education regarding how the blind child learns, interpretation of a specific child's development, or a demonstration to parents of various stimulation techniques to promote the child's growth. This could also mean providing remedial activities to correct the child's motor and behavioral problems or helping a parent to place the child in an appropriate nursery school. Specific interventions vary enormously, but the goal is relatively constant.

The third purpose of rehabilitation is to provide ongoing emotional support for parents and families. Most parents want to do what is best, but many do not know how. Parents' feelings of guilt, frustration, and inadequacy may interfere with their responses to the child. Perhaps no aspect can be more important to the blind child's future welfare than effective parent-child relationships.

ASSESSMENT

OPHTHALMIC

There are numerous procedures, tests, and specialized techniques used in an ophthalmic examination. Only a few of the basic assessments appear here to give a general idea of the content of an ophthalmic examination. (For a more complete discussion of visual assessment, see Robb [48].) An ophthalmic evaluation includes an examination of the appearance of the external and internal structures of the eyes plus tests of visual acuity and visual field.

The external appearance of the eyes, especially their position, size, symmetry, and movements is observed for abnormalities. Eyes that appear misaligned, disproportionate, asymmetrical, or unsteady may signal a visual disorder. The external structures, conjunctiva, cornea, sclera, and iris are visually examined for irregularities. Red-rimmed, encrusted, swollen, inflamed or watery eyelids suggest eye disease. The interior structures of the eyes are usually examined through the pupil with an ophthalmoscope, an instrument that magnifies and illuminates the structures. Tonometry measures intraocular pressure and is used to detect such conditions as childhood glaucoma. Retinoscopy, a method of measuring light reflected from the retina, is used to determine the amount of refraction needed.

In infants, routine vision testing involves elicited or observed visual fixation, visual tracking, pupillary responses to light, and blink responses to a threatening gesture. Infant visual acuity is variable and difficult to quantify. Reliable subjective testing of visual acuity is possible at about age 3. The child's disregard for objects in the peripheral fields can be tested, for example, by asking the child to grab the examiner's fingers as they are brought into view from behind the child's head.

Examples of common tests used to screen children for vision problems are the Screening Test for Young Children and Retardates (STYCAR) and the Snellen E. The STYCAR is particularly suitable for young or multiply impaired children. Depending on the child's chronological and mental age, the child is asked to name Snellen letters on a distance chart, to match letters on the distance chart with flashcards, to name common toys at varying distances, or to match toys observed at a distance with a duplicate set [51]. Various modifications of the Snellen E [37] are also available. In each, the child is asked to identify the direction of the "fingers" of the "E."

244

DEVELOPMENTAL AND EDUCATIONAL

The rationale for evaluation of the blind child is the same as for a sighted child: to screen for potential problems, to provide baseline information on which to measure progress, and to aid in treatment and educational planning. Prior to formal evaluation it is necessary to determine if there are concurrent problems, such as hearing loss or mental retardation, and the onset age, severity, type, and cause of the visual impairment. The child needs to be observed for any abnormality in posture, gait, hand function, balance, weakness, or abnormality in muscle tone or bulk. Subjective notes on the child's overall awareness, activity level, confidence, emotional expression, verbal expression, creativity, and purposefulness in behavior aid in the interpretation of other findings. Family history and observation of parent-child and child-peer interactions also provide important information for intervention programs.

Formal evaluation usually involves comparisons of a child's performance to a normative population or to a criterion. Normative populations may be large samples of either sighted or blind children. Criterion-referenced tests refer to the attainment of specific levels of performance. Normed tests are generally more helpful in determining a developmental diagnosis and service needs; criterion-referenced tests provide more useful information for individualized program planning. In either type of test, the behaviors measured may be elicited, spontaneous, or reported by the child's primary caretaker [33].

Standard developmental and educational tests as well as tests specifically designed for visually impaired children are used in both therapeutic and educational settings. Most standard developmental and educational achievement tests can be given to blind children with modifications in the method of administration. There is no consensus regarding whether it is best to employ tests designed for the sighted child or tests designed for the visually impaired child. Standard tests provide information about how the blind child compares to the sighted child, but they may underestimate the blind child's ability. Tests designed for the blind child probably give a better estimate of the child's ability, but they provide less information about how well the child functions as compared to his or her peers. In practice, both yield valuable information, and the decision rests on the use and the interpretation of the results.

Examples of common developmental assessments designed specifically for visually impaired children are the Maxfield-Buchholz Social Maturity Scale for Blind Preschool Children [39], The Oregon Project for Visually Impaired and Blind Preschool Children [8], and the Callier-Azusa Scale [55]). The Maxfield-Buchholz Scale, a revision of the Maxfield Adaptation of the Vineland Social Maturity Scale, is a developmental test normed on legally blind children that measures social competence of blind children aged from birth to 6 years in seven basic areas: self-help general, self-help dressing, self-help eating, communication, socialization, locomotion, and occupation. The Oregon Project is a criterion-referenced assessment and comprehensive curriculum guide that is appropriate for visually impaired children from birth to 6 years. The Oregon Project skills inventory is developmentally sequenced and organized into the areas of cognition, language, self-help, socialization, fine motor, and gross motor skills. The Callier-Azusa Scale is a criterion-referenced developmental scale designed to assess deaf-blind and multihandicapped children from birth to 9 years. It includes subscales of motor development, perception, daily living skills, language, and socialization. (For summaries of many of the tests appropriate for use with preschool and school-age visually impaired children, see Swallow [56] and Scholl [49].)

GROWTH AND DEVELOPMENT

GROSS MOTOR

In comparison to the sighted infant the blind infant's development patterns are uneven or atypical rather than simply delayed [14]. Movements that depend on reflex and neuromuscular maturation, such as head righting and posture, roughly parallel the sighted infant's growth; learned and self-initiated motor skills such as creeping and walking are often delayed [2]. Restricted experience, fear of discomfort, lack of visual motivation, absence of optical righting reactions, and inability visually to imitate probably account, in part, for gross motor differences.

Auditory stimuli entice the child to explore space by moving and contribute to the development of motor skills. Without vision, the coordination of prehension and hearing is delayed; the sighted child purposefully reaches for an object "on sight" between 5 and 6 months of age; intentional reach for an object "on sound cue" for the blind child may occur much later [20]. Search behavior on sound cue for the blind child depends on the development of the object concept, which usually occurs toward the end of the first year. Intervention programs designed to unite sound and touch may help narrow the gap between the gross motor achievements of blind and sighted children. Adequate parenting, physical and emotional contact, frequent position changes, assisted play, and multisensory toys enhance the achievement of object permanence and association of sound with an object in space.

As soon as the child learns to walk independently, he or she is taught the beginning skills for orientation and mobility. Orientation refers to the process of using the senses to establish one's position and relationship to all other significant objects. Mobility is the capacity, readiness, and facility to move about in the environment. Early mobility skills include techniques of human or sighted guide (skills to travel with a sighted person), trailing (establishing and maintaining a line of travel by using the fingers to "trail" the surface), and protective techniques (use of hand and arm in mobility to prevent injury) [27]. Readiness and maturity determine when an individual child learns these skills. However, in general at about age 2 or 3 years, the child is taught simple sighted guide

skills and trailing and progresses to advanced sighted guide skills and diagonal cane technique at about age 5 years [27]. Older children learn mobility systems for use outdoors and in unfamiliar places. The choice of mobility system (human guide, long cane, dog guide, or electronic travel aids) is individual and depends on personal preference, feasibility, cost, and availability of training. Many blind travelers use a combination of systems.

Visual, auditory, kinesthetic, and tactile information help children form concepts about themselves and their environments. The loss of vision may interfere with the development of body image and spatial concepts. The blind child with poor body image and spatial concepts may develop posture or gait disturbances [12]. Some common deviations include toeing-out feet, stiff-arm swing, wide-based or toe-heel gait, head drooping or turning, kyphosis, and pelvic or trunk tilts. Therapy activities aimed at improving body image and movement through space incorporate many planes of motion and are self-initiated. Modalities used to prevent or correct gross motor problems include scooter boards, carpeted tunnels, obstacle courses, jungle gym sets, tumbling mats, swings, ladders, etc. Regular physical fitness activities such as running, jumping, dancing, bicycle riding, tumbling, swimming, and balance activities such as beam walking and hopping also improve gross motor development. Blind children sometimes are afraid or hesitant with gross motor play activities and may need to be guided physically to learn these skills. For example, a child who is afraid of running may need to be taken by the hand and run in an open space.

FINE MOTOR
Vision mediates the developmental sequence that leads to coordinated use of the hands. The infant learns to engage the hands at midline, search, reach, grasp, release, and transfer objects through visual stimulation and visual motivation. In the absence of visual cues and incentives, blind infants tend to maintain non-

functional neonatal hand posturing (hands fisted at shoulder height, elbows flexed) longer than sighted infants [21]. From this position the blind child cannot develop fine motor control and tactile discriminatory skills. Since the blind child extensively uses the hands throughout life to interpret the physical world, fine motor development in childhood is particularly important.

The blind child needs games, toys, and activities that promote fine motor skills. Tactile discrimination develops through the child's interactive and exploratory contact with a variety of tactile sensations. Young infants can be assisted to hold the bottle, to play lap games, and to engage hands at midline. Babies who are too young to sit independently can be placed in a supported seat with a lap tray of toys or a toy tied to the chair. In this arrangement, the baby's random movements locate various sized, shaped, weighted, and textured toys that are easily retrieved. Children old enough to sit independently, however, should not be restrained by seats and playpens to allow them to explore the environment freely. Older children are encouraged to play with bead stringing, button boards, textured blocks, formboards, and the like.

COGNITION AND PERCEPTION

Infants learn fundamental cognitive and perceptual skills through sensorimotor experiences with the external world [46]. Vision impairments clearly reduce the variety and quantity of the visual sensory information, but the consequences of this loss to the cognitive and perceptual development of the blind child are a highly complex subject about which few broad generalizations can be made.

Controversy and inconclusiveness in the literature stem from a number of conceptual and methodological problems in the study of cognitive and perceptual differences between blinded and sighted children, and the accompanying theoretic issue of the role of vision in the development of perception and cognition. There is no unifying conceptual model to explain perception and cognition in the absence of vision; the application of models developed to explain cognition and perception with vision may be inappropriate models for the study of the blind child. It is difficult to separate the interactive effects of the blindness with deprivation in the physical or social environments that may be concurrent with the blindness. Heterogeneity among blind children on two variables of critical importance to the development of higher cortical and perceptual skills—age of onset of the blindness and residual vision—further confounds the study of cognitive and perceptual differences. Children who have had vision and children with residual vision are significantly advantaged in the achievement of perceptual and cognitive learning. Furthermore, the topic is inherently complex and has generated relatively little systematic study.

Most researchers have chosen to apply Piaget's theory of cognitive development to the study of the blind child. Hatwell's [26] application of Piaget's theory to blind children concluded that congenitally blind subjects show substantial delays in the achievement of cognitive development with the exception of verbal logical tasks. She maintained that the structure of cognitive development in the blind subjects, albeit delayed, was not qualitatively different from that of the sighted subjects. Using a Piagetian framework, Stephens and Grube [54] also found significant delays in the cognitive development of blind children; however, they demonstrated that after provision of developmentally appropriate experiences in reasoning, the blind subjects performed as well as the sighted subjects.

These conclusions of Hatwell and others who have similar findings are disputed. Warren [61] asserts that the findings of delays in cognitive development using Piagetian theory and tests are at best premature and he further proposes that remediation programs designed to minimize these reported delays are based on faulty assumptions. His statements are derived from challenges to the validity of experimental studies that compare blinded and sighted subjects within theoretic frameworks and tests developed to understand the developmental processes of sighted children. Blind children may develop at different rates and use different strategies that are not necessarily deficiencies and that need to be understood in order to develop successful intervention and education programs.

Vygotsky's theory of cognitive development [59, 60] may be more appropriate to the study of the blind child. Vygotsky believed in an intimate relationship between cognitive development and social interaction; what a child is capable of doing with the assistance of others might be more indicative of the child's mental development than what the child can do alone. The distance between the actual developmental level as determined by independent problem solving and the level of potential development as determined through problem solving under adult guidance or in collaboration with more capable peers are known as the "zone of proximal development." Vygotsky's zone of proximal development has important implications for the blind child. It emphasizes the need for a variety of appropriate social interactions to provide the scaffolding on which the child's intellectual capacities can build. Furthermore, Vygotsky's view of cognitive development may better explain why some blind children develop appropriately and others do not.

In a review of the literature on the blind child's perceptual development, Warren [61] concluded that in some areas blind children perform worse, whereas in other areas blind children perform better or the same as sighted children. Generally speaking, blind children perform the same as sighted children in perceptual discrimination abilities such as the perception of texture, weight, and sound. In higher-order integrative and complex perception such as form identification, spatial relations, and intermodality relations, the blind child performs less well than the sighted child [61]. These conclusions

were drawn primarily from studies of school-age children. There is very little information on the perceptual abilities of the preschool-age child.

Theory aside, most clinicians and educators would agree that the task of achieving cognitive and perceptual development is significantly more difficult for blind children, but that they will not necessarily be functionally limited in adulthood, or that the quality of their mental life will not necessarily be reduced. Nevertheless, learning opportunities and experiences for the blind child are likely to be less frequent and less spontaneous and are likely to require more attention, planning, and active organization. To develop successful cognitive and perceptual functions, the blind child, like all children, requires a variety and quantity of perceptual stimuli and exploratory and social experiences. Activities used to facilitate the blind child's perceptual and cognitive development focus on actual experience with objects and movement in a variety of sensory and social contexts. Gross and fine motor activities that facilitate physical development, therefore, also stimulate mental development. Games that teach body image are particularly important to the blind child's perceptual maturity. The child can learn to perceive the distance and direction of sound in group games or with various activities incorporating such items as bells, musical toys, and record players. Other examples of activities that promote cognitive and perceptual growth are lap games for babies, nested toys, water play, sorting games, busy boards, block play for toddlers, and playground sports and educational activities for school-age children.

PERSONAL AND SOCIAL DEVELOPMENT
Personal and social development are also controversial areas about which many theorists have written. Important differences between the blind and sighted child's social opportunities, experiences, and expectations may explain lags in emotional and social development. What these differences are and how they affect personal and social development are much less

248

clear. The organization of the blind child's personality is, however, probably more fragile than other areas of development [34]. Observers of blind children frequently comment on their passivity, compliance, and apparent lack of spontaneity or involvement. There is no inherent characteristic of blindness that would explain these observations; however, blindness does influence the dynamics of socialization that may affect personal and social development.

The blind child at all ages has a more difficult time forming social attachments and has fewer social experiences and fewer opportunities to learn and to demonstrate appropriate social behaviors. For example, learned social behaviors such as smiling are delayed, and usual modes of social contact such as eye contact are unavailable. Without the ability to communicate through vision and without visual information about the situation, the blind child may appear inattentive, unresponsive, or withdrawn, and may be hesitant or fearful. Social skills and manners are learned in part through imitation. Without visual information the child is disadvantaged in learning appropriate social behaviors and skills. Social expectations that are critical shaping forces in social behavior may also be affected. Scott [50] argues that the disability of blindness is a learned social role; the various attitudes and behaviors that characterize blind persons are acquired from well-intended service agencies for the blind through ordinary processes of social learning.

In early life careful nurturing of the parent-child relationship is essential to successful personal and social development. Parents need to be encouraged to hold and to handle the blind baby who needs more frequent physical and verbal contact than a sighted baby. Throughout the childhood a major effort needs to be made to ensure that the child participates fully in all the customary experiences of childhood—family events, playground activities, games, music, drama, parties, and so forth. Placement in a nursery school or preschool is usually indicated to help the child acquire sufficient experience in

groups. The setting of appropriate social expectations and the concomitant rewarding of appropriate and punishing of inappropriate social behaviors are critical to the child's success but are frequently difficult to determine. Within a carefully planned structure of opportunities and experiences, however, the child also needs sufficient freedom to explore and discover in order to obtain personal and social competence.

LANGUAGE

There is even less theory or research regarding the role of vision in, and the effects of blindness on, the development of language. The general trend of the literature suggests that language acquisition by blind children is delayed, but, in the absence of confounding factors, by about school age blind children acquire language competencies within normal ranges. For example, delays have been reported in phonologic development (i.e., less baby babbling), acquisition of concepts and meanings (i.e., prolonged echolalia), and in the development of morphology and syntax (i.e., more freewheeling and independent speech) [63]. Delays, however, are difficult to interpret. The blind child may use language strategies that are different from those of a sighted child but that do not constitute a language deficit [40].

The belief that the blind child's symbolic or cognitive capacity will always be compromised because the child does not have the sensory experience on which some concepts depend (e.g., understanding the meaning of color) is debatable. The view that words may be anchored to usable concepts even without the visual experience [35] contrasts with the view that the deficiency is real but perhaps inconsequential since most of language is nonvisual [62]. At this time, the deficiency (if indeed there is one) and whether or not it affects the adequacy of thought is not understood well enough to determine the functional significance.

Language disturbances observed in blind school-age children may not be attributable to blindness per se, but rather to emotional or environmental conditions that result because of the blindness. Language may be delayed if usual parent-child interactions with the baby are disturbed, that is, if parents fail to respond positively to the baby's early babbling, anticipate the child's needs, thereby inadvertently allowing the child to interact with only nonverbal cues, or talk for the child. Blind children whose early exploratory behavior with objects and people is restricted or limited may not have the sensory and emotional experiences on which language development depends.

The emphasis in language facilitation for the blind child is on the interactiveness of language learning with objects, experiences, and feelings in the daily life of the child. Language development is facilitated by rewarding the child's attempts at language; by naming objects the child touches; by relating concepts (e.g., soft) to different items; by encouraging the child to name, to repeat, to request, and to construct sentences; and by building vocabulary as the child increases his or her reserve of experiences and ideas. Early language is not facilitated, for example, by listening to television or radio as the child sits passively beside it; the child learns to ignore monotonous and confusing sound. Examples of specific activities that promote language growth include rhyming games, listening games, story telling, and puppet play.

ACTIVITIES OF DAILY LIVING
Because blind children cannot observe and imitate movements and actions, they may need more training than sighted children to learn skills of daily living. Blind children are sometimes poor feeders and slow to learn to bite and chew. Early introduction of solid foods and a varied diet help to prevent these problems. Blind children usually learn early to finger feed as part of mouthing behavior. Mouthing of objects lasts somewhat longer for blind children, but this should be allowed since the mouth is a discriminating sense organ that provides additional information to young children. Blind children who learn to hold their bottle make the

transition to cup holding fairly well. Spoon use is taught later by hand over hand assistance from an adult standing behind the child and guiding the hand, and by the use of tactile and verbal cues and praise. Heavy dishes with raised sides and the use of external cues, such as noting the edges of the placemat may help the child to learn to eat in a socially acceptable manner.

Toilet training a blind child requires some minor adaptations. A stool in front of the toilet seat that prevents the feet from dangling, or a small training chair with a toy attached, helps to comfort the child who may be afraid of sitting on the toilet seat. The child, if left too long on the chair, forgets the purpose. The chair should remain in one place so the child associates it with the toileting process; ideally this is in the bathroom, but other areas are acceptable. To encourage imitative behavior it may be necessary for the child to accompany the parent into the bathroom. Toilet training difficulty is often related to either physiologic immaturity or parental anxiety.

Dressing skills are also taught by physical guidance and tactile and verbal cues. Poor spatial and body-image concepts are a common cause of difficulty with dressing. Head control and proper spatial orientation may be lacking. In a sighted child, looking at the body helps promote good body alignment and orientation for dressing. The blind child may need to be taught to orient to the body part being dressed.

In addition, all the usual daily activities of adulthood need to be mastered in late childhood and adolescence such as money management, shopping, food preparation, home and child care, and career planning. These activities may require longer, somewhat modified training in order to learn, but in an emotionally and physically ready child, they are not usually a problem.

EDUCATION
Most children begin some sort of school program at about age 3, and many states have pro-

grams that begin even earlier. The blind child may be partially or totally integrated into the regular classroom depending on the child's specific abilities and the administrative practices of the particular school. General curriculum needs are the same for blind children as for sighted children, but teachers need to modify multiple aspects of most educational activities such as the presentation of the task, the time it takes the student to learn, the materials used, and the conditions under which it is taught. In addition, blind children require special training in Braille reading and writing, typing, orientation and mobility, activities of daily living, communication skills, and visual skills. Instructional approaches to teach visual skills include visual stimulation programs (developmental approach to providing visual sensory stimulation), visual efficiency training (training to take into account perceptual factors to aid in the development of functional vision), and visual use instruction (involving environmental adaptation to maximize vision, use of optical and nonoptical aids, and techniques to maximize the use of vision) [11]. Schools provide training in the activities specifically needed by the visually impaired student with special classes or tutors, resource rooms and equipment, and teacher-consultants to augment the classroom experience. If integration into the regular school is impossible or undesirable, day and residential special schools for the blind child are an option. (For a comprehensive presentation of education for the blind and visually impaired student, see Scholl [49].)

STEREOTYPED BEHAVIORS

Blind children often exhibit stereotypic, repetitive, or idiosyncratic behaviors. Some examples are body rocking, twirling or spinning, head banging or nodding, eye poking or fisting, exaggerated sniffing, prolonged hand watching, hand flapping, and finger flicking. Although the behaviors are loosely called "blindisms," they resemble the pathologic responses sometimes observed among institutionalized, mentally re-

tarded, emotionally disturbed, or autistic sighted children.

The behaviors are disturbing to parents and socially unacceptable. They give the child an appearance of maladjustment or of mental retardation and inhibit normal child-environmental interactions. Some such as eye fisting, which darkens and depresses the eyes, or head banging cause physical harm. The mannerisms disrupt communication and interfere with the child's ability to process efficiently available sensory information and cues.

There are many hypotheses about the causes of stereotypic behaviors. In general, they are thought to develop in response to inadequate sensory or social conditions including understimulation or experiential deprivation, disturbed parent-child relationships, or problems of adaptation, learning, and adjustment at transitional stages of development [52]. There are also several different theories about intervention programs to extinguish stereotypic behaviors. Much of the research on stereotypic behaviors, however, is conducted with severely autistic children and therefore may not be applicable to emotionally healthy blind children. Included among these theories are Bettelheim's psychoanalytic approach [6] and Lovaas' behavioral-social learning paradigm [38]. More recently, the sensory integrative approach developed by Ayres [5] to ameliorate neurologic dysfunction and to promote learning ability has been used in the treatment of stereotypic behaviors.

Behavior modification, in general, has been the most effective in eliminating persistent stereotypic behaviors in blind children. The assumptions of this approach are that the behaviors are learned and maintained through reinforcement. The goal of intervention is to substitute the stereotypic behavior with a socially appropriate adaptive behavior. It is better to anticipate and "redirect" a stereotypic behavior than to inhibit one in motion. Professionals often feel that the child old enough to understand should also be directly confronted regarding its inappropriateness.

PARENTS

Immediately following the birth of a blind child, all parents feel devastated and may experience some degree of shock, denial, grief, guilt, frustration, anxiety, anger, self-pity, and fear. Emotionally healthy parents eventually resolve these feelings and move gradually toward reorganization of their lives and long-term acceptance of the child. Parents may at various times have negative feelings toward the blind child, but these are usually short term or situation specific and are not disruptive to the parent-child bond.

Most parents want to do what is best for the child, but many do not know how. It is normal for them to feel somewhat inadequate to care for a blind child and to need information, practical advice, reassurance, and recognition of their competence as parents. An important task for parents early in the baby's life is for them to learn the special as well as the normal developmental needs of their baby [3, 41]. Their main problems are likely to be that they do not know how to set appropriate expectations or how to interpret certain behaviors of their blind child, and that they do not realize that the usual environment may need to be adapted to motivate the blind child.

There are some parents, however, who fail to make emotional contact and overtly or covertly reject their blind child. Examples of symptoms of abnormal parental reactions include inability to speak positively about the child, inability to be angry with or to discipline the child, absence of interest in the child's growth, inability to say the word *blind,* and lack of pleasurable contact with the child. These parents need a positive approach that reinforces their capacity to be effective parents and helps them to learn how to enjoy their child. It is important in these cases to emphasize the child's achievements to the parents, to relate achievements to the actions the parents have taken, and to impress on the parents their importance in the child's life.

AIDS AND EQUIPMENT

Toys

Important characteristics of toys for the blind child are that they are appropriate to the child's developmental age and that they capture the child's interest. Toys should be selected for tactile (texture, contour) and auditory (sound, pitch) diversity. Toys that depend on action by the child such as dangling bells and rattles for infants, push toys and bell blocks for toddlers, and Play-Doh, finger paints, kiddie cars, and musical instruments for preschoolers promote learning. Toys that stimulate imagination such as sand boxes and costumes are also desirable. Toys to be avoided are those that "do things" such as predominantly visual wind-up toys and toys that are perceptually or tactilely confusing such as model replicates, cutouts, and embossed picture books. Baby jumper seats should be used sparingly, if at all; blind toddlers may mimic the pleasurable bouncing sensation outside the seat. Baby walkers should not be used: Head injuries are caused by these devices; they encourage abnormal postural alignment and muscle development; and they may delay the onset of crawling or walking, the primary mode blind children have for exploring their environment.

Educational Aids

The blind student may require a wide variety of visual, auditory, tactile, as well as optical aids. Writing is assisted by a Braillewriter, or slate and stylus, felt tip pens, and bold or embossed lined paper. Aids to reading include Braille books, large-print books, "talking" books, closed circuit television that magnifies print on a screen, high-intensity lamps, and other electronic equipment. Math might require an abacus, "talking" calculator or other computation device, Braille ruler, and protractor. Typewriters, tape recorders, cassettes, and Braille watches also need to be available to the visually impaired student.

CONCLUSIONS

Perhaps the only trait that all blind children have in common is some degree of visual loss. The tendency of sighted individuals to assume behavioral similarities among blind children is potentially harmful to the child's development.

The apparent similarities among blind individuals are the result of complex social interaction, expectations, and perceptions rather than any real behavioral similarity. Within this context, professionals should strive to preserve the differences among visually impaired children, while eliminating the important differences between populations of blind and sighted children.

The overriding concern of all blind individuals is to be accepted by sighted persons in interpersonal relationships, community life, education, employment, and housing. Damaging stereotypes of the blind as defenseless, dependent, distant, solicitous, musical, courageous, and so forth prevent a natural integration of the blind with the sighted; nevertheless blind individuals must accept the fact that although people may at times seem unresponsive and insensitive to their needs, they must achieve behaviors and skills comparable to those of the sighted. The child who is accepted develops normally; the child who develops normally is accepted. Toward these ends, professionals have a dual responsibility: to promote healthy public attitudes about blind persons and to prepare the blind child for the demands of the world of the sighted.

REFERENCES

1. Action Committee on Myelodysplasia. Current approaches to evaluation and management of children with myelomeningocele. *Pediatrics* 63(4):663, 1979.
2. Adelson, E., and Fraiberg, S. Gross motor development in infants blind from birth. *Child Dev.* 45:114, 1974.
3. Als, H. Reciprocity and autonomy: Parenting a blind infant. *Zero to Three* 5(5):8, 1985.
4. Atkins, J. A., and Chapman R. L. Occupational therapy in a myelomeningocele clinic. *Am. J. Occup. Ther.* 29(7):403, 1975.
5. Ayers, A. J. *Sensory Integration and Learning Disorders.* Los Angeles: Western Psychological, 1980.
6. Bettelheim, R. *Truants from Life.* Glencoe, IL: Free, 1955.
7. Bradley, W. *Pathology and Pathophysiology of Inherited Neuromuscular Disorders.* Boston: Pediatric Rehabilitation, Tufts Research and Training Center, 1982.
8. Brown, D., Simmons, V., and Methuin, J. *The Oregon Project for Visually Impaired and Blind Preschool Children* (revised ed.). Medford, Ore.: Jackson County Education Service District, 1979.
9. Challenor, Y. B. Limb Deficiencies in Children. In G. E. Molnar (ed.), *Pediatric Rehabilitation.* Baltimore: Williams & Wilkins, 1985.
10. Colbert, A. P. Myelodysplasia. *Pediatric Rehabilitation.* Boston: Tufts Research and Training Center, 1982.
11. Corn, A. L. Low Vision and Visual Efficiency. In G. T. Scholl (ed.), *Foundations of Education for Blind and Visually Handicapped Children and Youth: Theory and Practice.* New York: American Foundation for the Blind, 1986.
12. Cratty, B. *Movement and Spatial Awareness in Blind Children and Youth.* Springfield, IL: Thomas, 1971.
13. Cutsforth, T. D. *The Blind in School and Society.* New York: American Foundation for the Blind, 1951.
14. Elonen, A. S., and Zwarensteyn, S. B. Appraisal of developmental lag in certain blind children. *J. Pediatr.* 65:599, 1964.
15. Eng, G. D. Diseases of the Motor Unit. In G. E. Molnar (ed.), *Pediatric Rehabilitation.* Baltimore: Williams & Wilkins, 1985.
16. Feingold, M., and Pashayan, H. *Genetics and Birth Defects in Clinical Practice.* Boston: Little, Brown, 1983.
17. Fienmann, N. L., and Takovac, W. C. Neurofibromatosis in childhood. *J. Pediatr.* 76:339, 1970.
18. Feiwell, E. Selection of appropriate treatment for patients with myelomeningocele. *Orthop. Clin. North Am.* 12(1):101, 1981.
19. Fraiberg, S. Blind Infants and Their Mothers: An Examination of the Sign System. In M. Lewis and A. Rosenblum (eds.), *The Effects of the Infant on its Caregiver.* New York: Wiley, 1974.
20. Fraiberg, S., Siegel, B. L., and Gibson, R. The role of sound in the search behavior of a blind infant. *Psychoanal. Study Child* 21:327, 1966.
21. Fraiberg, S., Smith, M., and Adelson, E. An educational program for blind infants. *J. Spec. Ed.* 3:121, 1969.
22. Goldenson, R. M. Muscular Dystrophy. In R. N. Goldenson (ed.), *Disability and Rehabilitation Handbook.* New York: McGraw-Hill, 1978.
23. Gordon, H. *Limb Deficiencies—Upper Extremity Training.* Boston: Tufts Research and Training Center, 1981.
24. Harris, J. Myelodysplasia: Orthopedic Management. *Pediatric Rehabilitation,* Boston: Tufts Research and Training Center, 1981.
25. Hatfield, E. M. Why are they blind? *Sight Sav. Rev.* 45:3, 1975.

26. Hatwell, Y. *Piagetian Reasoning and the Blind.* New York: American Foundation for the Blind, 1985.

27. Hill, E. W. Orientation and Mobility. In G. T. Scholl (ed.), *Foundations of Education for Blind and Visually Handicapped Children and Youth: Theory and Practice.* New York: American Foundation for the Blind, 1986.

28. Johnson, E. W. Pathokinesiology of Duchenne muscular dystrophy: implications for management. *Arch. Phys. Med. Rehabil.* 58:190, 1977.

29. Johnson, E. W. Types of Muscular Dystrophy. *Pediatric Rehabilitation.* Boston: Tufts Research and Training, 1981.

30. Jones, R. B. Needs of the pre-school visually handicapped child. *Trans. Ophthalmol. Soc. U.K.* 98:234, 1978.

31. Kirchner, C. *Data on Blindness and Visual Impairment in the U.S.: A Resource Manual on Characteristics, Education, Employment, and Service Delivery.* New York: American Foundation for the Blind, 1985.

32. Kleinberg, S. B. *Educating the Chronically Ill Child.* Rockville, MD: Aspen, 1982.

33. Knobloch, H., and Pasamanick, B. (eds.). *Gesell and Amatruda's Developmental Diagnosis* (3rd ed.). New York: Harper & Row, 1974.

34. Knobloch, H., Stevens, F., and Malone, A. *Manual of Developmental Diagnosis.* Hagerstown: Harper & Row, 1980.

35. Landau, B. Blind Children's Language is not "Meaningless." In A. E. Mills (ed.), *Language Acquisition in the Blind Child.* London: Croom Helm, 1983.

36. Lehrich, J. R. *Viral Diseases of the Central Nervous System.* Boston: Massachusetts General Hospital, 1982.

37. Lippmann, O. Vision of young children. *Arch. Ophthalmol.* 81:763, 1969.

38. Lovaas, O. I., Schreibman, L., and Koegel, R. L. A Behavior Modification Approach to the Treatment of Autistic Children. In E. Schopler and R. J. Reichler (eds.), *Psychopathology and Child Development.* New York: Plenum, 1976.

39. Maxfield, K. E., and Buchholz, S. *A Social Maturity Scale for Blind Preschool Children.* New York: American Foundation for the Blind, 1958.

40. McGinnis, A. R. Functional linguistic strategies of blind children. *J. Vis. Impair. Blind.* 75:210, 1981.

41. Mintzer, D., Als, H., Tronick, E. Z., et al. Parenting an infant with a birth defect: The regulation of self-esteem. *Zero to Three* 5(5):1, 1985.

42. Molnar, G. E. (ed.). *Pediatric Rehabilitation.* Baltimore: Williams & Wilkins, 1985.

43. Munsat, T. L. The Classification of Human Myopathies. In P. J. Vinken and G. W. Bruyn (eds.), *Handbook of Clinical Neurology.* Amsterdam: North-Holland, 1979.

44. National Society for the Prevention of Blindness. *Estimated Statistics on Blindness and Vision Problems.* New York: National Society for the Prevention of Blindness, 1966.

45. Norris, M., Spaulding, P. J., and Brodie, F. H. *Blindness in Children.* Chicago: University of Chicago Press, 1957.

46. Piaget, J., and Inhelder, B. *The Psychology of the Child.* New York: Basic, 1969.

47. Ribera, A. B. Myelodysplasia. In G. E. Molnar (ed.), *Pediatric Rehabilitation.* Baltimore: Williams & Wilkins, 1985.

48. Robb, R. M. *Ophthalmology for the Pediatric Practitioner.* Boston: Little, Brown, 1981.

49. Scholl, G. T. (ed.). *Foundations of Education for Blind and Visually Handicapped Children and Youth: Theory and Practice.* New York: American Foundation for the Blind, 1986.

50. Scott, R. A. *The Making of Blind Men: A Study of Adult Socialization.* New York: Russell Sage Foundation, 1969.

51. Sheridan, M. D. Vision screening of very young or handicapped children. *Br. Med. J.* 2:253, 1960.

52. Smith, M. A., Chethik, M., and Adelson, E. Differential assessments of "blindisms." *Am. J. Orthopsychiatry* 39:807, 1969.

53. Sousa, J. C., Gordon, L. H., and Shurtleff, D. B. Assessing the development of daily living skills in patients with spina bifida. Suppl. no. 37, Hydrocephalus and Spina Bifida. London: Spastics International Medical, 1978.

54. Stephens, B., and Grube, C. Development of Piagetian reasoning in congenitally blind children. *J. Vis. Impair. Blind.* 76:133–143, 1982.

55. Stillman, R. *Callier-Azusa Scale.* Dallas: Callier Center for Communication Disorders, University of Texas-Dallas, 1978.

56. Swallow, R. M. Fifty assessment instruments commonly used with blind and partially seeing individuals. *J. Vis. Impair. Blind.* 75:65, 1981.

57. Swanson, A. B. Clinical limb defects. *Clin. Symp.* 33(3):1, 1981.

58. Trefler, E. Myoelectics today. *AOTA Phys. Dis. News* 2(4):3, 1979.

59. Vygotsky, L. *Mind in Society.* Cambridge: Harvard University Press, 1978.

60. Vygotsky, L. *Thought and Language.* Cambridge: Massachusetts Institute of Technology Press, 1986.

61. Warren, D. H. *Blindness and Early Child Devel-*

opment (2nd ed.). New York: American Foundation for the Blind, 1984.

62. Werth, P. Meaning in Language Acquisition. In A. E. Mills (ed.), *Language Acquisition in the Blind Child.* London: Croom Helm, 1983.

63. Wills, D. M. Early speech development in blind children. *Psychoanal. Study Child* 34:85–117, 1978.

SUGGESTED READING

VISUAL DISORDERS

Fraiberg, S., and Fraiberg, L. *Insights from the Blind: Comparative Studies of Blind and Sighted Infants.* New York: Basic, 1977.

Harley, R. D. (ed.). *Pediatric Ophthalmology* (2nd ed.). Philadelphia: Saunders, 1983.

Hatwell, Y. *Piagetian Reasoning and the Blind.* New York: American Foundation for the Blind, 1985.

Mills, A. E. (ed.). *Language Acquisition in the Blind Child: Normal and Deficient.* San Diego: College-Hill, 1983.

Scholl, G. T. (ed.). *Foundations of Education for Blind and Visually Handicapped Children and Youth: Theory and Practice.* New York: American Foundation for the Blind, 1986.

Scott, R. A. *The Making of Blind Men: A Study of Adult Socialization.* New York: Russell Sage Foundation, 1969.

Warren, D. H. *Blindness and Early Child Development.* (2nd ed.). New York: American Foundation for the Blind, 1984.

SPECIAL ORGANIZATIONS

BIRTH DEFECTS

The National Foundation/March of Dimes, Box 2000, White Plains, NY 10602 is the major voluntary health organization devoted to the prevention and treatment of birth defects.

MUSCULAR DYSTROPHY

The Muscular Dystrophy Association, 810 Seventh Ave., New York, NY 10019 provides a multi-faceted service program about MD and related neuromuscular disorders.

NEUROMUSCULAR DISEASES

The Spina Bifida Association of America, 343 South Dearborn Avenue, Chicago, IL 60604 provides information and resources on this disorder.

The National Ataxia Foundation, 4225 Golden Valley Rd., Minneapolis, MN 55422 provides for service, prevention education, and research. It works in conjunction with the Friedreich's Ataxia Group in America, P.O. Box 1116, Oakland, CA 94611 to provide education, research, and patient care for the different types of ataxia.

VISUAL DISORDERS

There are many local, state, and national, private and public organizations that provide information, service, and materials to visually impaired children and their families, professionals, and the public. Only a few of the larger national organizations are listed below. For further information on organizations, contact the American Foundation for the Blind, local human service directories, phone directories, and government offices.

American Foundation for the Blind, Inc., 15 West 16th St., New York, NY 10011 Phone: (212) 620-2000

American Printing House for the Blind, P. O. Box 6085, 1839 Frankfort Ave., Louisville, KY 40206 Phone: (502) 895-2405

Library of Congress, National Library Service for the Blind and Physically Handicapped, Independent Ave. at First St. East, Washington, DC 20540 Phone: (202) 287-5000

National Association for Visually Handicapped, 22 West 21st St., New York, NY 10010 Phone: (212) 889-3141

National Society for the Prevention of Blindness, 500 East Remington Rd., Schaumburg, IL 60173-4557 Phone: (312) 843-2020

10 Medical Disorders

Martha K. Logigian

This chapter addresses the medical disorders of childhood that are most frequently seen in pediatric rehabilitation programs. These conditions often require the input of an interdisciplinary team of professionals who focus not only on the disease process, but on the physical and emotional growth and development of the child, and the development of coping strategies in the family. Many of these conditions have generic issues and problems; thus, knowledge of the disease process assists the therapist in forming a treatment strategy. Exercise and developmental activity to the child's tolerance and that the condition will allow are commonly included in the therapy program. Specific concerns are addressed under individual conditions.

ASTHMA

Asthma affects 11.4 percent of all children with chronic disease under 17 years of age [39]. It is a pulmonary condition in which intermittent episodes of coughing, wheezing, and shortness of breath at rest or with normal physical activities occur in response to a multiplicity of stimuli, usually in association with a hyperresponsive condition of the bronchi. It is manifest physiologically by widespread narrowing of the bronchial tubes and can change in severity spontaneously or with medical therapy [27]. Recurrent attacks can result in permanent lung damage and an excessive burden on the heart.

Severe attacks can be exacerbated by autonomic responses as a result of the child's panic. Emergency medical care is usually required in severe attacks (status asthmaticus) to prevent respiratory failure and anoxia.

Asthma is the most common chronic disease of childhood, with an estimated 2 to 4 percent of the population and 2 million under the age of 16 having the disease [2]. The onset is typically between 3 and 8 years of age. There have been many theories of what causes asthma, among them psychological sequelae and allergens. However, it is currently believed that through a complex physiologic process, the bronchial tubes are unable to react to various irritants in a normal manner [29]. Many factors can precipitate an asthma attack such as allergens, stress, infection, pollution, cold, and exercise.

Medical management for asthma involves the use of various medications and in some situations, allergy testing and avoidance of allergens. Most medication is aimed at preventing asthma attacks. Specific medications, such as adrenaline, are administered in emergency situations to reverse the bronchial obstruction, that is, increase bronchial dilation and allow movement of air into and out of the lungs. If the attacks are difficult to control, the use of bronchodilators or oral medication, or both, may be required for longer periods of time [20, 27].

Rehabilitation management focuses on teaching the child breathing exercises and relaxation techniques. The latter can be helpful in case of a severe attack, as panic and anxiety may worsen the situation, and if the child can relax, hyperventilation may be avoided.

With this disease, physical endurance may be affected, and excessive exercise may facilitate breathing difficulties. School authorities may need guidance for children with asthma to determine activity tolerance. In addition, absence from school, usually a few days at a time, is common. Teachers should provide a home program for the child during these absences so that the child does not fall behind in school [19].

If the asthmatic child is sensitive to certain allergens, the home, school, and play environments may need adaptation. Cooperation and compliance by the child and family are critical for the successful management of asthma. In addition, they should be augmented through patient-parent education and the teaching of self-management skills (e.g., the child learns to avoid specific allergens) [36]. Fortunately, studies indicate that there is a spontaneous remission of asthma symptoms in 20 to 40 percent of children with asthma at 10- to 20-year follow-up [9].

BURNS

Childhood burns often result from a child's curiosity and playful exploration. However, Binder [3] points out that 80 percent of burned children live in stressful environments or have a premorbid history of behavior problems. Home environments of young children are often unsafe or the providers contribute to the event through negligence or abuse. Older children with emotional problems, particularly boys, have an increased risk of accidents. Table 10-1 presents common burns of childhood. Three times more boys than girls are burned above the age of 9, yet there is no difference between sexes for children under 9. Of the more than 2 million burns that occur annually, approximately one half involve children. Of these children, 100,000 require hospitalization and approximately 6000 die annually. Flames account for approximately 44 percent and hot liquids for 30 percent of all thermal injuries [24].

According to the American Burn Association, burns are classified as minor, major, and critical (Table 10-2), based on size and age (Fig. 10-1), and depth of the burn (Table 10-3).

Minor burns are generally treated on an outpatient basis with a topical agent and dressing to prevent infection. If the burn is located near a joint, active assistive range of motion is indicated. If the hand is burned, splinting and follow-up care may be required [3].

The child with moderate-to-major injury is stabilized in the emergency room. First-aid pro-

TABLE 10-1. Burns of childhood

Age	Cause	Body areas
6–36 mo	Scalding: hot liquid splash Hot bath water, negligence, or abuse	Head, face, shoulder, arm, upper trunk One or both lower extremities, buttocks, perineum, lower abdomen
9–24 mo	Electric burns from chewing on electrical cord	Mouth, lips, commissures, tongue, alveolar ridge
12–36 mo	Contact burns from touching stove, radiator, iron, hotplate Contact burn: child abuse; placement on hot object	Palms and fingers Hands, feet, buttocks
6–14 yr	Flame burns from playing with matches, gasoline, fire crackers, etc.	Face, anterior neck and trunk, hands, arms, thighs
Adolescent boys	Electric burns from playing around high-tension power source	Entrance most frequently upper extremities; exit anywhere

Source: From H. Binder. Rehabilitation of the Burned Child. In G.E. Molnar (ed.), *Pediatric Rehabilitation*. Baltimore: Williams & Wilkins, 1985. Copyright © 1985, the Williams & Wilkins Co., Baltimore.

TABLE 10-2. Triage of burn patients

Triage to	Minor injury: outpatient treatment	Major injury: admit to burn unit of general hospital	Critical injury: admit to burn center
Children			
Partial thickness	<10% TBSA	10–15% TBSA	>15% TBSA
Full thickness	< 2%	2–10%	>10%
Adults			
Partial thickness	<15%	15–30%	>30%
Full thickness	< 2%	2–10%	>10%
Age		Patient <2 yr with minor injury	Patient <10 yr with major injury
Involvement of hands, face, feet, perineum	Never	Minor injury with involvement	Major injury with involvement
Electrical injury	Never	Desirable	Preferred
Chemical injury	Never	Desirable	Preferred
Frostbite	Never	Desirable	Preferred
Inhalation injury	Never	Desirable	Preferred
Major associated medical illness	Never	Desirable	Preferred
Associated fractures, multiple trauma	Never	Desirable	Preferred

TBSA = total body surface area.
Source = From R.E. Salisbury, N.M. Newman, and G.P. Dingeldein, Jr. (eds.). *Manual of Burn Therapeutics*. Boston: Little, Brown, 1983. P. 4.

Area	Birth–1 yr	1–4 yr	5–9 yr	10–14 yr	15 yr	Adult	Partial thickness 2°	Full thickness 3°	Total
Head	19	17	13	11	9	7			
Neck	2	2	2	2	2	2			
Anterior trunk	13	13	13	13	13	13			
Posterior trunk	13	13	13	13	13	13			
Right buttock	2½	2½	2½	2½	2½	2½			
Left buttock	2½	2½	2½	2½	2½	2½			
Genitalia	1	1	1	1	1	1			
Right upper arm	4	4	4	4	4	4			
Left upper arm	4	4	4	4	4	4			
Right lower arm	3	3	3	3	3	3			
Left lower arm	3	3	3	3	3	3			
Right hand	2½	2½	2½	2½	2½	2½			
Left hand	2½	2½	2½	2½	2½	2½			
Right thigh	5½	6½	8	8½	9	9½			
Left thigh	5½	6½	8	8½	9	9½			
Right leg	5	5	5½	6	6½	7			
Left leg	5	5	5½	6	6½	8			
Right foot	3½	3½	3½	3½	3½	3½			
Left foot	3½	3½	3½	3½	3½	3½			
						Total			

FIG. 10-1. Lund-Browder chart for burn estimate, showing percentage of body area involved (birth through adulthood). (From R. E. Salisbury, N. M. Newman, and G. P. Dingeldein, Jr. [eds.]. *Manual of Burn Therapeutics.* Boston: Little, Brown, 1983. P. 3.)

TABLE 10-3. Classification of burn depth

Degree	Possible cause	Appearance and Texture	Sensation	Course
FIRST DEGREE				
Superficial layers of epidermis destroyed; vasodilation	Ultraviolet exposure: sunburn, ultraviolet light; low-intensity flash	Redness only—will blanch with pressure and refill; no blistering; minimal or no edema; normal texture	Hyperesthesia; sensitive to temperature; slight pain; tingling	Complete recovery within 5–10 days; peeling
SECOND DEGREE				
Superficial layer of skin destroyed; partial thickness	Contact with hot liquids; scalds; flash flame	Large, thick-walled blisters may increase in size; redness around blistered area; normal-to-firm texture	Painful; hyperesthesia; sensitive to heat and cold	Recovery in 16–21 days; some scarring; wound will heal by itself if nothing causes further damage
DEEP SECOND DEGREE				
All but deep layers of dermis destroyed; capillary permeability	Scalds; flame	Usually no blister formation; mottled reddened base; broken epidermis; weeping surface; edema; firm texture	Very painful; may be anesthetic during first few days but sensation will return as tissues recover	Infection may convert to third degree; crust will develop and when removed tiny pigskinlike areas will be seen, and will heal very slowly; most hypertrophic scarring results from deep second-degree burns
THIRD DEGREE				
Full-thickness destruction; coagulation of protein	Flame; electrical; contact with hot objects	Usually brownish, may be white, black, or red; no blisters, or if present, thin-walled and will not increase in size; broken skin with fat exposed; edema; firm or leathery texture	Painless; insensitive to pin prick; danger of shock	Regeneration of skin not possible, cannot heal by self; eschar sloughs; grafting is necessary; scarring, loss of contour and function result; time to heal depends on whether grafts take
FOURTH DEGREE				
Tissue under skin destroyed; may include fascia, muscle, tendon, bone, subcutaneous tissue	Flame; electrical; prolonged contact with hot objects	Muscle, tendon, bone may be exposed; infection may soon intervene; edema	Painless	Early debridement necessary to establish adequate drainage; grafting necessary; takes months to heal
Char	Flame; deep electrical	Black skin; leathery texture	Painless	Should be excised early; amputation of limb probably necessary

Source: From M. Logigian (ed.). *Adult Rehabilitation: A Team Approach for Therapists.* Boston: Little, Brown, 1982. P. 153.

cedures are provided, and the severity of the wound is determined. Subsequently, the child is transferred to a specialized burn treatment unit for further medical treatment. Respiratory care is provided including maintenance of a patent airway. Fluid replacement therapy is initiated to prevent hypovolemic shock. Intravenous medication is given for pain and to prevent infection. Intravenous hyperalimentation may begin on the third or fourth posttrauma day to deal with the significant metabolic drain produced by the burn. If the child can eat, supplemental foods are provided and a high-caloric, high-protein diet with supplemental vitamins and iron is maintained.

Wound care begins as soon as the immediate life-threatening conditions are addressed. Wounds are cleansed, loose tissue is removed, and a topical antibacterial agent is applied. Positioning (Table 10-4) and splinting (Table 10-5)

TABLE 10-4. Positioning to prevent deformity

Area burned	Resulting deformity	Position of prevention
Neck		
Anterior aspect or circumferential	Flexion contracture of neck	No pillow under head
Posterior aspect (only)	Extensor contracture of neck	Prone—pillow under upper chest to flex cervical spine; supine—small pillow under neck
Axilla		
Anterior	Adduction and internal rotation	Shoulder joint in abduction (100–130°) and external rotation
Posterior	Adduction and external rotation	Shoulder in forward flexion and 100–130° abduction
Pectoral region	Shoulder protraction	No pillow; shoulders abducted and externally rotated
Chest or abdomen	Kyphosis	As above and hips neutral (*not* flexed)
Lateral trunk	Scoliosis	Supine, affected arm abducted
Elbow (anterior surface or circumferential)	Flexion and pronation	Arm extended and supinated
Wrist		
Total or volar surface	Flexion	Splint in 15° extension
Dorsal surface	Extension	Splint in 15° flexion
Hip (includes inguinal and perineal burns)	Internal rotation, flexion, and adduction; possible joint subluxation if contracture severe	Neutral rotation and abduction and maintain extension by prone position or *pillow under buttocks*
Knee (popliteal surface or circumferential)	Flexion	Maintain extension, using posterior splints or suspend heels with plastic heel protecting boots. *No pillows* under knees while supine or under ankles while prone
Ankle	Plantar flexion if foot dorsiflexor muscles are weak or their tendons are divided	90° dorsiflexion with splint if possible rather than foot board

Source: Taken with permission from *Nursing the Burned Patient*, I. Feller and C. Archambeault-Jones. Ann Arbor, Mich.: National Institute for Burn Medicine, 1973.

TABLE 10-5. Splints

Area	Position	Splint
Neck and chin	Extension	Neck conformer
Anterior trunk	Extension (shoulder retraction)	Body jacket with neck conformer or halo neck splint
Lower extremity	Knee extension	Three-point extension splint or posterior knee pan splint
Ankle/toes	Foot neutral plantar flexion	Foot drop splint, anterior ankle conformer
Axilla	90° shoulder abduction, elbow extension	Airplane splint or axilla conformer
Elbow	Extension	Three-point extension splint or pan splint
Wrist/hand	20°–30° wrist extension, 50°–70° MCP flexion, full extension PIP/DIPS, abduction/extension thumb	Resting pan splint

[3, 5, 25] are initiated within the first 24 to 48 hours. The burn can be cared for using the exposure method or dressing of the wound, surgical excision, and grafting of the burn site. In general, all full-thickness burns are grafted [15].

Hydrotherapy can be used for wound cleansing and during range of motion. This modality is particularly useful in treating children with burns because it minimizes the discomfort of handling. Immersion in water eases the removal of dressings and encourages movement through play with favorite toys.

As the child progresses from the critical/emergent to the acute phase of burn rehabilitation (as scar tissue begins to form), preventing functional loss is of major importance. An exercise program at this time focuses on stretching of healing skin; maintaining range of motion, motor coordination, strength, and endurance; and promoting functional independence [30].

Children often exhibit increased pain reactions during exercise, which may be due to fear, apprehension, or lack of understanding of the importance of movement. Play can be the best means of eliciting active motion and enabling increased control and success experiences [30]. This can include group activities such as ball toss or individual games such as "Simon Says."

Active participation in dressing changes, grooming, and other functional activities is important for children to maintain ego development during this stressful time. Ambulation is encouraged as early as feasible. Special attention is given to a gait program because children have a greater tendency for assuming comfortable positions and need additional guidance in correct posture and movement patterns [30]. Individual and group play activities, circular walker, bicycles, and tricycles provide incentives for walking.

In addition to exercise and activity, every effort is made to decrease hypertrophic scar formation. Early scar control is crucial to obtain optimal long-term results and thus should start as wound healing begins and continue until the healed tissue is flat, soft, and supple, and light pink, white, or brown [32]. Scar control often involves the use of various techniques and materials that enable application of external pressure on the scar area (Table 10-6).

The rehabilitative/reconstructive phase can take several years of in- and outpatient care. During this time, the exercise and functional activity program continues as does scar control efforts. Reconstructive surgery may be recommended.

TABLE 10-6. Orthotic materials used for burn scar control

Name (source)	Characteristics	Uses
Compression wraps Elastic wraps 2-, 3-, 4-, 6-, ½ length, double length (any medical company) Elset (Tubiton House, Medlock St., Oldham 011 3HS, England)	Effective compression; proper width conforms well to irregular body parts; easy to vary tension; rubber deteriorates on exposure to oils. Nylon bandages cut into fragile tissue; laundering is time consuming. Very soft, flexible elastic fabric; conforms for stump wraps and finger wraps	Gradient pressue wrap; most pressure at distal point with support to most proximal point. Spiral or figure of eight wrap to any body part Early compression when little tension is tolerated
Tubular products Elastic net Tubigauze (Scholl Hospital Products Division, 213 W. Schiller St., Chicago, IL) Tubigrip elastic bandage (Tubiton House) Compressogrip (Fred Sammons, Box 32, Brookfield, IL 60513)	Open mesh net; conforms to regular body parts; cuts into tissue if no interface is present, due to swelling around fibers in mesh. Rib weave stockinette covered with latex rubber yarns introduced into the fabric in continuous lengths; shaped support bandage available for arms and legs; friction to tissue diminished if applied from applicator; Tubigrip: 33% rubber and 67% cotton and is therefore more effective to maintain compression because rubber is elastic; Lycra or Spandex products change in compression after 30-min stretch due to viscoplasticity of synthetic fibers; laundering is easier than elastic wraps; fabric may roll at proximal edge and cause decubiti	Secure gauze bandages; may slightly reduce swelling; allows individual bandaging of fingers Compression of any cylindrical body part, particularly effective in applications involving knee or elbow because bandage does not gather in joint space. One to three layers may be used to achieve adequate pressure; several sizes may be combined for cone-shaped body parts
Commercially produced individual garmets Jobskin garments (Jobst, Box 653, Toledo, OH 43694) Elastic garments (Bioconcepts, 7324 N. 71st St., Scottsdale, AZ 85253) **Pre-sized garments.** Tubigloves (Tubiton House): Jobst pre-sized standard glove; Isotoner gloves	Gradient pressure lycra garments individually fitted to specific body measurements. Jobskin elastic pressure covers are engineered to apply physiologically correct counterpressure to newly formed scar tissue Bioconcepts garments are also individually fitted to specific measurements Costly; deteriorate from exposure to oils, detergent, or heat; fabric synthetic and viscoplasticity causes compression to relax after 30 min. Presized garments may be used to toughen	Head and face: hood; neck: turtleneck, soft collar; Chest and arms: vest with sleeves; Legs: stocking torso and two-leg stocking with panty Any combination of areas can be compressed with these garments. Concave areas need inserts or overlay for extra pressure

Material	Comments	Uses
(Aris, 417 5th Ave., New York, NY 10016); Tubigarments (Tubiton House)	tissue for final individual garment; frequently fit is less than ideal	
Insert or overlay materials (preformed)		Inserts or overlay to increase pressure on scars; especially effective if beveled for concave areas such as breast and buttock cleavage. Protection at irritated skin creases. Finger web spreaders
Adhesive-backed foams Reston (3M) Spenco padding (Spenco Med Products, Inc., P.O. Box 8113 Waco, TX 76710) Poly cushion (Fred Sammons) Vigilon (C. R. Bard, Inc., Berkeley Hts., NY 07922)	Soft padding may be stuck to garment, patient's shoe, etc; may cause excessive sweating. May macerate tissue due to moisture collection; may collect bacteria if patient's hygiene is not meticulous. Cut with scissors. Prolonged drying time if laundered	
Open cell foam Alimed (Alimed, 172 W. Newton, Boston, MA 02118) Cushion foam Backpacker's mattress Tubifoam and arthropads LMB finger pressure wraps (LMB, Hand Rehab Products, Inc., P.O. Box 1181, San Luis Obispo, CA 92406)		
Closed cell polyethylene sheets, aliplast, plastazote	Resilient, light weight, flexible, fairly durable, cut with scissors, can be heated and molded to patient	Shoe inserts, support for neck foam collars. Temporary "wraparound" knee extension splint
Orthopedic felt, 1/4-in., 1/2-in. (any medical company)	Polyester felt can be washed and dried. Cut with tin snips or felt shears. Does not usually cause sweating. Can sew to garments or secure with pocket	Beveled inserts or overlays
Insert materials (liquid with catalyst) Otoform K (WFR Aquaplast Corp., P.O. Box 215, Ramsey, NJ 07446)	Silicone-type material cures in 5 min with catalyst. Viscous enough to set up without running to edges. Moderately flexible when set up	Beveled inserts especially effective in thumb webs

TABLE 10-6 (CONTINUED)

Name (source)	Characteristics	Uses
Silicone Medical elastomer 382 (Dow Corning Corp., Medical Products, Midland, MI 48640)	Liquid silicone sets up with stannous octoate catalyst; may cause excessive sweating. Odor controlled somewhat by boiling elastomer. Conforms to all irregularities.	Postoperative dressing over interface for skin grafting (½ elastomer, ½ prosthetic foam)
Prosthetic foam Q7-4290 (Dow Corning)	Expands 7 times when mixed with catalyst. Forms open cell foam. Odor may be offensive. Conforms perfectly to scar.	Positioning splint especially for hands of children. Hand web expanders. Insert or overlay adhered to tee-shirt or tubular elastic
Strapping material Velfoam Beta pile Duravel (LMB) Polyester wicking (Fred Sammons)	Soft nap; easy to secure with Velcro	Splint strapping, finger web spreaders, beveled insert or overlay for scars
Low-temperature plastic K-splint (Sammons) Polyform (Rolyan, P.O. Box 555, N93-W14475 Whittaker Wax, Menomonee Falls, WI 53051)	Plastic material. Easily removable. Secure with elastic wrap, tubular elastic, or straps. Bonds with heat. Washable. Hard, smooth surface at room temperature. Cut with scissors at 70°C (140°F). Shape conforms perfectly to patient and to raised scars. May need silicone or sponge insert to keep pressure on raised area. If perforated, may retain bacteria. Scars may grow into perforation if no interface is used. Swelling of tissue at perforations may cause itching	Draping plastic, insert or overlay to prevent or stretch contractures, static or dynamic splinting materials
Orthoplast isoprene (Johnson & Johnson Products, Inc., Chicago, IL)	Synthetic rubber, smooth, relatively stable surfaces at room temperature. Cut with scissors and mold at 60°C (130°F). Does not conform exactly to scar. Must be stretched with some pressure to conform. Bonds with surface clean and heat. Washable. Easily removable	Used as above. Usually does not require insert for scar compression because plastic does not conform accurately to scar
Casting materials Splints Rolls	Variety of plaster widths and set-up times; becomes warm during set up. Can be fit for total contact pressure to scars; must be applied over interface, e.g., webril	Total-contact splint must be removed with cast cutter. Impression material for positive cast of neck

266

High-temperature plastics	Stable to 350°F; must be cut warm or cut with saw or moto-tool. Must be vacuum formed or shaped by hand over plaster cast of body part. Tissue can be observed through splint. Tissue must be observed for contact dermatitis. Washable. Easily removable	Transparent face and neck orthosis. Inserts or overlays in circumscribed scar areas. Individual splints to compress areas needing more pressure than circumferential elastic can provide without impairing circulation or nerve function
Cellulose acetate butyrate (Eastman Kodak) Uvex		
Polycarbonate "Lexan"		
"Tufak" (any plastic company)		
Thermovac-clear or Suralyn (U.S. Manufacturing, 180 N. San Gabriel Blvd., P. O. Box 5030, Pasadena, CA 91107)		
Tenite Butyrate Aquaplast-clear (WFR Co.)	Polycarbonate bubbles if not dehydrated at 250°F for 6 hr	

Source: From S. V. Fisher and P. A. Helms (eds.). *Comprehensive Rehabilitation of Burns.* Baltimore: Williams & Wilkins, 1984. Copyright © 1984, the Williams & Wilkins Co., Baltimore.

During the acute phase, the pain, isolation, and strange environment of the hospital can create confusion, panic, and anxiety in children. They may feel real or imagined guilt associated with the cause of the burn. Regression is a common phenomenon as the child is unable to sort out these feelings. The child may become disruptive or manipulative on the unit. Psychiatric intervention becomes of critical importance for the child and family [6].

The long-term emotional damage of a major burn may be as severe as the physical damage. The disfigurement of burns can be catastrophic. Young children often focus on the immediate discomfort and pain of the burn. As long as dependency needs are met by parents and staff, they experience fewer long-term problems than older children [6]. However, the burn wounds, pressure garments, and restrictive movements can give the child a strange appearance, which presents difficulties, especially for the school-age child. The older child may be able to cope while in the protective environment of the burn unit, yet have difficulty with the outside world. Peers significantly influence the developing self-image of the adolescent, and the changes in appearance and abilities may bring on fears of rejection and despair. Therapists and teachers can help the child by gradually enabling experiences outside the burn unit. Trips to other parts of the hospital, visits from friends and classmates, or a day trip to a favorite site can help decrease the child's anxiety.

Family support during this traumatic time is very important. The family can assist in meeting the needs of the child through frequent visits and by making favorite toys, books, and food available. Yet parents need support as well to learn to care for the burned child and to prepare for the future. Circumstances surrounding the burn injury may pose difficulties, especially if the burn injury involves abuse or neglect. If this situation exists, staff must deal with their feelings of anger toward the family so that optimal care can be provided.

Play experiences, particularly for the younger child, can be valuable therapeutic interventions. Through the use of art, music, and games, the child is encouraged to share feelings and learn about upcoming procedures such as surgery or wound care. One such activity is play with a Surgi-doll, which has dressings and splints similar to those of the child [22].

As the child may need lengthy hospitalization, a hospital school program should begin as soon as possible. It provides some normalcy [19] and enables the child to keep up with classmates. The hospital teacher needs to establish a regular schedule that coordinates with activities of the burn team. Learning about the child's limitations and abilities helps to reinforce appropriate behavior and skills. Contact should be maintained with the home school, and home visit prior to the child's discharge from the hospital can be useful. Follow-up communication with the school teacher and child eases the transition for the burned child from hospital to home and back to school [17]. As the child grows, vocational counseling may be helpful.

CANCER

Cancer is the second major cause of death in children. With the emergence of chemotherapy to augment surgery and radiation as treatment modalities, death is no longer the inevitable outcome in all cases, but it continues as a threat for most with the disease. Many different types of cancer have been identified in children, the most common being leukemia (Fig. 10-2).

What causes cancer and why cells become malignant are questions that remain unanswered. However, in an attempt to find the answers, many areas are under investigation such as environmental exposure to carcinogens. Scientists have found that children of mothers who have taken various drugs during pregnancy (e.g., diethylstilbestrol [DES]), have an increased risk of cancer. Viruses, exposure to physical (e.g., asbestos) and chemical (e.g., drugs, pollutants) carcinogens, familial predisposition, and chromosomal aberrations are

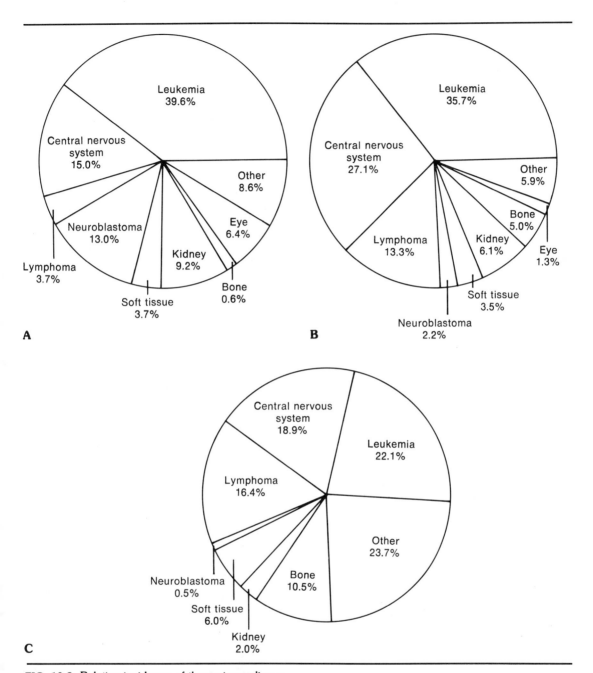

FIG. 10-2. Relative incidence of the major malignancies in children. A. From birth–5 yr. B. From 5–10 yr. C. From 10–15 yr. (From A. J. Altman and A. D. Schwartz. *Malignant Diseases of Infancy, Childhood, and Adolescence.* Philadelphia: Saunders 1978. P. 3.)

among other causes under investigation. Until etiologic answers are found, health care workers must be knowledgeable of the potential cancer risks so as to provide accurate information to families coping with a child with cancer [1, 11, 37].

CANCERS COMMON IN CHILDHOOD

Leukemia is the term used for a group of diseases in which there is uncontrolled proliferation of white cell precursors that fail to mature and accumulate in the bone marrow, blood, and tissue. They inhibit the production of normal red blood cells, white cells, and platelets. This results in anemia, significantly lowered resistance to infections, and thrombocytopenia. Thus, the early symptoms include pallor, fatigue (of anemia), joint pain (associated with leukemic involvement of the bone), fever (associated with infection), and petechiae or purpura (bleeding).

Eighty percent of leukemia in children is acute lymphoblastic leukemia (ALL). It has a peak incidence between 2 to 6 years of age and is more common in boys. This type of leukemia may have central nervous system involvement (infiltration of meninges by leukemic cells) and gonadal leukemia. The treatment for this type of cancer involves chemotherapy, radiation therapy, and bone marrow transplantation. Sixty percent of the children with this type of leukemia have a 5-year complete remission.

Acute nonlymphoblastic leukemia (ANLL) accounts for 15 percent of leukemia in children. This type includes acute myeloblastic (AML), acute promyelocytic (APML), acute myelomonocytic (AMML), acute monocytic, and acute erythrocytic leukemia. Central nervous system involvement is also seen with this form of leukemia. Chemotherapy and bone marrow transplantation are the treatment modalities used. Sixty to eighty-four percent achieve a 9- to 16-month remission with treatment. With bone marrow transplantation there is a 60 percent chance of long-term remission.

The remaining 5 percent of childhood leukemia is called chronic myelogenous leukemia (CML). Two forms of the disease occur, an adult form that is more common in 10- to 12-year olds, and a juvenile form that has a peak incidence in 1- to 2-year olds. The adult form is slightly more common in boys. Chemotherapy and bone marrow transplantation are the treatment modalities used in this form of leukemia. The adult form of CML has a 25- to 30-month survival rate; the juvenile form has a 6-month survival rate.

Lymphoma includes Hodgkin's disease and non-Hodgkin's lymphoma. Hodgkin's disease is a malignancy of the lymphoid system. Sixty to ninety percent of those with the disease have cervical adenopathy. Other symptoms include anorexia, weight loss, malaise, lethargy, fever, night sweats, and pruritus. Staging is used to determine the extent of the disease when it is diagnosed. Treatment includes radiation therapy and chemotherapy. Survival for more than 5 years is expected depending on the stage of the disease and histologic type (e.g., stages I and II have a 90 percent survival rate, while stage III has an 80 percent survival rate).

Non-Hodgkin's lymphoma is a malignant tumor originating in any lymphatic tissue in the body. It is more common in boys from infancy through adolescence, with a slight increase from 5 to 8 years of age. It has a rapid onset and progresses quickly. Signs and symptoms depend on the sites involved (Table 10-7). Some centers recommend staging to determine the extent of the disease when diagnosed. Chemotherapy, radiation therapy, and possibly surgery are the treatments of choice. Ninety percent enter complete remission with treatment and seventy-six percent survive 5½ years.

Wilms' tumor is a neoplasma of the kidney found in infants and young children. It is a large, rapidly growing tumor, usually noticed due to abdominal swelling or palpation of an abdominal mass. Staging of the disease has been done by the National Wilms' Tumor Study. Surgery is the treatment of choice, with radiation and chemotherapy if indicated. Stage I

TABLE 10-7. Sites of involvement at diagnosis and sites of metastasis in NHL according to primary site

Primary site	Sites of involvement at diagnosis		Metastatic sites	
	Most common	Other	Most common	Other
Abdomen	Kidney Peripheral nodes Liver Pleura Para-aortic nodes Bone marrow	Testicles Mediastinum Tonsils Ovaries CNS	Bone marrow Primary site CNS Pleura Chest wall Kidney Peripheral nodes Liver	Testes Para-aortic nodes Spleen Bone Nasopharynx
Mediastinum	Peripheral nodes Pleural effusion Liver Bone marrow Kidney Para-aortic nodes Heart (pericardium)	Lungs Tonsils Bone Subcutaneous tissue	Bone marrow Primary site CNS Spleen Liver Kidneys	Subcutaneous tissue Testes Bowel Nasopharynx Orbital cavity Pleura
Peripheral node	Bone marrow Mediastinum Para-aortic nodes Bone Kidney	Subcutaneous tissue Nasopharynx Liver Spleen Prostate	Primary site Bone marrow CNS Liver Bowel Spleen	Subcutaneous tissue Mediastinum Lungs Orbital cavity Kidneys Skeletal Testes
Nasopharynx	Bone marrow Para-aortic nodes Abdomen	CNS	Bone marrow CNS	

Source: From Association of Pediatric Oncology Nurses, *Nursing Care of the Child with Cancer*. Boston: Little, Brown, 1982. P. 113. Original data from N. Wollner. In M. B. Twomey and R. Goods (eds.), *The Immunology of Lymphoreticular Neoplasms*. New York: Plenum, 1978.

tumors of favorable histology have an excellent prognosis. Most children with the tumor have a 90 percent chance of long-term survival. Histology, tumor weight, positive lymph nodes, and the patient's age are predictors of relapse.

Neuroblastoma is a malignant neoplasma from embryonic neural crest tissue. It originates from the adrenal medulla or sympathetic ganglia along the craniospinal axis. This type of tumor includes neuroblastoma, ganglioneuroblastoma, ganglioneuroma, phenochromocytoma, and neurofibroma. Fifty percent of the cases occur in children under the age of 2. The most common presenting sign is an abdominal mass. Neuroblastomas disseminate early to the bones, lymph nodes, liver, and subcutaneous tissue. Staging of the disease has been suggested. Surgery is the treatment of choice, with radiation therapy and chemotherapy carried out to control metastases. Survival is inversely correlated with the age of the child at the time of diagnosis. Age of the child, stage of the disease, time of diagnosis, and tumor location influence prognosis. Overall 32 percent survive 2 years disease-free.

Soft tissue sarcomas include rhabdomyosarcoma, 53 percent, and nonrhabdomyosarcoma, 47 percent. Primary sites in children for rhabdomyosarcoma are head/neck, extremities, genitourinary tract, retroperitoneal area, gastrointestinal/hepatobiliary tract, intrathoracic area, perineum, and anus. The disease peaks in 2- to 6-year olds for head/neck and genitourinary tract tumors, and in adolescence for males for genitourinary tract tumors. These are highly aggressive tumors with early infiltration and distant metastasis. Signs and symptoms vary according to the location and histology of the tumor and metastasis. Staging of the disease has been accomplished by the Intergroup Rhabdomyosarcoma Study.

Surgery, radiation, and chemotherapy are the treatment modalities involved. Survival of approximately 5 years depends on the extent of the disease at the time of the diagnosis: stage I has a 96 percent survival rate, stage II has an 80 percent survival rate, stage III has a 75 percent survival rate, and stage IV has a 2-year survival rate, depending on site of primary tumor (tumors of the orbit have an overall good prognosis), tumor histology (alveolar tumors usually are more extensive), and age, (1- to 7-year olds have the best cures).

Nonrhabdomyosarcomas are less common sarcomas of childhood and adolescence. They are more common in adults, but the prognosis is better for children, often requiring surgery alone (Table 10-8).

TABLE 10-8. Soft-tissue sarcomas in childhood

Tumor	Common primary sites	Peak age at diagnosis	Prognosis
Fibrosarcoma	Extremity	< 5 yr	Excellent (83–92% survival) with surgery alone
		10–15 yr	60% survival at 5 yr (similar to adult series)
Neurofibrosarcoma	Extremity, abdomen, trunk		Strongly related to stage. Very good for stage I, II; poor for stage III and IV
Leiomysarcoma	Retroperitoneum vascular tissue, gastrointestinal tract		Nongastrointestinal tract tumors, prognosis is good. Gastrointestinal tract: high incidence of metastases.
Liposarcoma	Extremity, retroperitoneum	0–2 yr, 2nd decade	Very good with complete excision
Synovial sarcoma	Extremity (lower > upper)		Similar to adult studies: 45–70% 5-yr survival
Hemangiopericytoma	Extremity, retroperitoneum, head and neck		Young children: excellent with surgery alone. Older children, similar to adults 30–70% survival at 5 yr
Alveolar soft part sarcomas	Extremity		Survival: 80% at 2 yr, 56% at 5 yr, 47% at 10 yr. No long-term cures known.
Primitive neuroectodermal tumors	Chest wall, extremity, pelvis	Not known	Related to stage. Long-term prognosis not known at present.
Extraosseous Ewing's sarcoma	Paravertebral extremity	2nd and 3rd decades	60% long-term survival. Prognosis related to stage.

Source: J. S. Miser and P. A. Pizzo. Soft tissue sarcomas in childhood. *Pediatr. Clin. North Am.* 32(3) June, 1985.

Malignant bone tumors include osteosarcoma and Ewing's sarcoma. The prevalence of bone cancer increases with the age of the child. Signs and symptoms include pain, swelling, and restricted function in the involved area. There may also be fever, anemia, and weight loss. A bone biopsy is done to confirm the diagnosis. A common metastatic site is the lung.

Osteosarcoma is a primary bone tumor from the mesenchymal cells. It is more common in males, and 75 percent of the cases occur from 10 to 25 years of age. It affects the epiphyseal growth areas of the long bones. Fifty percent involve the distal femur and proximal tibia. The next most common site is the proximal humerus. The disease has a gradual onset with pain a common symptom. Surgery, and if necessary chemotherapy, is the therapy provided. If no treatment occurs, within 6 to 9 months, metastases occur usually in the lungs. With treatment there is a 50 to 60 percent 5-year survival rate.

Ewing's sarcoma is usually found in males, 5 to 15 years old. It is a primary bone tumor from the bone marrow space and presents pain of increasing severity. It affects the long bones of an extremity or the trunk and the flat bones of the pelvis or ribs. Metastases are usually to the lungs and multiple other bones. Radiation therapy is the treatment of choice, and in some instances an exercise program is provided, with chemotherapy as indicated. The Intergroup Ewing's Sarcoma Study indicated disease-free survival at 172 weeks for 58 percent of the children studied.

Brain tumors are most frequent in 5- to 10-year-olds with a slight increase in males. This type of cancer involves an expanding mass (tumor) within a closed container (skull), the result being an increase in cranial pressure. Thus the signs and symptoms are headache, emesis, papilledema, seizures, and visual problems. A computed tomography (CT) scan is used for diagnosis. Surgery, radiation therapy, and chemotherapy are all used in the treatment. Prognosis depends on the type of tumor, grade of the malignancy, and location. For example, one study of children with astrocytomas predicted a survival rate (5 years) for 65 percent of grades I and II; tumors occurring in the brain stem have a 12 percent survival rate. Recurrent malignant primary brain tumors have an extremely poor prognosis. The following is a list of the more common brain tumors in children:

Astrocytoma	Most frequent in cerebellum, can occur in brain stem and cerebral hemospheres; grades I to IV
Medulloblastoma	Arises from primitive neuroepithelial cells, disseminates via cerebrospinal fluid pathways predominantly in the cerebellum, fourth ventricle, and brain stem.
Ependymoma	Arises from primitive neuroepithelial cells of the ventricles, common below tentorium, disseminates via cerebrospinal pathways
Craniopharyngioma	Benign neuroepithelial tumors, yet malignant behavior due to continuity with vital structures; involves craniopharyngeal canal; common in sella turcica
Glioblastoma	Histologically high-grade astrocytoma; 12-month survival following radiation

Retinoblastoma, the most common eye tumor in children, is usually diagnosed by the age of 5. The presenting symptom is leukokoria. The child may also exhibit strabismus, inflammation of the eye, and frequent second malignancies. Treatment can involve surgery, radiation, photocoagulation, cryotherapy, and chemotherapy. There is an 80 to 90 percent survival rate, and 70 to 80 percent retain some vision in the treated eye.

CARE OF THE CHILD WITH CANCER

Advances in the treatment of cancer in children have led to dramatic improvements in survival. However, treatment modalities affect malignant and healthy cells. Thus, toxicities can be experienced by many organ systems immediately following treatment, whereas others may occur months or years later.

Few situations require more knowledge and understanding than the physical care of the child with cancer [34]. Bone marrow suppression, immunosuppression, and infections result from the cancer itself or the complications and side effects of treatment. Almost any system in the body can be involved and demand specific care for the prevention and management of these problems.

Adequate nutrition is essential so that the child can fight off infection, tolerate chemotherapy, and control anorexia. Nausea, vomiting, diarrhea, and gastrointestinal bleeding may occur with chemotherapy and radiation. Among the intervention strategies for these problems are proper positioning of the child, intravenous fluids, and good oral hygiene. Sensitivity by the team toward keeping the environment pleasant, particularly during mealtimes, and free of noxious stimuli, and the presentation of special foods, such as ice cream and milk shakes, can also be helpful.

Hygiene is extremely important, since the skin is the body's natural barrier against infection [34]. Irradiated skin can be dry and scaling, requiring a lubricating agent if radiation therapy is complete. Lesions, bleeding of the skin, and epistaxis can develop from chemotherapy and radiation, which demand immediate attention to contain infection from the child's own body flora.

Bone and joint pain, fractures, amputation, and immobility are among the musculoskeletal problems caused by the cancer or its treatment.

Each requires specific therapeutic intervention and careful physical handling by the members of the health care team.

Increased cranial pressure and seizures often result from certain types of cancer. These situations call for specific medical intervention, special physical handling of the child, as well as environmental changes. Minimizing bright lights and loud noises, for example, may make the child more comfortable. Support and reassurance to the child and family can also be helpful.

Pain can be experienced relative to the disease and may be exacerbated by fear and anxiety about the cancer and its treatment. For some families, pain is a constant reminder of increased morbidity and death, thus interfering with normal family function [9]. Young children may not be able to describe the pain and its location, instead they cry or rub a painful area. The inability to express the pain phenomenon to enable assistance increases the feelings of frustration, helplessness, and guilt families experience.

In addition to medication, surgery, and radiation used in controlling pain, various therapeutic methods can also be useful such as heat, massage, and relaxation techniques. Providing information, support, and an attitude of acceptance of the child can help alter the pain experience and thus make it more bearable [14].

The adjustment of the family to a child's having cancer and its treatment is a difficult one. With the support and encouragement of all the members of the team and time, the initial shock of the diagnosis can be overcome. In most cases, acceptance of treatment and adaptation to change and predicted outcome will also occur.

The theoretical framework provided by Kubler-Ross and adapted by Hall, Hardin, and Conastser is useful in the assimilation and adaptation process [14]. This framework involves stages of loss; the first stage includes denial, when there may be rejection of diagnosis; unwillingness to talk about it; euphoria; restlessness; and anxiety. During this stage the development of positive coping mechanisms, validation of reality, clarification of feelings of the parents, and normal family routines should be encouraged. Anger is the next stage. This is typically expressed as overt anger of abusive language, derogatory comments, and physical display of anger or covert anger of complaining, ingratiating behavior, or denial of unpleasant situations. Intervention can include helping the family identify the cause of their anger and providing consistent, truthful information and reassurance. Bargaining is the third stage. The family may overcompensate or have rigid compliance with health measures believing this will guarantee a cure. A review of the facts of the situation and the encouragement of intrafamily support may be useful in this situation. Depression usually follows next, with a decreased interest in the environment, alterations in daily activities, and increased demands on staff. The child and family should try to develop a consistency in activities of daily living, and the family should offer praise for the child's efforts.

The final stage is acceptance. At this time the child and family can discuss the condition and treatment openly and recognize that there may be times when behavior from the previous stages will be exhibited. The team continues to provide consistent information, positive reinforcement, and asks the family to help others in their adjustment process.

Following the initial diagnosis and treatment, the next stressful period is remission. Early counseling can prevent major problems at this time. Particular attention must be given to the maintenance of normal family patterns, relationships among family members and friends, and school attendance [21]. The child may have misapprehensions about the disease. Reactions to a changed body image, for example, hair loss, caused by the disease may be felt by the child and peers. "The child needs a great deal of support upon reentering the home and school environment" [14]. The school teacher should be informed of the situation, and an explanation to peers and classmates may be helpful.

The terminal period for those who succumb to the disease presents another set of challenges. Issues of pain control, nutrition, and symptom management require careful attention. The well-being of the family system needs frequent monitoring. Lansky notes,

The death of the child is always accompanied by shock and confusion, regardless of the intervention and preparation. Normal grief is a long-term process and, consequently, follow-up should be prolonged. The most acute grief often begins several months after the death and may last up to 2 years with sporadic recurrences thereafter. Reassurance to the family that this is normal is an important aspect of intervention.

LATE EFFECTS OF CANCER

Cardiomyopathy, congestive heart failure, and pericarditis can be the late effects of cancer treatment experienced by the cardiovascular system. The endocrine system can be affected with late abnormalities manifested in the hypothalamic-pituitary axis, thyroid gland, and gonads. The gastrointestinal system late sequelae are hepatic injury following chemotherapy and radiation therapy and chronic enteritis secondary to radiation therapy. The musculoskeletal system can be affected, especially from radiation: It damages areas of bone growth such as in vertebral bone, resulting in scoliosis, and epiphyseal growth in long bones, resulting in asymmetrical deformities. The nervous system can experience long-term neurotoxicity, which may be manifested as an encephalopathy, peripheral neuropathy, or neuropsychological and intellectual dysfunction. The major late effects on the lungs are interstitial pneumonitis and pulmonary fibrosis and on the urinary tract, radiation nephritis and chronic cystitis [4]. Each problem area demands special attention and individualized therapeutic intervention.

As a result of long-term survival, individuals previously treated for cancer in childhood are at risk for developing a second malignancy—17 percent by 20 years. However, although chemotherapy and radiation therapy are potentially teratogenic, there is no indication of a deleterious effect in the offspring of cancer patients who have completed all treatment prior to pregnancy. Careful follow-up of patients with cancer is needed to document adverse late effects, to identify etiologic agents, and to alter treatment to give the least toxic therapy without sacrificing the quality or duration of survival [4].

CARDIAC DISORDERS

The two major classifications of cardiac problems in children are congenital heart disease (CHD) and rheumatic heart disease (RHD). CHD is the result of genetic factors (e.g., those associated with Down's syndrome), environmental factors such as the mother's exposure to radiation or drugs during pregnancy, or parasites (particularly in Third World countries). Congenital cardiac defects include patent ductus arteriosus, ventricular or atrial septal defect, or aortic stenosis. The child with a defect can experience fatigue, shortness of breath, and cyanosis. A heart murmur, abnormal heart rate, or heart failure can develop and worsen as the child gets older. However, medical management of the CHD controls the symptoms until improvement occurs or cardiac surgery will be tolerated. Most defects can be corrected or the symptoms alleviated with cardiac surgery [12, 28].

RHD is the term used to describe the permanent heart damage that can result from rheumatic fever (RF). RF begins with a strep bacterial infection, which is typically manifested by a sore throat. Approximately 90 percent of sore throats are viral in origin; however, 10 percent are streptococcal bacteria, and those of the beta-hemolytic (group A) strain cause RF. Most children with strep throat experience fever, sore throat, and large tender cervical lymph nodes. The disease is commonly treated with penicillin.

If not treated, 3 percent of the cases develop RF. Fifty percent of those who develop RF and are untreated develop RHD [8].

The presentation of RF is 1 to 3 weeks post–strep throat and the child will experience:

Major symptoms
   Heart murmur (develops from carditis)
   Skin rash (erythema marginata)
   Subcutaneous nodules (chorea)
Minor symptoms
   Arthralgias (tender, swollen joints)
   Prolonged P-R interval
   Family history of RF
   Elevated sedimentation rate
   Elevated white blood cell count
   Positive C-reactive protein

T. Duckett Jones developed the Jones Criteria, which state that if the child has two major or one major and two minor criteria, one can be reasonably assured that the child has RF [8].

RF demonstrates a specific arthritis involving pain in large joints (elbows, knees, ankles, wrists). It is called migratory polyarthritis because it moves to many joints and is often accompanied by a red rash with sharp margins, subcutaneous nodules, and a heart murmur. Chorea typically occurs late (approximately 6 months after onset) in the course of the disease. These involuntary, slow, rhythmic movements and incoordination persist for several months and then disappear.

In approximately half of all cases of RF, carditis develops, and the heart valves are inflamed and thickened, leaving scar tissue when they heal. The resultant valve abnormalities such as regurgitation or stenosis can cause the valve flaps not to open easily, as wide as they should, or to close properly.

The most common reason for the heart murmur is mitral or aortic regurgitation. Regurgitation indicates that the valve has become deformed in such a way that it will not close properly. Thus blood leaks backward into the chamber (regurgitates). In two thirds of the children who develop a heart murmur, the murmur disappears in 1 to 2 months. The remaining one third have murmurs that continue. If the leakage from the valve is severe, enlargement of the left ventricle and left atria can occur with time. This situation ultimately causes pulmonary edema and congestive heart failure. The right ventricle is put under a strain, enlarges, and fails. With this enlargement the electrical conduction system does not work properly.

Stenosis, which is a clacification of the valve, interferes with an adequate blood supply passing through the valve. Cardiovascular consequences of valvular defects depend on which valves are affected and how they are affected. Serious valvular defects are corrected by surgery to repair or replace the diseased valve. Valve replacements play an important role in the management of patients with stenosis, when clinical symptoms of cardiac decompensation, shortness of breath, or angina affect the performance of activities of daily living.

Treatment for those who develop carditis is a 2-month course of steroids. If the individual has only the arthritis, treatment with aspirin is indicated with 2 to 3 weeks in the hospital and is continued for about 3 months at home. Penicillin is also given to treat any remaining strep in the throat. It is continued on a daily basis often for 20 years or an entire lifetime if there is severe heart damage. RF will recur if the person has another strep throat in 25 percent of the cases and can lead to further heart involvement/damage. The incidence of RF decreases after age 20, with a dramatic fall after age 30 [8].

For those children who have had RF with no heart involvement, there are no restrictions on activities. Those with heart involvement (RHD) have a life expectancy and activity limitations equivalent to the severity of the RHD. Alterations in the child's routine may be required to accommodate limitations on activities. For example, some children may require a shortened school day combined with home teaching, a modified physical education program, daily rest periods, and special snacks.

With many cardiac disorders, parents, teachers, and therapists may overprotect the child, fearing a worsening of the condition should the child become overexcited or stressed. However, typically the child will exhibit shortness of breath or fatigue as a result of overexertion, not further cardiac complications. Thus, the child should be encouraged in as normal a life-style as possible, allowing the child to limit, set, and take responsibility for following the daily medical regime. This allows independence and enables the child to develop normally. Fortunately, in recent years the number of cases of RF in the United States has fallen dramatically, due to increased use of throat cultures to detect strep throat and early treatment of those with strep throat [23].

CYSTIC FIBROSIS

Cystic fibrosis (CF) is a hereditary disease with an estimated incidence of 1 in 2000 births. There is a 1 in 4 chance of a child having the disorder if both parents are carriers. It is the most common, lethal genetic disease of white North Americans, involving not only the mucus-secreting glands of the pancreas and lungs, but all exocrine glands [26].

Children with cystic fibrosis experience infection and abnormal mucus secretion, which gives rise to chronic, progressive obstructive lung disease, which is ultimately fatal [7]. Dysfunction of other exocrine glands produces pancreatic insufficiency, which interferes with the digestive enzymes needed for food absorption, intestinal obstruction, gallstones, and biliary cirrhosis. Common symptoms of the disease include excessive sweating, heat sensitivity, wheezing, coughing, lack of endurance, poor weight gain or loss of weight, and bulky, foul-smelling stools. Children with the disease tend to be of small stature with thin extremities and a barrel chest.

Cystic fibrosis is usually diagnosed early in life because the child has frequent respiratory infections or fails to thrive. A sweat test is done to measure salt content of perspiration because an elevated sodium and chloride content of the sweat is a diagnostic hallmark of the disease [7].

Greater efficacy of treating infections and pancreatic disorders and improved nutrition have contributed to the significant increase in life expectancy for a child with CF. Every effort is made to prevent recurring respiratory infections through the use of antibiotics and aerosal therapy, breathing exercises, and postural drainage to decrease the amount of mucus in the lungs. Vitamins, enzymes, and a high-protein, low-fat diet are prescribed, and frequent meals are provided to aid in food absorption [13].

Rehabilitation management focuses on maintaining or improving the efficiency of lung function so that the child can grow, play, and work as normally as possible. The child and parents are taught mechanical techniques of draining the bronchial passages and how to improve the efficiency of breathing by means of coughing, postural drainage, and breathing exercises [26, 35].

Coughing is essential for pulmonary hygiene. It is the normal way the body prevents the buildup of secretions in the lungs. Sputum is brought up from the bottom of the lungs, where the bronchial tubes are small, into the large trachea and mouth. Children with cystic fibrosis must be encouraged to produce a productive cough, not a forced or strained one. Parents need to reinforce a positive attitude toward coughing, as the child may be embarrassed about coughing in social situations.

Used in conjunction with aerosol therapy, postural drainage is one of the most important forms of therapy. With careful positioning, a therapist uses chest clapping to encourage the patient to cough up as much sputum as possible.

People with breathing or respiratory difficulty develop the habit of using accessory muscles for respiration. The use of these muscles results in abnormal, inefficient respiration and poor posture. Breathing exercises are designed to improve respiration, ventilation, and posture. For example, the child lies down on the back with as many pillows as is comfortable. Placing one hand on the stomach, just under the rib cage, the child breathes in and raises the stomach, so that the hand goes up, then breathes out as slowly as possible while the stomach and hand go down. To make the breathing exercises more of a game, a favorite toy can be placed on the stomach instead of the hand and then let the toy go up and down. The child can blow out a candle and try to flatten the flame for as long as possible without blowing out the flame. Or, if in good condition, the child can play a wind instrument and other blowing games. In all of these exercises, the child is taught to breathe out longer than to breathe in, to ensure that all the air is out before starting a new breath.

Children with breathing difficulty tend to use the muscles of the neck and upper chest to aid in breathing. When these muscles are used over a prolonged period, poor posture develops, with rounded tight shoulders, a forward thrust of the head, and a lumbar lordosis. Exercises designed to improve posture by strengthening the muscles of the abdomen, back, shoulder, and neck should be done daily.

All forms of activity should be encouraged within the child's ability to aid in preventing the accumulation of secretions in the lungs. Running and active play can often do more to help raise sputum than other forms of therapy. Among the activities suggested are swimming, running, ball throwing, badminton, ping pong, bicycle/tricycle riding, baton twirling, weight lifting, acrobatics, and dancing [35].

A shortened life span is expected for children with CF, although now, with improved medical care, some survive into young adulthood. Families need support in coping with the stresses and responsibilities of this dreaded illness. Research on a variety of childhood chronic illnesses, including CF, has consistently underscored the importance of the family context as a mediator of adjustment. Family members should be involved in the patient's ongoing physical care in ways to facilitate problem solving, decision making, and management concerning disease-related stress [26].

The child/adolescent may experience adjustment problems as a result of the physical inadequacy caused by the disease and isolation due to hospitalizations or being homebound from frequent respiratory infections or medical complications. Emotional support of the child and an environment that encourages as normal development as possible aid the child and family in coping with the disease. Comprehensive care of children and adolescents with CF should address the mastery of anxiety about the disease and its treatment, understanding and compliance with the medical regimen, integration of the illness into family life, reconciliation of family needs with those of the child with CF, and adaptation to hospital, school, and peers [26].

CF presents children and families with similar problems (hospitalizations, frequent physician visits, physical deterioration) to those faced by many with a chronic illness. Early identification of the problems and therapeutic intervention aid in the development of appropriate coping strategies.

Given the long-term nature of the disease, relationships with health care personnel are particularly critical. A change in personnel can be traumatic and requires adjustment on the part of the child and family. Likewise, emotional stress can be experienced by the practitioner as a formerly healthy child deteriorates. Recognizing and accepting the changes in the chronically ill child help the health care worker to provide continued support for the child and family.

DIABETES

Diabetes is a heterogeneous group of diseases that arises between the genetic constitution of the individual and specific environmental factors. There are two major types of the disease: maturity-onset type and juvenile-onset type, both having long-term complications that vary among individuals. Juvenile-onset diabetes represents about 10 percent of all cases and usu-

ally develops in persons under 20 years of age, with an abrupt onset [31].

The disease is characterized by a marked decline in the number of beta cells in the pancreas, which leads to a deficiency of insulin and an elevation of glucose in the blood. The lack of insulin accelerates the breakdown of the body's fat reserve. This results in the production of ketones and acids that lower the pH of the blood and produce diabetic ketoacidosis that can result in death. Injections of insulin are necessary to regulate the blood glucose level, thus this more severe form is referred to as insulin-dependent diabetes [31]. The long-term complications of diabetes are many and result in disorders that affect many organ systems.

Insulin shock (hypoglycemia) is the reaction to an excess of insulin, and diabetic coma (ketoacidosis) is the result of insufficient insulin. These are the two primary problems teachers and therapists must recognize in the child with diabetes. Other complications usually do not occur in childhood if the disease is managed appropriately [33]. Table 10-9 lists the symptoms of these conditions that can be used to identify a critical situation at school, home, or play.

HEMOPHILIA

The term *hemophilia* means "love of blood." It is a genetic bleeding disorder in which the clotting system is not working well. It affects 1 in 5000 males born each year, 20,000 in the United States and 400,000 worldwide. The disease is sex-linked, recessive, carried on the X chromosome, and thus transmitted from mothers to sons (50 percent). Fifty percent of the daughters will be carriers [10]. Those with the disease do not bleed more easily but bleed longer, that is, platelets form; however, there is incomplete clotting. The problem that develops is bleeding internally (intracranial bleeds in severe hemophiliacs) and into weight-bearing joints: knees, elbows, ankles, hips, and shoulders, in order of prevalence [16].

There are two types of the disease, hemophilia A, or classic hemophilia, presents a

TABLE 10-9. Symptoms of diabetic coma and insulin shock

	Diabetic coma	Insulin reaction
History	Insufficient or omitted insulin Infection Dietary indiscretion Gastrointestinal upset	Excessive insulin Unusual exercise Too little food
Onset	Slow, hours–days	Sudden, minutes
Skin	Flushed, dry, hot	Pale, moist, cool
Behavior	Drowsy	Excited
Breath	Acetone	Normal
Respirations	Air hunger	Normal to rapid, shallow
Blood pressure	Low	Normal
Vomiting	Present	Absent
Hunger	Absent	Present
Thirst	Present	Absent
Urinary sugar	Large amount	Absent in second specimen
Response to treatment	Slow	Rapid

Source: From E. Ivimey, Diabetes notes from lecture. Boston: Boston University, 1978.

factor VIII deficiency (AHG deficiency). Hemophilia B, or Christmas disease, has a factor IX deficiency (plasma thromboplastin component deficiency). Classification is based on level of circulating coagulation factor in the plasma. In children with mild hemophilia, the plasma coagulation factor ranges from 6 to 50 percent, and they only bleed with severe trauma or surgery. Those with moderate disease have a factor that ranges from 1 to 5 percent, and they bleed with mild trauma. Those with severe hemophilia, who account for 20 percent of the hemophiliac population, have a factor of less than 1 percent, and they bleed spontaneously with no known trauma [5, 10].

The clinical presentation is rarely in infancy. It is more commonly identified following a tooth eruption, laceration of tongue, or bruises from falls. Hematuria is seen in 7 percent of the cases between the ages of 5 and 10. Hemarthrosis begins around age 4, and about 10 percent of adolescents with the disease have arthropathies [10]. Joint problems that develop in hemophiliac arthropathy typically go through an acute phase of synovitis (joint tenderness and swelling as a result of a fresh bleed). Subsequently, the subacute phase involves synovial thickening and vascularization of the synovial membrane with a propensity for more bleeding. Thus, muscle wasting, chronic pain, joint destruction, and osteoporosis develop as chronic hemarthrosis. The old form of medical treatment for the disease was to give fresh blood. Now, medical treatment includes fresh-frozen plasma, cryoprecipitate, factor VIII or IX concentrates, immunosupressant agents, and analgesics (avoid salicylates).

Rehabilitation management includes exercise, splints, recreational activities, and psychosocial support. In designing the exercise program, limb circumference and leg-length discrepancy are assessed. Before designing the program, the therapist must be aware of the child's clotting factor, state of the bleed, and inhibitors. Goals are to decrease the deformity and pain and to evaluate the child for a supportive device. Knees, elbows, and ankles are the major locations for bleeding, which occurs from the synovium. The child complains of a bubbly, tingling feeling in the joint. Joint swelling, decreased range of motion leading to flexion, and increases of joint space from more bleeding occur. Immobilization of the joint may be required, depending on the severity of the bleed. Isometric exercises may be beneficial particularly during a flare. Once the flare is no longer active, resistive exercises and range of motion (to prevent contracture from frequent bleeds) can begin. Postural exercises are also included in the therapy program to correct secondary scoliosis due to uneven weight bearing.

Splints are frequently used to immobilize a joint during an acute flare. The most commonly used is that to immobilize the knee. In addition, night splints may be recommended in the chronic stage of the disease to avoid further bleeding.

Competitive and contact sports are discouraged [16]. Noncompetitive and noncontact sports such as walking and bicycling are allowed, as are tennis and golf if there is no elbow involvement. Jogging may be allowed if the quadriceps and hamstrings are of normal strength. Swimming may also be encouraged provided diving and playing in a shallow pool are not allowed due to the risk of injury.

Children with hemophilia and their families require psychosocial support and genetic counseling about the disease. Overprotection of the child may be normal, and parents and teachers must temper their own fears with the knowledge of the consequences of the risks allowed [19]. With appropriate medical and rehabilitation management, most of these children now have a normal life expectancy.

SICKLE CELL ANEMIA

The term *sickle cell anemia* includes sickle cell anemia, sickle cell–hemoglobin C disease, and sickle cell–beta thalassemia. It is an inherited disease of the blood, which is characterized by a prevalence of sickle-shaped red blood cells. These cells are more fragile and inflexible than normal red blood cells. These characteristics of the cells account for the vaso-occlusive complications and hemolytic anemia of the disease [38]. A vaso-occlusive crisis is very painful. The sickle cells become permanently trapped in the circulatory system, which causes circulatory stasis and hypoxia. Tissue necrosis and pain (painful crisis) result from extensive occlusion. The usual consequences of a vaso-occlusive crisis are mild, yet repeated episodes can cause changes in psychosocial behavior and progressive organ failure [38]. Painful abdominal crises do occur in children, although the more common type of pain is musculoskeletal pain. These transient episodes, which can last from days to weeks, are the result of ischemic damage to the tissue. Some crises are precipitated by fever, infection, dehydration, or exposure to cold.

Anemia is secondary to abnormal fragility and rigidity of the sickle cells. Three types of anemic crises are common to the disease. The first, splenic sequestration, may occur in complement with a viral syndrome. Weakness, pallor, and an enlarging abdomen develop rapidly, and hypovolemic shock can occur due to massive pooling of blood in the spleen. An aplastic crisis or suppression of erythroid production is the second type. This occurs during or after an infectious illness. Hemoglobin falls rapidly due to the short life span of the cells as erythroid production is inhibited by infection. The third type is a hyperhemolytic crisis, characterized by a sudden increase in scleral/icterus, pallor, and fall in hemoglobin. Acute bacterial infections and exposure to certain drugs have been implicated in this type [38].

Other complications of the disease involve the central nervous system, cardiovascular system (frequent in children with the disease), genitourinary tract, pulmonary function, hepatobiliary system (hepatomegaly), ocular manifestations, skeletal system (avascular necrosis of the femoral head), skin (skin ulcers), and obstetric/gynecologic complications.

The classic course of the disease is extremely variable, with some patients having one crisis every few years and others having weekly or monthly crises. In between painful crises, the patient is symptom-free. Vaso-occlusive and anemic crises are seen often in the young; adults experience complications of chronic anemia and organ failure. In general, those with hemoglobin C and beta thalassemia have a milder course of the disease [38].

It is estimated that 1 in 400 black persons in the United States has sickle cell anemia, and 1 in 10 is a carrier of the trait. Carriers of the trait are asymptomatic. To inherit the disease, a child must inherit the trait from both parents, and then there is a 1 in 4 chance that each child will have the disease. The greatest frequency of the disease is in geographic areas where malaria is endemic, because there is a protective effect of the sickle cell trait against fatal malarial infections [38].

Lack of physical endurance, delayed maturation, short stature, frequent infections, fever, pain, and anemia are common problems for these children. However, they should be allowed to participate in normal activities to their ability. If the child is forced to miss school during a sickle cell crisis, a home school program should be provided so that no time is lost at school. Due to delayed maturation, social development is a critical area, particularly as the child enters adolescence. It is important to encourage participation in nonphysical extracurricular activities as a means of developing avocational and vocational activities and social skills. Parents and offspring must receive genetic counseling, and attention should be focused on the psychosocial effects of this chronic illness and hospitalization. Adequate nutrition and good dental care are critical. Pain management and infection control are important medical concerns. Transfusion therapy and antisickling agents may be a part of the medical regime. With the prevalence of the disease, it is important to recognize the impact this situation can have on future generations. However, with appropriate medical management, a child with sickle cell anemia can expect to have a normal life span.

REFERENCES

1. Altman, A. J. (ed.). Pediatric Oncology. *Pediatr. Clin. North Am.* 32(4):June, 1985.
2. American Lung Association, 1980 Bulletin.
3. Binder, H. Rehabilitation of the Burned Child. In G. E. Molnar (ed.), *Pediatric Rehabilitation.* Baltimore: Williams & Wilkins, 1985.
4. Byrd, R. Late effects of treatment of cancer in children. *Pediatr. Clin. North Am.* 32(3):835, June, 1985.
5. Clark, S. K., and Logigian, M. K. Burn Rehabilitation. In M. K. Logigian (ed.), *Adult Rehabilitation: A Team Approach for Therapists.* Boston: Little, Brown, 1982.
6. Cromes, G. F. Psychological Aspects. In S. V. Fisher and P. A. Helm (eds.), *Comprehensive Rehabilitation of Burns.* Baltimore: Williams & Wilkins, 1984.
7. Davis, P. B., and Kaliner, M. Autonomic nervous system abnormalities in cystic fibrosis. *J. Chronic Dis.* 36(3):269, 1983.
8. Dye, R. Rheumatic Heart Disease. Notes from lecture. Boston: Spaulding Rehabilitation Hospital, 1976.
9. Ekwo, E., Kim, J. O., Dusdieker, L., et al. Prognostic factors predicting control of chronic asthma symptoms in children receiving prophylactic bronchodilator therapy. *J. Chronic Dis.* 37(4):263, 1984.
10. Eng, G. *Hemophiliac Arthropathy.* Boston: Tufts Research and Training, 1982.
11. Fochtman, D., and Foley, G. E. (eds.). *Nursing Care of the Child with Cancer.* Boston: Little, Brown, 1982.
12. Graham, T. P. When to operate in the child with congenital heart disease. *Pediatr. Clin. North Am.* 31(6):1275, 1984.
13. Gurwitz, D., et al Perspectives in cystic fibrosis. *Pediatr. Clin. North Am.* 26(3):603, 1979.
14. Hall, M., Hardin, K., and Conastser, C. The Challenges of Psychological Care. In D. Fochtman and G. V. Foley (eds.), *Nursing Care of the Child with Cancer.* Boston: Little, Brown, 1982.
15. Hartford, C. E. Surgical Management. In S. V. Fisher and P. A. Helm (eds.), *Comprehensive Rehabilitation of Burns.* Baltimore: Williams & Wilkins, 1984.
16. Hemophiliac Care Center. Notes from lecture. Boston: Brigham and Women's Hospital, 1985.
17. Hunter, W. M. The Schoolteacher in the Burn Center. In R. E. Salisbury, N. M. Newman, and G. R. Dingeldein (eds.), *Manual of Burn Therapeutics.* Boston: Little, Brown, 1983.
18. Ivimy, E. Diabetes notes from lecture. Boston University, 1978.
19. Kleinberg, S. B. *Educating the Chronically Ill Child.* Rockville, MD: Aspen, 1982.
20. Landau, L. I. Outpatient evaluation and man-

agement of asthma. *Pediatr. Clin. North Am.* 26(3):581, 1979.

21. Lansky, S. B. Management of stressful periods in childhood cancers. *Pediatr. Clin. North Am.* 32(4):625, 1985.

22. Levinson, P., and Ousterhout, D. K. Art and play therapy with pediatric burn patients. *J. Burn Care Rehabil.* 1(1):42, 1980.

23. Levinson, S. S., et al. The Chicago rheumatic fever program: a 20 plus year history. *J. Chronic Dis.* 35(3):199, 1982.

24. MacMillan, B. G. Burns in children. *Clin. Plast. Surg.* 1(4):633, 1984.

25. Malick, M. H., and Carr, J. A. *Manual of Management of the Burn Patient.* Pittsburgh: Harmarville Rehabilitation Center, 1982.

26. Matthews, L. W., and Drotar, D. Cystic fibrosis—a challenging long term chronic disease. *Pediatr. Clin. North Am.* 31(1):133, 1984.

27. McFadden, E. R., and Feldman, N. T. Asthma: Pathophysiology and clinical correlates. *Med. Clin. North Am.* 61(6):1229, 1977.

28. Nadas, A. S. Update on congenital heart disease. *Pediatr. Clin. North Am.* 31(1): 153, 1984.

29. Neijens, H. J., Duiverman, E. J., and Kerrebijn, K. F. Bronchial responsiveness in children. *Pediatr. Clin. North Am.* 30(5):829, 1983.

30. Nothdurtt, D., Smith, P. S., and LeMaster, J. E. Exercise and Treatment Modalities. In S. V. Fisher and P. A. Helm (eds.), *Comprehensive Rehabilitation of Burns.* Baltimore: Williams & Wilkins, 1984.

31. Notkins, A. L. The causes of diabetes. *Sci. Am.* 241(5):62, 1979.

32. Rivers, E. A. Management of Hypertrophic Scarring. In S. V. Fisher and P. A. Helm (eds.), *Comprehensive Rehabilitation of Burns.* Baltimore: Williams & Wilkins, 1984.

33. Rosenbloom, A. L. Primary and subspeciality care of diabetes mellitus in children and youth. *Pediatr. Clin. North Am.* 31(1):107, 1984.

34. Sauer, S. N., Atwood, P., and Sohner, D. The Challenges of Physical Care. In D. Fochtman and G. V. Foley (eds.), *Nursing Care of the Child with Cancer.* Boston: Little, Brown, 1982.

35. Schwartz, R. H. *A Guide to the Physical Management of Cystic Fibrosis.* Rochester, N.Y.: Strong Memorial Hospital, 1970.

36. Schwartz, R. H. Children with chronic asthma: care by the generalist and the specialist. *Pediatr. Clin. North Am.* 31(1):87, 1984.

37. Stagner, S. (ed.). Cancer in Children. In D. Fochtman and G. V. Foley (eds.), *Nursing Care of the Child with Cancer.* Boston: Little, Brown, 1982.

38. Vichinsky, E. P., and Lubin, B. H. Sickle cell anemia and related hemoglobinopathies. *Pediatr. Clin. North Am.* 27(2):429, 1980.

39. U.S. National Health Survey (1959–1961). *Illness Among Children.* Washington: U.S. Department of Health, Education and Welfare.

SUGGESTED READING

BURNS

Clark, A. M. Thermal injuries: the case of the whole child. *J. Trauma.* 20(10):823, 1980.

Kibbee, E. Life after severe burns in children. *J. Burn Care Rehabil.* 2(1):44, 1981.

Malez, M. P. Teaching children about matches: control of fireplay. *J. Burn Care Rehabil.* 2(3):163, 1981.

Project Burn Safety. *Protect Someone You Love.* Boston: U.S. Consumer Product Safety Commission, BURNS, 1978.

11 Psychosocial Disorders

Judith D. Ward

The goal of rehabilitation, the development of skills needed to function within one's environment, can be applied to the treatment of psychosocial disorders. However, the total treatment of children with psychosocial disorders also may involve one or more of the psychotherapies and social intervention where the child's environment becomes the focus of change. Thus, an integrated approach to treatment is necessary.

ANXIETY DISORDERS

The anxiety disorders are those disturbances of behavior due to anxiety that interfere with social and academic performance. The American Psychiatric Association's *Diagnostic and Statistical Manual of Mental Disorders (DSM III)* [1] describes three categories of childhood anxiety disorders:

1. Separation anxiety disorder
2. Avoidant disorder of childhood or adolescence
3. Overanxious disorder

Children with *separation anxiety disorder* suffer extreme anxiety about being separated from family, familiar surroundings, or familiar associates [1]. They will not go away to camp, sleep over at a friend's house, or even go on school trips [73]. They worry about future events that may separate them from their families, and sometimes they develop somatic complaints when anticipating separation.

When they are away from home they get homesick, or they worry that something will happen to loved ones while they are away [1]. Sometimes separation anxiety takes the form of panic attacks, nightmares, or fear of the dark. These children can be very demanding of those to whom they are attached, requiring constant attention, even refusing to sleep alone [1]. School phobia is a common form of separation anxiety [48].

The age of onset of separation anxiety is before age 18 and can be as early as preschool age. It often follows some form of stress: the loss of a significant person or pet, or a change of environment [1]. It is equally common in boys and girls [2]. Children with this disorder come from close, caring families, but the significance of the family pattern in the disorder is unknown [1]. Kanner [48] proposes that this behavior is encouraged by the mother in response to her own neurotic needs.

Children with *avoidant disorder* are detached or timid to such an extent that it interferes with social functioning. Although they desire close relationships with family and familiar people, they shrink from interaction with strangers [1]. Some children appear aloof, shunning normal play activities and social interactions; some seem to be daydreamers [21]. Other children are obviously timid—inhibited around strangers, soft spoken, and unassertive [1]. Avoidant disorder is more common in girls and has its onset during the early school years [2].

The anxiety of *overanxious* children is less specific than in the other anxiety disorders. These children worry excessively about future events, their past or future performance, and what people will think of them. They are easily embarrassed and often seek reassurance from others; they may worry about their own health or the health of others; and, they may have psychosomatic complaints. It is equally com-

mon in boys and girls who are characteristically conscientious and overly conforming and who tend to come from families where there is a great deal of concern about performance [1].

Feelings of insecurity underlie each of the anxiety disorders. These children have fears about their ability to cope with life. This is manifested in the overanxious child's worries and perfectionism. In the case of children with separation anxiety, the fears may be focused on one situation, such as in school phobia, or the fears may be more diffuse with anxiety about engaging in any unfamiliar activity or leaving the usual environment. In the avoidant disorder the individual's insecurity may be camouflaged by aloofness, but it is there. Children with separation and avoidant disorders handle their feelings of insecurity by avoiding anxiety-producing circumstances. They may be perfectly happy with family, in familiar situations. However, fear of separation and avoidance can seriously limit the child's opportunity for developmental life experiences and can lead to increased insecurity.

Children learn about themselves and their abilities by interacting with others, playing, participating in school, and taking risks. They test themselves against the world. If their interactions with their friends, family, and the environment are fun, rewarding, and successful, they feel competent and are ready for new challenges. If their experiences are frustrating, scary, or unrewarding, they are less apt to feel competent and open to new experiences. Children with anxiety disorders do not feel competent and often avoid interactions that might build self-confidence.

ETIOLOGY

Often the interaction of *multiple factors* underlies anxiety disorders. From this perspective, the child most vulnerable to an anxiety disorder is temperamentally predisposed, experiences traumatic life events, and has parents who reinforce the maladaptive characteristics or foster hostility and incompetence.

PSYCHODYNAMIC FACTORS

The psychodynamic theories about the cause of anxiety disorders emphasize the intrapsychic conflict underlying the behavior. The anxiety and avoidant behaviors are seen as symptoms of repression and inhibition.

Horney [42] explains anxiety disorders (neuroses) in terms of repressed hostility engendered by poor parenting practices combined with a lack of genuine parental warmth and affection. The lack of warmth is camouflaged by the parents' claim to be acting in the child's best interest. Often the parents arouse hostility by unjust reproaches or inconsistent behavior such as overindulging and then rejecting the child. They interfere "with the most legitimate wishes of the child, such as disturbing friendships, ridiculing independent thinking, spoiling its interest in its own pursuits, whether artistic, athletic or mechanical—altogether an attitude of the parents which if not in intention nevertheless in effect means breaking the child's will" [42].

These children become inhibited and anxious. They feel inadequate and thus overly dependent on the parents, which contributes to more compliance and anxiety. Children who are frequently criticized feel they have to earn their parents love and respect. They show this by being perfectionistic and self-critical. They are anxious about their performance and feel that they are failures, even when they do well [21].

TEMPERAMENT

Children who develop anxiety disorders tend to be sensitive and shy and may be temperamentally more vulnerable to the development of anxiety disorders.

Temperament refers to the behavioral style of an individual. Thomas, Chess, and Birch [75], in their longitudinal study of infant development, identified nine temperamental characteristics found in infancy that describe the child's behavioral style (Table 11-1). These characteristics are descriptions of behavior. There is no good or bad temperament, but there are certain characteristics that fit better in certain circumstances. Thomas and colleagues [75] noted certain constellations of temperamental characteristics that made children either difficult or easy to raise: Easy to raise children were positive in their initial reaction to new situations and adapted easily. They were regular and predictable in their hunger, sleeping, and toileting habits. Their reactions were easygoing, and their moods were positive.

Difficult to raise children had negative responses to new stimuli and were slow to adapt.

TABLE 11-1. Categories of temperamental characteristics

Activity level is the *frequency, tempo,* and *level* of motor activity typical of the child.

Rhythmicity is the *regularity* of repetitive biologic functions: sleeping, eating, bowel and bladder functions.

Approach or **withdrawal** refers to the child's *initial* response to new people, procedures, or things.

Adaptability is the child's *eventual adjustment* to new situations.

Intensity of reaction is the *energy* in the child's response to stimuli, regardless of whether it is a positive or negative response.

Threshold of responsiveness is the *level of stimulation* required to evoke any response from the child.

Quality of mood refers to the predominating mood.

Distractibility "refers to the *effectiveness* of extraneous environmental stimuli in interfering with or altering the direction of ongoing behavior"

Attention span is the *length of time* the child spends at a particular activity. **Persistence** is how long the child pursues an activity in the face of *obstacles* or difficulties.

Based on A. Thomas, S. Chess, and H. G. Birch. *Temperament and Behavior Disorders in Children.* New York: New York University Press, 1968.

They were irregular in biologic functioning, and their reactions were intense and frequently negative. Twenty-three percent of the children studied, who developed behavior problems, were temperamentally difficult children [75].

ENVIRONMENT

Although some children with anxiety disorders are probably children who are not adaptable, who withdraw from new circumstances, and who are highly responsive to the reactions of those around them, an individual's temperament does not necessarily shape his or her destiny. The environment is an equally important influence.

Behavior is shaped by the environment. Temperamental characteristics can be *modified or reinforced* by the way children are raised. If a child's first reaction to new stimuli is avoidance, it can be reinforced by an overprotective parent who unintentionally makes matters worse. On the other hand, the parent who understands that the child is slow to warm up to new experiences will expose the child to gradual, small doses of the new stimuli and help the child overcome his or her initial reaction.

Children who are not temperamentally predisposed can also develop anxiety disorders through *traumatic experiences*. Those who have suffered from illness or injury may not develop confidence in themselves, and these feelings of inadequacy can lead to avoidance of usual childhood activities or a general sense of insecurity [21]. The loss of a loved one or a major change in the environment can have a negative effect on the child's development of confidence and mastery.

Children also learn from the behavior of those around them (*modeling*). Overprotective parents can instill fear in their children [21] and reinforce feelings of inadequacy and dependence by restricting opportunities to test abilities and develop the confidence acquired by successfully meeting challenges. This can become a vicious cycle where avoidance increases insecurity and leads to more avoidance.

Neglected children may also lack success experiences because they have not been taught the skills necessary to succeed physically or socially. The development of self-esteem is a complex process of learning and testing skills through play, work, and social interaction. Children need to meet with success, but in the process, they need to be allowed to make mistakes. Meeting challenges builds confidence. Interference with any of the elements in the process can lead to insecurity and anxiety about one's own capabilities and can lay the groundwork for an anxiety disorder.

DIAGNOSIS

Diagnosis of an anxiety disorder is usually based on interviews of the child and parents. The psychiatrist or social worker takes a history of general health, the child's physical and social development, and the problem behavior. Other information gained through interviewing and observation is a description of temperament, attitudes and behaviors related to school, and social and play behaviors [5]. Psychologists and occupational and recreational therapists may take part in this initial gathering of information, which is pooled and becomes the basis for the diagnosis made by the psychiatrist.

The causal factors related to the problem need to be clarified so that treatment will be appropriate. Causal factors include

1. *Precipitating factors* are those that "trigger" [21] the disorder. For example, a bad grade on an exam may be the last straw, precipitating school phobia in a child who was already feeling inadequate and anxious [5].
2. *Predisposing factors* are preexisting conditions that make a person vulnerable to a disorder, under certain circumstances [21]. These can include temperament, illness, injury, or environmental circumstances [5].
3. *Reinforcing factors* are those circumstances that maintain the condition [2, 5]. If the child with school phobia is allowed to stay home from school and receives extra attention and

special treats, the avoidant behavior is reinforced.

4. *Protective factors* [2] are those positive aspects of the situation that can be used to ameliorate the problem. These can include the motivation and strengths of the child and the willingness of the family to help.

Additional assessments will reflect the frame of reference of the therapists involved.

ASSESSMENT AND TREATMENT

Psychotherapy
Psychodynamic psychotherapy uses the relationship between the therapist and child for assessment and treatment [5]. There are many techniques of psychotherapy. Psychoanalytic therapists are extensively trained in methods of exploring the unconscious. They use the processes of transference and interpretation to uncover and resolve unconscious conflict. Other psychotherapists (psychiatrists, clinical psychologists, psychiatric social workers) may not delve as deeply into unconscious material. Through their relationship with the child they provide the opportunity for expression and discussion of problems. Assessment is an ongoing process in psychotherapy. As the child interacts with the therapist information is gained about the problem.

From the *psychodynamic perspective,* the "root of the problem [is] the child's submission and denial of his self" [60]. Therapy helps the child get in touch with him- or herself, by encouraging talk about problems, giving the child undivided attention, and listening without criticism. The therapist encourages the child to express feelings and ideas without feeling ashamed or guilty [60]. This may be the first relationship with an adult that is based on respect and acceptance, and through such a relationship, the child gains self-acceptance and self-esteem [5, 60].

Psychotherapy with children differs from that with adults in several ways: First, adults usually seek a therapist on their own initiative, in response to a problem; children do not seek treatment, and they may not view their treatment needs in the same way as the referring adults [61]. Children are much more dependent on their families and their environment than adults [61]. The child needs to know that the therapist will not be taking sides with the parents [18] and that the therapy sessions are confidential [61]. Finally, children's personalities are more flexible than adults; they are less repressed, their defenses are less ingrained, and thus, they may change more quickly [18].

The therapist needs a strong knowledge of normal child development. Sometimes parents perceive behavior as a problem when, in fact, it is normal for the child's age. The form of psychotherapy depends on the developmental level of the child [61]. Young children may not be verbal enough to talk about their feelings and problems. Often, child psychotherapists use play as a medium of communication and expression for those who are too young or too anxious to talk freely.

Behavior Therapy
Behaviorally oriented therapists focus on the specific maladaptive behaviors of the child, without much emphasis on the psychodynamics of the disorder. Through interviews with the child and family and observation of the child, the problem behaviors are identified and target behaviors specified (see the discussion of behavioral assessment under Conduct Disorders, later in this chapter).

In *behavioral treatment,* motor, social, or academic skills are taught if the child's maladaptive behavior is based on skill deficits. Parents are taught behavioral intervention skills to augment or reinforce therapy, and, if they lack knowledge of child development or parenting skills, these are taught. Children with overanxious disorder, where excessive worry or somatic complaints are the predominating symptoms, are taught relaxation techniques. If the child has the symptoms of separation anxiety or avoidance disorder, the focus of treatment is on the devel-

TABLE 11-2. Developmental task groups

Group	Abilities needed by child	Goal of group	Therapist's role
Parallel: A gathering of individuals working or playing in the presence of one another, with little sharing of the task	Some work or play skills Minimal toleration of presence of others	Develop ability to work or play near others Develop awareness of others Some verbal and nonverbal interaction	Provide material and toys for activity Help child feel safe and accepted Reinforce group interaction
Project: Children involved in a short-term activity where there is some cooperation or competition. The emphasis is on the activity, not the interaction	Awareness of others Some ability to interact with others verbally or nonverbally	Opportunity to test relationship with others Learn to seek and give assistance in work, play, or games	Provide short-term activity requiring interaction of two or more people for completion Meet child's safety and belonging needs
Egocentric-cooperative: A group engaged in relatively long-term activity, planned and implemented by the group. Group based on "enlightened self-interest." "The individual recognizes that his rights will be respected only through respect for the rights of others" [15]	Able to cooperate and compete when love and safety needs are met by therapist Able to plan and implement activity	Develop ability to participate in a group activity by cooperating in planning and implementing task with minimal intervention of therapist Learn to respect rights of others Learn to meet esteem needs of others	Reinforce cooperation, disregard quality of end product Meet love and safety needs Give minimal task assistance
Cooperative: A homogeneous group, often of the same sex, in which members gather together out of enjoyment of one another. Group members trust one another enough to express feelings honestly. The activity is less important that the group interaction	Trust in group members	Open expression of feelings Ability to meet the needs of group members	Help child find compatible friends, perhaps get group started, then withdraw Can act as "advisor"
Mature: A heterogeneous group where the task and need satisfaction are of equal importance. Group members select, plan, and implement activities. Group provides "an opportunity for exploration, practice, and reinforcement of a variety of membership roles" [15]	Old enough (usually adolescence) to understand group process Can cooperate with others and can contribute to the task	Develop ability to assume a variety of group roles, both task roles and social/emotional roles	"Co-equal group member" [15] Helps members identify membership roles May model roles

Source: Based on A. C. Mosey. *Three Frames of Reference for Mental Health.* Thorofare, NJ: Slack, 1970.

opment of skills and behaviors that will enable the child to approach and cope with the feared situations.

School phobia is the most commonly reported childhood fear treated by behavior therapists [38]. A form of *systematic desensitization* is used to overcome the fear and avoidance found in school phobia. It combines approaches to eliminate avoidance behavior while counterconditioning the fear response. Counterconditioning is the development of a desirable response (relaxation) in the place of an involuntary, undesirable one (anxiety).

First, the individual is taught relaxation techniques. Then, the therapist and client develop a list of fearful stimuli, which are ranked in order of the degree of anxiety they arouse. Next, counterconditioning takes place by a series of exercises in which the client is asked to imagine phobic situations while maintaining a state of relaxation.

Therapists have adapted systematic desensitization for younger children who do not seem to benefit from imagining phobic events in preparation for meeting the feared situation in real life [39]. Most desensitization therapy for young children takes place in vivo (in real life).

Some therapists report that children have trouble learning to relax [57], others report success in teaching relaxation techniques [39]. Hatzenbuehler and Schroeder [39] conclude that while children may be able to learn to relax, it is difficult for them to sustain the relaxation response when confronting the feared stimuli in vivo. Instead of teaching the child to relax, some therapists use emotive imagery. They ask the child to imagine pleasant or funny situations while involved with fear stimuli.

Children will often overcome their fears if they see another child of their own age engaged in the feared situation (*modeling*). The child who is shy with strangers is less reluctant to approach a strange adult if he or she sees friends doing it. The timid child will wait until a bold friend pats the dog before he or she will.

Models show children how, where, and when to perform, and the consequences of the model's actions encourage or discourage imitation. Studies have shown that the more the model is like the individual, the easier it is to identify with the actions: Weight-reduction programs use former fat people as leaders; recovered drug addicts and alcoholics work with substance abusers. Children do best if the models are close to their own age [38] and show that, although they are afraid, they can cope [56].

Activity Therapies
Recreation, art, music, and occupational therapists have much to contribute to the treatment of the anxious child. Children often resist the "talking therapies." They do not see how psychotherapy relates to their lives. They want to live in the present and forget about unpleasant past experiences [31]. They would rather have fun than dredge up their fears and traumas. Children learn by doing, and the therapist who uses activities as the basis of treatment is providing a nonthreatening environment that is like the real world of children.

The anxious child needs the opportunity for expression, development of coping skills, and enhancement of self-esteem and feelings of competence. Music, dance, play, sports, and art are excellent ways to facilitate expression. Therapy can be unstructured where the child chooses the mode of expression or structured to bring out specific emotions. For some children, the simple expression of emotion is enough to relieve anxiety. Therapy used to provide an emotional outlet is called release therapy.

Release therapy gives the child the chance to ventilate bottled-up feelings of anger, guilt, and anxiety [39]. Through play, art, music, etc., the child acts out feelings that have been repressed. Release therapy differs from psychoanalytic play therapy because the therapist does not interpret the child's behavior. The only goal is to express disturbing emotions and thus relieve tension [17].

Release therapy is suitable for children who have anxiety (for example, nightmares) due to a specific traumatic experience [17, 42]. Usually children work through frightening experiences during play or by talking about them, without the help of a therapist. But some children do not, either because the event was extremely fearful or the precipitating factor was one of a series of stresses and became the "last straw" [42]. Very young children may not be able to talk about their frightening experiences.

Release therapy can be an end in itself or one aspect of activity therapy. When using it, the therapist takes care that the child does not get hurt in the process and makes it clear that acting-out behavior is not being encouraged outside the therapy situation [17].

Using carefully selected, supervised activities, therapists *develop new skills or enhance existing skills*. The therapy situation offers an environment that is physically and psychologically safe for the child to practice skills without fear of failure. Helping the anxious child to feel safe enough to try new activities and form new relationships is a great challenge to the therapist. Activities are presented at a level that will ensure success and yet be challenging enough so the child will experience a genuine feeling of accomplishment when successful. Anxious children have low self-esteem and may not recognize their accomplishments. They may feel like failures even when they have done well.

Group activities help anxious children develop social skills if the social interaction is carefully graded. Mosey [58] has described the developmental hierarchy of task groups (Table 11-2). Children with avoidance disorder can work their way through these group situations, gaining confidence and skill at each level. Initially, the very shy child may need individual sessions to develop trust in the therapist before joining a group led by that therapist [58].

Self-Esteem

Self-esteem is built through an accumulation of therapeutic experiences. The attention and respect therapists give the child; the opportunity for self-expression, where feelings are accepted as valid; and the acquisition of new skills all contribute to the child's self-confidence and feelings of self-worth. Giving children the opportunity to make decisions and take initiative is important in building self-esteem. Letting them choose the activity, lead an exercise, or set up a room for a group activity are ways that the therapist shows respect and confidence in children. The therapist needs to recognize when to control the therapy situation in order to ensure the child's success and when to stand aside and allow independence and the assumption of responsibility.

Family

As in most disorders of childhood, treatment involves the family as well as the child. Sometimes parents lack knowledge about normal development and child rearing, and this would be the focus of help [5]. Sometimes the child's problems reflect marital conflict, lack of communication, or family chaos. Family therapists, psychologists, or psychiatric social workers help families deal with these issues.

ANOREXIA NERVOSA

Anorexia nervosa, or nervous loss of appetite, is a disorder in which young women starve themselves in an obsession to become thin. The loss of weight is not due to any apparent organic disease or the unavailability of food. It is not found in groups where there is a real threat of starvation [10]. Anorectics are typically young, female, and come from middle- or upper-class families where food is plentiful [10, 23, 45].

The age of onset is between 12 to 18 years [1] although it can first occur as late as 30 years of age [6]. It is found in 1 in 250 females who are between 18 and 25 years of age [1].

Anorexia nervosa is diagnosed when there is a loss of at least 25 percent of body weight in the absence of a known physical illness; an intense fear of becoming fat, even while losing weight; a disturbed body image (feeling fat although emaciated); and a refusal to maintain normal body weight [1].

Casper and Davis [14] describe the course of anorexia nervosa as having three phases with characteristic symptoms and dynamics for each phase. *Phase I: prodromal phase* is the period before weight loss, when certain events occur that lead the future anorectic to become preoccupied with herself and to decide that her unhappiness is due to her weight or physical development.

Phase II: developing anorectic attitude is the time when the girl starts dieting and feels better about herself as she starts to lose weight. The anorectic attitude is the fear of eating that develops in this stage [14]. Although they deny it, anorectics become obsessed with food and develop rituals around the little food they eat [10]. Their tastes are often bizarre, but they usually avoid carbohydrates, preferring low-calorie foods and liquids [14].

They exercise relentlessly or frantically engage in school or work activities [23]. This hyperactivity is amazing in light of their starvation. People who are starved usually are lethargic and irritable. Anorectics feel happier and more energetic as they lose weight and gain a feeling of power over their bodies [14]. Along with the exhilaration of power comes the fear of losing control of their eating. Some lose control and binge, then vomit and use laxatives to "cleanse" themselves. During this period, the anorectic denies she has a problem, although she may be preoccupied with food and unable to concentrate on other things [14].

Phase III: starvation effects become evident. Although the anorectic is not concerned about her emaciation, she may reluctantly admit that something is wrong as the other effects of starvation become evident. With the loss of 25 to 50 percent of normal body weight, she feels weak, dizzy, develops insomnia, amenorrhea, hypothermia, and hair and skin changes [14]. In this phase she may attempt to eat or try to stop vomiting, but she is still afraid of losing control and becoming fat [14].

If patients will accept treatment during phase II, they can be treated as outpatients, but they will require hospitalization if they reach phase III [14]. Hospitalization may seem desirable because it interrupts family conflicts around eating, but the decision about hospitalization is based on the severity of starvation and the emotional climate of the home, as well as the availability of a facility with experience with anorexia nervosa [11].

It becomes critical to treat the starvation of patients in phase III. Anorexia nervosa can end in death. Irreversible tissue damage can result from starvation, and those who engage in vomiting and purging can suffer severe disturbances in the electrolyte balance [10, 11, 63].

ETIOLOGY

The cause of anorexia nervosa is uncertain. If it is *organic,* the most likely area for problems would be the hypothalamus [6, 63]. Hormone studies indicate that there is hypothalamic dysfunction, but it is not known if the hypothalamic dysfunction is caused by starvation or other stress, or both, or if the hypothalamic dysfunction causes anorexia [6].

The *psychological theories* of etiology include those that view it as due to learned behavior and those that stress more psychodynamic factors. Girls suffering from anorexia have common characteristics of low self-esteem, feelings of helplessness [65] and overcompliance to the expectations of others [10, 11, 23]. Anorectics are repeatedly described as being good children, obedient, well mannered, high achievers who never caused problems [10, 63]. They are perfectionistic and industrious [10] and have often been provided with many educational and cultural opportunities [10, 23]. Bruch [10] describes their families as being success, achievement, and appearance oriented.

As children, they go to extraordinary means to please others, without regard for their own feelings or wishes. Bruch [10] tells of the child who, on discovering her hidden Christmas present, began to express her desire for it, although she had not the slightest interest in it.

These "perfect" children become adolescents who have been so compliant that they feel they have no identity of their own. They have lived their lives trying to please others, and now that it is time to become independent, they are out of touch with themselves. They do not know what they feel or think and do not have the inner resources or the sense of autonomy to be successful adolescents or adults.

Anorexia may begin like any other adolescent diet, but the anorectic becomes so obsessed with her diet and weight because she perceives this as one area in her life which she can control [10, 11, 66, 78]. The dieting starts, and with the weight loss and rigid adherence to deprivation and exercise, develops a sense of power and control of life. The compliant child becomes rigidly stubborn in the pursuit of thinness. She becomes secretive and sneaky about not eating. When emaciation becomes noticeable to others she denies it and claims to feel fat. She refuses food and denies that she is hungry. Anorectics will look in the mirror and still not "see" their skeletal appearance [10, 11].

Frequently the diet starts when there is a change in their lives [10] such as death or illness of a friend or relative; change in the family constellation through birth or divorce; or a change in environment due to moving or going away to college [23]. Life changes or dissatisfaction with one's figure are considered precipitating events rather than direct causes of anorexia nervosa.

DIAGNOSIS AND ASSESSMENT

The procedures for diagnosis and assessment are like those described earlier in anxiety disorders. Typically, anorectics will not have trouble with work or school performance since they tend to be perfectionistic and achievement oriented [34]. Their leisure and social activities may be restricted if they are preoccupied with diet and exercise to the exclusion of other activities, and they may avoid social activities associated with food [34].

Bailey [4] notes that when anorectic patients respond to leisure surveys, they show a low frequency of leisure activities and little awareness of their own needs and values. Self-attitude surveys show them to have "dramatically lowered self-esteem" [4]. Although they have high verbal and cognitive functioning, their group interaction skills are diminished. They perform best on tasks that are very structured [4].

TREATMENT

Much of the occupational therapy literature on eating disorders [4, 33, 34, 55] emphasizes the importance of mutual agreement between therapist and patient in the establishment of treatment goals. An important objective in the treatment of anorexia is the development of a sense of autonomy and effectiveness. The manner in which treatment goals are established sets the tone for this philosophy.

The approaches used for treating anorexia nervosa depend on the frame of reference and discipline of the treating professional. Bemis [6] has classified the various models of treatment as psychodynamic, family interactional, behavioral, and medical.

Psychodynamic Approach

Therapists using the psychodynamic approach view anorexia as a symptom of ego deficits in which the anorectic does not feel a sense of effectiveness or self-respect [10, 11, 65, 78]. The objectives of the psychodynamic approach are to develop ego skills [78], correct defective self-perception [6, 10, 11], and to develop interpersonal skills [6]. Therapy focuses on the development of a "valid self concept and the capacity for self directed action" [10] rather than on interpretation of behavior. This is done by helping the patient identify who she is, what she feels, and what she wants. The patient is active in the treatment process. Self-initiated behavior is recognized and encouraged [10, 11].

Occupational therapists can help the anorectic with self-expression by using expressive media such as art, crafts, and movement to help the patient identify and express feelings [34]. Because of their great need for control and perfect performance, anorectics are uncomfortable with unstructured activity. Bailey [4] discusses how a medium such as ceramics, which can be graded from slip casting (controllable outcome) to coil construction (unstructured) can help patients learn to tolerate imperfection and gradually learn to express themselves more freely.

The anorectic strives for control in reaction to a deep-seated sense of ineffectiveness. This is perhaps the most important concept for the therapist to remember. McColl, Friedland, and Kerr [55] have made some interesting and sobering observations of their anorectic patients' responses to occupational therapy activity. The therapists used activities such as knitting, calligraphy, and beadwork, assuming that successful completion of an activity would contribute to an increased sense of effectiveness. This assumption held for the early stages in the treatment of anorexia; however, later in treatment, the patients did not seem to gain satisfaction or feelings of effectiveness from their "prolific and excellent performance on activities. . . . Instead they regard the successful completion of activities as somewhat irrelevant . . ." [55]. With anorectics, the important part of the activity is not the end product, but the opportunity to consciously choose and make decisions about their activities [55]. The sense of personal effectiveness gained through autonomous decision making is the goal of activity therapy.

Family Interactional Approach
Those employing family interactional therapy view anorexia as a symptom of dysfunctional family patterns with the conflict over the anorectic serving as a means to avoid the real issues [10]. Crisp and colleagues [23] found that over half of the 102 female anorectic patients they studied had disturbed relationships with their parents, which often related to the parents' problems with each other. It is not known if family problems are caused or exaggerated by the stress of living with a child with anorexia nervosa [6]. Although there is no typical family pattern, many families are appearance and achievement oriented [10] and hide poor marital relationships behind a facade of normality [23]. Not all children in achievement-oriented families develop anorexia. Bruch [10] feels that the anorectic families are less sensitive to the child and interfere with the development of autonomy. In therapy, the anorectic may idealize the family and be unable to articulate family pathology [66].

Behavioral Approach
Behaviorists view anorexia as learned behavior that is explained, variously, as a means to gain attention; a phobic avoidance of getting fat; or a social role, modeled by a friend or relative [6]. One study of the friends and relatives of anorectic college students found that they admired the anorectic's self-control and discipline in dieting [9].

Most behavioral programs focus on weight gain and techniques such as goal setting, behavioral contracting (see conduct disorders later in this chapter), and social reinforcement. Contracts can take place between doctor and patient or the child and her parents, but behavioral approaches are better controlled in an inpatient treatment setting [63]. The hospitalized anorectic is usually restricted to bed rest and is allowed activity only when she shows a predetermined weight gain or consumes a specified amount of food. The curtailment of activity conserves calories and also allows activity to be used as a reinforcer for adherence to a dietary regime. Even in the hospital, the anorectic will try to undermine the program by secret vomiting, exercising in bed, or hiding food if she panics about weight gain or fears losing control of eating. Sometimes psychotropic drugs are used to help control anxiety [51, 54, 78].

Cognitive therapy is a behavioral technique that addresses the individual's illogical beliefs about food and weight. Some typical beliefs are that food is bad [33], fat is bad, or that the anorectic must be a perfect person [67]. In cognitive therapy the patients are helped to identify this irrational thinking and to see the effect it has on their behavior. This is often done in a group situation where anorectics learn to examine and change their faulty patterns of thinking.

Anorectic patients experience a great deal of stress on a weight-gain program, which they need to learn to manage. Increasing social skills and widening their social networks [67] can give patients support and relieve stress. Learning relaxation techniques helps lessen the effects of stress.

Through cognitive therapy anorectics learn to manage stress by identifying what kinds of thoughts might precipitate a binge or a fasting regimen. By anticipating these thoughts and the events that trigger them, the patients can plan how to intervene in the faulty thought process. They are also taught to anticipate and not to overreact to setbacks in their control of their eating disorder.

Some programs for the treatment of anorexia nervosa include psychotherapy for treatment of the psychological problems and behavioral interventions for weight gain and skills training. These two approaches can be coordinated for maximum effect. For example, as the patient, through psychotherapy, learns to identify needs and becomes more comfortable with self-expression, she can become involved with assertiveness training (a behavioral approach). *Assertiveness groups* serve not only as forums for practicing assertiveness skills, but also show the anorectic that she is not alone with her problem of self-assertion. Work in the assertiveness group can help the patient function better in family therapy by helping her anticipate and rehearse (role play) assertive ways to participate in family interactions [4].

Medical Treatment

Even those therapists who believe that the psychodynamic roots of the problem must be treated before the patient can be considered improved agree that productive work on building up the ego cannot occur while one is experiencing the effects of starvation [10, 11, 66]. Thus, the treatment of starvation comes first. For inpatients with life-threatening weight loss, marasmus, and low serum potassium levels who cannot gain weight by more conventional approaches, hyperalimentation may be necessary [53]. Hyperalimentation is the intravenous infusion of nutrients that rapidly restores nutritional balance.

Not all anorectics will require hyperalimentation or tube feeding. Some will eat when it is explained that they can work more effectively on their psychological problems if their malnutrition is corrected. They need to be reassured that they will not be forced to gain too fast and become fat [11].

Many feel that the psychotherapist can work more effectively if the monitoring of the diet is separate from, but concurrent with, psychotherapy. This keeps the therapist out of the battle over eating and enables therapy to focus on self-esteem and the development of autonomy [11, 66].

OUTCOME

It is difficult to assess the long-term adjustment of the anorectics since follow-up studies use different criteria to define recovery [6]. A single episode of anorexia nervosa with a full recovery is most common, but mortality rates are reported at between 15 and 21 percent [1]. Anorectics who binge and purge (bulimia) have more chronicity [23, 63, 74]. They also have a higher incidence of depression and suicide [74].

CONDUCT DISORDERS

A large part of the psychiatric population of older children and adolescents consists of those with conduct disorders [5]. These children fail to conform to the norms of society and disregard the rights of others. Nine percent of males and two percent of females under age 18 have a conduct disorder. The onset is before puberty in males and, usually, postpubertal for females [2].

The antisocial behavior of children with conduct disorders may include lying, stealing, fighting, destroying property, setting fires, and physical aggression toward people and animals. In order to be diagnosed as a conduct disorder, the pattern of antisocial behavior must be present for at least 6 months [2]. The American Psychiatric Association's *Diagnostic and Statistical Manual of Mental Disorders (DSM-IIIR)* [2] classifies conduct disorders in three categories: solitary aggressive type, group type, and undifferentiated type.

Children with the solitary aggressive type of conduct disorder violate the rights of others through acts such as vandalism, assault, rape, or fire-setting [1, 5]. They have not formed social bonds with others; they show no guilt or anxiety about their aggressive acts; and often they make no attempts to conceal their acts from others. They are not loyal, and they do not form lasting friendships [1]. Children with the group type of conduct disorder lie, steal, and run away from school or home. Although aggression may be present, they are capable of social attachment and experience guilt or anxiety [1, 2]. The undifferentiated type of conduct disorder, which is the most common, has a mixture of antisocial behaviors that do not fit into either of the other two categories [2].

ETIOLOGY
Children who experience rejection or whose family life is disrupted by multiple foster home placements or institutionalization are most likely to develop conduct disorders [5]. These are children whose social development has been impaired.

Children learn culturally determined behaviors through the example set by role models with whom they have an emotional attachment. Social learning and conscience development begin in early infancy through a process of dependence on, and identification with, the primary caretaker, usually the mother. This socialization process begins with bonding, the attachment that occurs between infant and mother through continual interaction as the mother meets the child's physical and emotional needs [5].

As children mature they learn right and wrong through the example of those around them and by being rewarded for prosocial behavior and punished for antisocial behavior. When there is a close attachment to parents, children want to please them, and the child's positive behaviors are reinforced by the pleasure they elicit from the parents.

The socialization process can be disrupted or impaired in a number of ways. Bonding may not be strong if the mother is unresponsive to the child's needs, if she does not recognize the needs of the child, or if she is unable to adequately fulfill them. Sometimes mothers do not have knowledge of human development or nurturing practices. If the mother is depressed or ill, or if she is preoccupied by socioeconomic pressures, she may not be adequately responsive to the child. Children who are institutionalized often do not receive the care they need for their emotional development [5]. Individuals whose emotional needs are not met in infancy and childhood do not learn to form interpersonal bonds. They lack the capacity for empathy, and because they do not connect emotionally with others, they do not feel guilty or remorse when they hurt others.

Even where bonding takes place, the socialization process may be inadequate if parents are inconsistent or harsh in their responses to the child. Children will not learn socially acceptable behavior if such behavior is not consistently reinforced. This can happen with overindulged children, as well as those who are abused or neglected [5].

Socialized children are capable of developing relationships with others, forming empathy and loyalty. They internalize the standards of behavior of those around them [15]. If their primary role models are delinquent or deviant, they will learn delinquent or deviant behavior.

Sometimes there is an organic basis for the impaired development of social behavior. Antisocial behavior is more common in children with brain damage, but most children with conduct disorders are not brain damaged [5].

Aggressive behavior is associated with many factors. Undersocialized children do not develop the capacity to form emotional ties and do not feel guilt or remorse over aggressive acts. They are often quite egocentric and do not accept responsibility for their actions. If they express regret over their acts, it is for the purpose of ameliorating punishment rather than because they are remorseful [18].

Socialized children may also be aggressive. Aggressive behavior may be learned from the behavior of role models (deviant socialization), or aggression may be inadvertently reinforced by parents, teachers, or others [64]. The "neurotic delinquent" [18] is one whose aggression is a reflection of anxiety and insecurity, rather than a lack of socialization. The acting-out behavior serves to discharge or externalize unconscious psychological conflict [15]. Some children who have neurologic impairments or attention deficit disorder are impulsive and aggressive. They may know the norms of acceptable behavior but are unable to adequately control their impulses.

ASSESSMENT

With the exception of the child whose acting-out behavior is based on a neurosis (see Anxiety Disorders, earlier in this chapter), traditional psychotherapy has proved to be ineffective in treating conduct disorders [5, 68]. The most effective treatments are based on social learning theory using behavioral management techniques. Thus, assessment follows a behavioral frame of reference.

The goal of assessment is to identify excessive noxious behaviors and deficit prosocial behaviors and to determine the environmental factors that precipitate and maintain the child's antisocial behavior. In addition to antisocial behaviors, the assessment will commonly show a high rate of aversive behaviors such as running, jumping, teasing, crying, whining, and yelling.

The assessment of environmental factors that cause and maintain antisocial behavior is as important as the identification of the child's target behaviors. Usually, parental child-rearing practices become the focus of the environmental assessment. The interchange between parents, siblings, and the child is examined to identify antecedents and consequences of target behaviors. If problems are most severe at school, the academic environment becomes the focus of assessment. Much of the information is gained through interviews with the child, family members, and teachers and through direct observation of social exchanges.

The antisocial behavior and aggression of the child with a conduct disorder may be reflections of inadequate development of social skills. When assessing social skills, one can identify specific behaviors that are needed for successful social functioning within specific circumstances. Then the individual can be observed for the presence or absence and the quality of these behaviors. Dodge and Murphy [25] have proposed a model for assessing social competence that analyzes three major aspects of social behavior: (1) decoding and interpreting social cues from the environment, (2) deciding how to respond to social cues, and (3) enacting the behavioral response to social cues.

Studies show that aggressive children and adolescents tend to interpret other people's behavior as hostile, and this biased interpretation is related to other deficits in decoding environmental cues. These deficits may include an inadequate search for or incomplete attention to social cues [25]. Also, aggressive children are not able to generate a variety of possible responses to social cues [25, 49]. Their behavioral repertoire may be limited because they lack knowledge of various alternatives of behavior, or they impulsively act on the first response that comes to mind [49]. The identification of the impaired aspects of social competence will help in the formulation of intervention strategies.

The goal of assessment is to clearly define the behaviors that are to be the target of intervention. These target behaviors are described in terms of their intensity, the frequency and time of day in which they are occurring, and their antecedents and consequences. A description of parental responses to the child's behavior also becomes part of the baseline data that are collected.

TREATMENT

In all types of conduct disorders, the common problem is a high frequency of disruptive, noxious, antisocial behaviors [1]. These behaviors are the primary target of intervention using *behavior modification techniques*. According to social learning theory, human behavior is learned through interaction with the environment. A reciprocal relationship between the individual and the environment exists, where the environment influences action and action influences the environment [13]. When a bully intimidates peers into doing his or her bidding, the compliance of the peers reinforces the bully's behavior. Patterson and colleagues [64] describe this pattern of behavior as coercive because the child's "noxious responses" control others through negative reinforcement. Socially aggressive behavior is learned gradually, by an accumulation of such incidents [64]. The primary goal of therapy is to intervene in the process by systematically and consistently punishing noxious behavior and systematically and consistently reinforcing prosocial behavior.

When possible, it is important to have parents involved in treatment. They can be taught to recognize how they may be reinforcing antisocial behavior, and they can learn methods of intervention.

A common method used by therapists in assisting parents is the use of the behavioral contract, a written statement about the privileges and responsibilities of two or more people. It is an effective vehicle of treatment for older children and adolescents and their families.

A written contract structures interpersonal exchanges by describing *who* will do *what,* to or for *whom* and *when* [77]. It describes behavior in specific, attainable actions and specifies the reinforcers and who will supply them.

Often, problems between parents and children are caused or exacerbated by faulty communication. The process of formulating a contract requires and fosters communication and negotiation. The contract is developed through a series of exercises in which family members identify which behaviors need to be changed, the priorities for behavior change, and which reinforcers can be used (Fig. 11-1). Contracting is based on the assumption that there is reciprocity in social interaction [77]. Contingencies are negotiated between parent and child based on what each wants and what is possible for each to give.

The contract provides a vehicle for parents to learn to provide the child with reasonable punishment and positive reinforcement. It also facilitates the development of negotiation skills [64].

Whether the child is being treated in a residential setting or at home, the behavioral treatment methods are the same. The treatment program is highly structured because children with aggressive conduct disorders are less responsive to social reinforcers and require more concrete methods of reinforcement [64]. Patterson and colleagues [64] have found that aggressive children are less responsive to punishment than other children, and they often react to scolding or nagging by escalating their noxious behavior. Thus parents or caretakers need to learn other modes of discipline.

Patterson and colleagues [64] teach parents to refrain from nagging or scolding. Instead, parents are to *immediately* punish *every* occurrence of *targeted* negative behavior. They are instructed to name the behavior being punished so the child will be clear about what actions are unacceptable. There is to be no argument

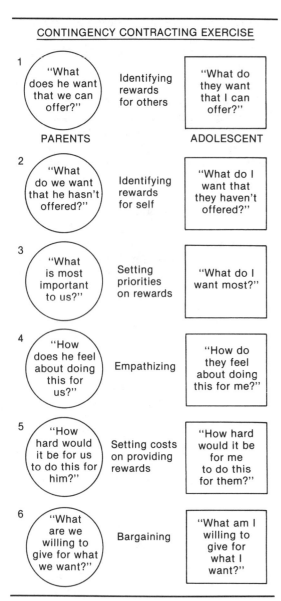

CONTINGENCY CONTRACTING EXERCISE

PARENTS		ADOLESCENT
1. "What does he want that we can offer?"	Identifying rewards for others	"What do they want that I can offer?"
2. "What do we want that he hasn't offered?"	Identifying rewards for self	"What do I want that they haven't offered?"
3. "What is most important to us?"	Setting priorities on rewards	"What do I want most?"
4. "How does he feel about doing this for us?"	Empathizing	"How do they feel about doing this for me?"
5. "How hard would it be for us to do this for him?"	Setting costs on providing rewards	"How hard would it be for me to do this for them?"
6. "What are we willing to give for what we want?"	Bargaining	"What am I willing to give for what I want?"

FIG. 11-1. Contingency contracting exercise. (From L. Weathers and R. P. Liberman. Contingency contracting with families of delinquent adolescents. *Behav. Ther.* 6:360, 1975.)

about punishment: These children can lure parents and therapists into arguments about punishments, which is a form of coercive behavior to escape punishment. The contract helps eliminate arguing because it specifically describes target behaviors, defines the punishment, and helps parents stand firm in their discipline.

Exclusion and *response-cost time-out* are useful consequences of aggressive behavior. The child is not allowed to participate in certain enjoyable activities or a valued possession or privilege is removed if undesirable targeted behaviors are demonstrated. *Overcorrection or restitution* procedures (see description in Chapter 3) are also useful techniques with aggressive children [13, 64].

Family members need to learn to *reinforce positive behaviors*. Often the aggressive child is so obnoxious that positive behavior is overlooked or taken for granted. Parents are trained to acknowledge and reward good behavior [64].

Skill Development and Problem Solving
A secondary characteristic of conduct disorders is deviant socialization or undersocialization. Thus, another aspect of treatment is *social skill training*, also called psychoeducational therapy. Goldstein [37] defines social skill training as "the planned, systematic teaching of the specific behaviors needed and consciously desired by the individual in order to function in an effective and satisfying manner, over an extended period of time, in a broad array of positive, negative, and neutral interpersonal contexts." Social skill training is much like behavior therapy: It is planned and systematic. Specific behaviors are targeted for development, and they are defined in observable, measurable terms [37].

An important aspect of social skill training is learning to problem solve. The aggressive individual's inability to interpret social cues and generate a variety of nonaggressive alternative responses is considered a cognitive problem-solving deficit. *Cognitive problem-solving* programs address these deficits by teaching youngsters *how* to think about interpersonal problems [36]. Children are taught how to consciously and systematically go through the steps in the problem-solving process [36]:

1. Identifying or defining the problem
2. Identifying or gathering related information
3. Examining and evaluating the possibilities of actions/alternatives
4. Selecting a course of action
5. Acting
6. Evaluating the consequences of that action

The problem-solving approach is taught and then practiced by using games and other structured activities. This approach helps impulsive youngsters become more reflective. For children whose only response to conflict is aggression, this process helps them think about other nonaggressive behavioral options (alternative-solution thinking). It also helps them think about how their actions affect others (consequential thinking) [36].

It may be necessary to develop specific skills to enhance the problem-solving process. Participants may need to learn how to listen, and how to ask questions or ask for help. Part of defining the problem situation in interpersonal conflict includes identifying one's own feelings and understanding the feelings of others [37].

Some of the strategies used for problem solving and social skill training are didactic instruction in the method, role modeling of prosocial behavior, and role playing in situations analogous to common aggression-arousing situations. The presentation of movies, written scenarios, or enacted conflictual situations, followed by discussion and role playing of possible behavioral alternatives help develop alternative thinking and decision-making skills [49].

Treatment Settings
The setting for treatment depends on the child's home environment and the nature and serious-

ness of the behavior problems. When family circumstances are poor and the child's behavior is serious and persistent, residential treatment, in a group home, special school, or foster home may be desirable [5]. However, Chamberlain and Steinhauer [15] caution that, while families need support and occasional relief from these children, long-term separation can exacerbate the condition. Residential treatment is a last resort; work with children and families in their natural environment is the preferred approach.

If the family is unable to invest the time and energy required for intervention, the child may be treated in a residential, academic, or foster home setting. The procedures are the same regardless of the setting. The program is planned and supervised by a person trained in behavioral management procedures and implemented by those who are in regular, close contact with the child.

SUBSTANCE ABUSE
The National Institute on Drug Abuse sponsors the research program, *Monitoring the Future: A Continuing Study of the Lifestyles and Values of Youth,* which studies the prevalence and trends of drug use by American high school seniors [44]. From 15,791 to 18,924 high school seniors respond to questionnaires each year. The survey of the class of 1984 (Fig. 11-2) shows that 93 percent of the students had used alcohol, 70 percent had used cigarettes, and 55 percent had used marijuana. Most of the students using any of these substances had their first experience with them before they were in high school [44] (Table 11-3). About 43 percent reported that at some time they had used illicit drugs such as hallucinogens, cocaine, opiates, stimulants, or sedatives and tranquilizers that were not prescribed [43]. According to the National Institute on Alcohol Abuse and Alcoholism [62], almost 20 percent of 14- to 17-year-olds seriously abuse alcohol. And, 10,000 people age 16 to 24 are killed in alcohol-related accidents each year.

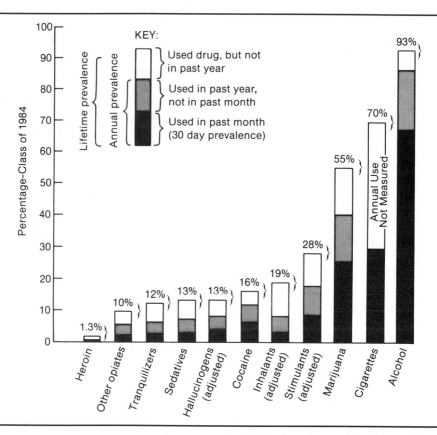

FIG. 11-2. Prevalence and recency of drug use in the class of 1984. (From L. D. Johnston, P. M. O'Malley, and J. G. Bachman. *Use of licit and illicit drugs by America's high school students 1975–1984*. National Institute on Drug Abuse. DHHS Publ. No. [ADM] 85-1394. Washington, DC: Government Printing Office, 1985. P. 20.)

While it may be inevitable that most adolescents will experiment with drugs or alcohol, parents and professionals are concerned with the circumstances contributing to drug use and the characteristics of youth who are more prone to go from experimentation to abuse.

PATTERNS OF ABUSE

The earlier individuals are introduced to alcohol and marijuana, the more likely they are to add other illicit drugs to their repertoire, and the more likely they are to become involved in drug dealing and criminality [46].

Kandel [46] has studied the developmental stages of adolescent drug involvement. Based on analyses of longitudinal and cross-sectional data, she has identified four stages of drug use: "Adolescents' involvement in drugs appears to follow certain paths. Beer and wine are the first substances used by Youth. Tobacco and hard liquor are used next. The use of marijuana rarely takes place without prior use of liquor or

TABLE 11-3. Grade of first use for 16 types of drugs, class of 1984

Grade in which drug was first used	Marijuana	Inhalants[a]	Amyl/butyl nitrites	Hallucinogens[a]	LSD	PCP	Cocaine	Heroin	Other opiates	Stimulants[b] (adjusted)	Sedatives	Barbiturates	Methaqualone	Tranquilizers	Alcohol	Cigarettes (daily)
6th	4.3	1.3	0.6	0.1	0.1	0.5	0.1	0.0	0.2	0.5	0.4	0.2	0.1	0.2	10.4	2.9
7–8th	14.1	3.1	1.5	1.2	0.7	0.5	0.7	0.2	0.8	3.1	1.8	1.4	1.0	1.4	22.4	5.9
9th	13.6	2.7	1.7	2.5	2.0	1.3	2.3	0.4	2.3	8.9	4.2	3.2	2.6	3.5	23.6	5.1
10th	11.2	2.9	1.7	3.0	2.1	1.2	3.4	0.3	2.5	7.9	3.8	2.9	2.5	2.5	18.4	4.2
11th	7.3	2.0	1.3	2.6	2.1	1.0	5.0	0.2	2.3	4.9	2.1	1.5	1.6	3.1	12.0	2.5
12th	4.4	2.4	1.3	1.2	1.0	0.5	4.6	0.2	1.6	2.6	1.0	0.7	0.5	1.7	5.9	1.4
Never used	45.1	85.6	91.9	89.3	92.0	95.0	83.9	98.7	90.3	72.1	86.7	90.1	91.7	87.6	7.4	78.0

Note: This question was asked in two of the five forms (N = approximately 5700), except for inhalants, PCP, and the nitrites, which were asked about in only one form (N = approximately 2800).

[a] Unadjusted for know underreporting of certain drugs.

[b] Adjusted for overreporting of the nonprescription stimulants.

Source: From L. D. Johnston, P. M. O'Malley, and J. G. Bachman. *Use of Licit and Illicit Drugs by America's High School Students 1975–1984.* National Institute on Drug Abuse. DHHS Publ. No. (ADM) 85-1394. Washington, DC: Government Printing Office, 1985. P. 66.

tobacco, or both. Similarly, the use of illicit drugs other than marijuana rarely takes place in the absence of prior experimentation with marijuana."

One drug is not substituted for another at each stage of involvement. Most drug users are multiple drug users [19, 26]. This does not mean that all adolescents who drink will go on to other drugs, but it is very likely that those who use "hard" drugs started with alcohol.

Donovan and Jessor [26] used data from two nationwide surveys of high school students to identify the level of alcohol use that leads to involvement with illicit drugs. They characterized drinking behavior as abstention, nonproblem drinking, and problem drinking. Students who abstain from alcohol also abstain from illicit drugs. Those who engage in nonproblem drinking either use no illicit drugs or (about 10%) use only marijuana. Problem drinkers, those whose drinking interferes with personal and social adjustment and who are frequently drunk, are also more involved with illicit drugs.

FACTORS IN ABUSE

Explanations for why youths use drugs vary according to the professional discipline of the theorist and the population of the drug users who are the subject of their research. Drug abuse is found in all segments of American society, and a multitude of factors play parts in the initiation, continuation, and cessation of drug use.

With the exception of the abuse of prescription medication, the initiation of drug use usually occurs between the ages of 13 and 25 [52]. In order for initiation to occur, the substance must be available in an environment where peers and role models are tolerant of drug use. Smith [70] points out that although illicit drugs can be found at most schools, they are not available to all students: "Availability depends on who the adolescent or preadolescent knows and how he or she is perceived by potential suppliers. If friendship groups include users, availability is greater, and the likelihood of use

is increased; so is the likelihood of very early initiation of use."

Experimenting with drugs is probably not preventable and Amini, Salasnek, and Burke [3] claim that people who use drugs experimentally are different from those who abuse drugs. Drug use at an early age usually reflects difficult family relationships, and the earlier the age of initiation, the more likely it is that the individual is disturbed [40]. Impulsivity, depression [69], low self-esteem [72], and self-destructiveness [40] are all characteristics of individuals who are prone to misuse drugs.

Drug abuse is one way in which disturbed adolescents deal with their problems. For some, drug abuse is part of a larger picture of juvenile delinquency and self-destructive behavior [40]. It is not just exposure to drug users that leads to drug abuse. Youths who initiate use of illicit substances are already "presocialized" to do so [52]. Rebelliousness and nonconformity are the characteristics most often cited of those who start using drugs at an early age and who are likely to increase drug usage. Some individuals do not support the traditional norms and values of society and have a greater toleration of deviance [29, 32].

The roles of parent and peer influence on drug use are not clear [35]. Although in adolescence there is normally a shift from parental influence to that of peers, adolescents do not reject all the values and attitudes of their parents [47]. Kandel [47] has found that both parents and peers can have a strong influence on adolescents, but they influence different domains. Peers influence current life-styles, and parents influence values and future life goals.

Kandel [47] notes that, although peers are more influential than parents in the use of drugs, parental behavior can moderate peer influence. For instance, the initiation of the use of marijuana is more influenced by peers than parents. But, the transition from marijuana use to other illicit drugs is related to parental behavior [47]. Initiation into the use of hard liquor is related to its use by peers and the quantity and frequency of parental drinking [35].

Adolescents with strong family ties, whose parents make an effort to meet their emotional needs are less likely to use marijuana. Parenting styles also influence drinking behavior. "Laissez-faire" parenting or a parental approach that is limiting and overcontrolling increases the probability of adolescent drinking [35].

Although peers have a great deal of influence on the drug use of their friends, it is not clear the extent of influence parents have on their child's choice of friends. Glynn [35] says that drug users seek drug users as friends. And Kandel [47], in her study of adolescent friendships, found that adolescents who share certain characteristics, including use of marijuana, are more likely to become friends.

The use of opiates is associated with disruptive family life where economic deprivation is common. Many opiate users live in urban slums where heroin is readily available. Here, the delinquent and drug subculture can easily have a stronger influence on the child than families that are preoccupied with the struggle to survive [16]. Juvenile opiate addicts tend to be depressed. They expect to fail, are easily frustrated, and are overwhelmed by a sense of futility [16]. Coleman [22] found that in heroin-addict families, there are an unusual number of deaths. Stanton [71] also identified death and loss through separation in a high proportion of addicts' families. Stanton views drug use as a reflection of the family's fear of separation and a means of the addict remaining dependent on the family, while appearing to be independent.

ASSESSMENT

Blum and Singer [7] present a framework for assessing adolescent abusers based on the theory that drug abuse is part of a pattern of social deviance. Their framework addresses six categories of theories about social deviance: socialization and value development, institutional

provision and opportunity, peer group, family, theories about personality and self-image, and biogenic factors.

Socialization and value development theories attribute deviancy to a lack of internal social values or negative socialization. Those who lack values are vulnerable to stress and are easily influenced by situations around them. Negative socialization refers to those who have social values that are in conflict with the values of the larger society [7].

Institutional provision and opportunity theory stresses the lack of employment and educational and other institutional opportunities, which interferes with development of successful social skills. *Peer group theories* emphasize the role of peers in influencing social behavior, and *family theories* focus on family dynamics. *Personality theories* look at factors such as self-esteem, depression, and learning as important contributions to social deviance. And finally, consideration is given to *biogenic factors,* those neurologic or genetic effects on behavior [7].

The interaction of a number of these factors probably contribute to drug abuse, but by assessing the individual in each category, a more comprehensive picture becomes evident. Treatment goals or preventative measures can be established for each domain identified as a problem. Within this framework a variety of professional disciplines may be involved in evaluation and treatment planning.

TREATMENT

For adolescents whose drug use reflects anxiety or depression, *individual therapy* addressing these issues may be appropriate (see anxiety disorders section for more on treatment of anxiety). Often individual therapy is one part of a treatment program that includes peer group or family therapy, or both.

Amini and colleagues [3] believe that adolescents who abuse tolerance-type drugs (amphetamines, barbiturates, opiates, and glue) have such a weak ego structure that they cannot, initially, benefit from individual psychotherapy. They believe that residential treatment where the individual becomes a member of a therapeutic community and deals with issues of trust and intimacy comes first.

Residential Programs

Many residential treatment programs are based on the characteristics of a *therapeutic community*. The concepts associated with a therapeutic community arose in mental hospitals with the recognition that patients are influenced by their social environment and that the passivity of the sick role does not prepare for discharge from the institution.

In a therapeutic community the social environment is the vehicle of therapy. Patients (residents) are involved in daily living activities that maintain the functioning of the program: cooking, cleaning and maintenance work, as well as participation in program decision making. Participants work closely with each other, and isolation is discouraged [27]. The everyday interaction of residents is used in group therapy and community meetings. A great deal of social and emotional intimacy occurs although sexual contact is taboo. The residents of the community are as active as the staff in treatment. Self-help and peer help is expected. A high value is placed on communication, honesty, and group cohesiveness. Less distinction and more communication takes place between residents and professional staff than is usually found in the hierarchy of the medical model.

Therapeutic communities tend to be most appropriate for those adolescents who have never developed the emotional and social skills to live in the larger society. These adolescents are often addicted to opiates. They have failed in school and are unemployed. They come from chaotic families and have never developed a feeling of competence. They lack a sense of direction, are easily frustrated, and have great difficulty problem solving [30].

The therapeutic community is designed not only to eliminate drug abuse, but to develop the ego strength and skills necessary to function in the community at large. Responsibility for one's own behavior is a critical philosophic approach with addicted individuals [24]. The development of responsible behavior is considered more important than insight-oriented therapy.

Typically drug addicts have a great deal of difficulty with authority figures and difficulty with intimacy and interpersonal relationships [30]. Thus peers who are veterans of the program are sometimes used as "bridges" [24] between newly admitted residents and staff. The development of peer relationships is an important developmental task of adolescence, and the emphasis on peer help is especially relevant for teenage drug abusers.

In therapeutic communities for adult addicts, a great deal of confrontive exchange between patients or between staff and patient occurs. Those who work with adolescents caution that this confrontive approach needs to be modified with adolescents [24, 30]. Although their lying and manipulative behavior needs confrontation, "young people have not lived long enough, or solidified enough of themselves, that their defenses are impregnable" [24].

The residential treatment environment for addicts is very structured. Rules are explicit and unbendable. Filstead and Anderson [27] give the four rules of their program: (1) no drugs or alcohol, (2) no violence, (3) no sex, and (4) residents must report rule violations to the community. Their facility does not have locked doors, and they have found them to be unnecessary.

Some therapeutic communities do daily urine analysis for the detection of drug use [24]; others do urine tests if substance abuse is suspected [27]. It is critically important that illicit substances are not used by residents. Not only do they completely subvert the goals of the program, but they undermine the confidence residents have in the staffs' ability to detect deceit and protect the abusers from themselves. In most programs broken rules result in expulsion from the program.

Residential programs for children and adolescents require a complex offering of services. Developmental needs must be addressed. Not only do these children have drug problems, but they are in the formative years where the foundation must be laid for adult life. Programs must be available for education and prevocational and social skill development. Healthy role models are important. A 1 hour per day session with a professional counselor is inadequate for the problems of institutionalized children. Staff must teach skills and be with the children in work and recreation [27]. It is the daily mundane interactions that build trust, respect, motivation, and the courage for the addict to develop and change.

Outpatient Programs

Filstead and Anderson [27] describe an extensive *outpatient program* for youths who are highly motivated and whose families are willing to be involved in treatment. These adolescents must not have physical or psychiatric difficulties. They must be willing to abstain from drugs and alcohol, and they must not have a history of failure in an outpatient program in order to be considered for outpatient rather than residential treatment.

The three-phase program is 20-weeks long and involves group work, with peers and with the family; individual therapy; and participation in a program such as Alcoholics Anonymous. If the individual fails to attend the program, uses drugs or alcohol, or exhibits violent behavior, their participation in the program is terminated, and residential treatment is recommended [27].

Family Involvement

Many outpatient and residential treatment programs require *family involvement* in therapy. Family dynamics often maintain drug-taking behavior, even if they were not involved in initiating it [76]. Often, in the drug abuser's family there is conflict between the parents and overinvolvement between the drug user and one parent [28]. The close parent may make excuses for the child's behavior. One goal of therapy is to help the parents become closer as a couple, forming a "united front" in dealing with the drug abuser [28]. Without placing blame, the therapist helps parents identify ways in which they may have been maintaining the child's drug abuse.

Control is an important issue, especially with adolescents. Typically, patterns of both overcontrol and undercontrol emerge in drug abuser's families. Understandably, when parents become aware of their child's drug use, some respond with strict monitoring of every move the child makes. They worry about the influence of peers and check the child's room for drugs. This can exacerbate the problem. On the other hand, parents may not be clear about rules for the child, or they may be inconsistent in enforcing rules. One parent may undermine the authority of the other [28].

The therapist helps the family members negotiate and establish realistic rules and identify those areas where control might be lessened. It is important to discuss the consequences of rule infringement before problems occur so that parents will not overreact to misbehavior. The therapist provides support for parental consistency while encouraging appropriate independence, peer involvement, and responsibility in the adolescent. "The therapist needs to search for competence, looking for areas of untapped strength and resources of the individual, as well as demonstrating to the family that each member has more skills and breadth than the family perceives" [28].

Medical Management

Before the problems that underlie drug-taking behavior can be tackled, the individual should be drug-free. In the case of physical dependence to an addictive substance, this may require inpatient medical supervision.

Narcotics, barbiturates, alcohol, and the minor tranquilizers produce physical dependence if taken regularly over time (Table 11-4) [1, 21, 41]. Hofmann [41] explains that physical addiction occurs only if the individual consumes the

TABLE 11-4. Drug characteristics

Drug classification	Desired effect	Other effects	Physical dependence	Tolerance	Withdrawal symptoms
Narcotics Opium Morphine Codeine Heroin Methadone	Relief of pain, relief of tension and anxiety, euphoria, sedation, treatment of heroin dependence (methadone)	Dizziness/orthostatic hypotension, itching, vomiting, dysphoria, constipation, miosis (contracted pupils), CNS depression	Yes	Yes	4–8 hr after last dose: rhinorrhea, lacrimation, nausea, vomiting, diarrhea, chills and perspiration, dehydration, CNS excitability, increase blood pressure, muscle twitching and spasms
Central nervous system depressants Alcohol Barbiturates Nembutal Seconal Amytal Tuinal	Tension reduction, euphoria, release inhibitions, sleep, sedation	Incoordination, reduced visual acuity, reduced pain perception, slow reaction time, impaired judgment, impaired concentration, vomiting, stupor	Yes Yes	Yes Yes	Tremor, weakness, perspiration, agitation, nausea, vomiting, seizures (in some), hallucinations, tachycardia, may result in death
Other Quaaludes Valmid Placidyl Doriden			Yes	Yes	
Antianxiety drugs Miltown Librium Valium		Lethal with alcohol (antianxiety drugs)	Yes	Yes	Similar to alcohol
Volatile hydrocarbons cements, glues, paint removers, cleaning fluids, lighter fluids	Euphoria, delusions, hallucinations, distorted perceptions, giddiness	Slurred speech, ataxia, nausea, vomiting, photophobia, diplopia, tinnitus, unconsciousness, hypoxia, death	No	Yes	

Drug	Desired effects	Adverse/acute effects	Physical dependence	Psychological dependence	Withdrawal symptoms
Hallucinogens LSD Mescaline Peyote Psilocybin	Altered perception: color, shape, distance, body image; depersonalization; illusions; warped time sense; philosophic, egocentric thinking; euphoria	Impaired judgment, panic, confusion, depression, toxic psychosis, megalomania, paranoia, flashbacks	No		
Phencyclidine (PCP)	Euphoria, grandiosity, slowed time sense	Agitation, anxiety, lability, synesthesia, nystagmus, ataxia, slurred speech, high blood pressure, stupor, toxic psychosis			
Marijuana Hashish	Relaxation, euphoria, intensified perceptions, slow time perception, preoccupation with stimuli, depersonalization apathy	Increased appetite, tachycardia, dry mouth, dysphoria	No		
Stimulants Amphetamines Benzedrine Methadrine Dexedrine Cocaine	Elation, grandiosity, loquacity	Agitation, hypervigilance, tachycardia, high blood pressure, nausea, vomiting, chills, perspiration, impaired judgment, aggression, delusions, hallucinations	Yes/no (opinions vary)	Yes	Depression, fatigue, disturbed sleep, increased dreaming

Source: Based on data from references [1, 21, 41].

309

drug at such a regular interval that the effect of the drug never completely wears off. Children and young adolescents rarely have the opportunity to maintain this level of intake. However, medical supervision of detoxification is important if addiction is present.

Although adolescents consider opiates more dangerous than sedatives [43], the withdrawal symptoms from sedatives are more rigorous, and the combination of alcohol and sedatives can be fatal [20]. Youths also consider sniffing volatile solvents as a babyish activity [41], yet sniffing can result in death or damage to peripheral nerves, bone marrow, liver, and kidneys [20].

Management of intoxication, detoxification, and medical complications of drug use often takes place in a general hospital where help for the psychosocial problems is not available. Young people whose abuse of drugs requires medical treatment should be referred for therapy.

PREVENTION

The main concern with drug abuse in youth is that it occurs at a time when the groundwork is being laid for adulthood. Important decisions are made in adolescence about educational and employment objectives. New roles are assumed. Youths who abuse drugs are less likely to complete their education and are more likely to be unemployed [52]. Thus, much of the thrust of research on adolescent drug abuse has been in the area of identifying factors contributing to drug abuse in order to develop programs of preventative intervention.

Prevention programs fall into two general categories: those that give information in order to affect attitudes and values and those aimed at developing social skills and expanding activities [50].

Education programs are based on the premise that people would not abuse drugs if they knew the consequences of using drugs. Some programs, in addition to giving information about drugs, encourage participants to examine their values and the relationship between their belief system and drug use. Theoretically, individuals who understand themselves can make responsible decisions about drugs [59].

Except for cigarette use, these approaches have not proved very effective [59] because they do not account for the many factors associated with drug abuse [29]. They do not teach coping skills [29], and they presuppose that people are rational in their approach to substance use [59].

Programs for *skill development* are based on the theory that drug abuse is a symptom of psychosocial problems and drugs are used to relieve anxiety, achieve popularity, status, or self-esteem and in imitation of role models [8]. It is believed that youngsters who have healthy egos will not need to turn to drugs. Thus, developing skills that will enhance personal competence and self-esteem will prevent the need for drugs.

Families of children who are in the early stages of drug use or who have academic and behavioral problems have been the focus of skill training. These families learn problem-solving techniques, contingency contracting, and communication skills [12].

A variation on skill development programs is the approach that uses activities that offer the kind of experience drugs might provide. For instance, if an individual is a thrill seeker, he or she learns to climb mountains. If peer acceptance is a motive, group activities or group therapy are used [72].

Identifying a target population for prevention programs is a challenge. There are numerous factors that predispose the individual to drug abuse: availability, peer use, early experimentation, parental substance use, and family relationships. Rebelliousness and delinquent behavior may also be precursors of drug abuse. Bry [12] suggests that when attempting to identify youth at risk, instead of searching for the most important predisposing factor, one should identify those who must deal with the greatest number of these factors [5].

Choosing the appropriate program for the

target population is an additional issue. Successful programs need to be analyzed to identify why they were successful and how they were implemented. A lot of work still needs to be done in the area of prevention [50].

REFERENCES

1. American Psychiatric Association. *Diagnostic and Statistical Manual of Mental Disorders* (3rd ed.). Washington, DC: APA, 1980.
2. American Psychiatric Association. *Diagnostic and Statistical Manual of Mental Disorders* (3rd ed. rev.). Washington, DC: APA, 1987.
3. Amini, F., Salasnek, S., and Burke, E. L. Adolescent drug abuse: Etiological and treatment considerations. *Adolescence* 11:281–299, 1976.
4. Bailey, M. K. Occupational therapy for patients with eating disorders. *Occup. Ther. Ment. Health* 6:89, 1986.
5. Barker, P. *Basic Child Psychiatry* (3rd ed.). Baltimore: University Park, 1979.
6. Bemis, K. M. Current approaches to the etiology and treatment of anorexia nervosa. *Psychol. Bull.* 85:593, 1978.
7. Blum, A., and Singer, M. Substance Abuse and Social Deviance: A Youth Assessment Framework. In R. Isralowitz and M. Singer (eds.), *Adolescent Substance Abuse: A Guide to Prevention and Treatment.* New York: Haworth, 1983.
8. Botvin, G. J. Prevention of Adolescent Substance Abuse Through the Development of Personal and Social Competence. In T. J. Glynn, C. G. Luekefeld, and J. P. Ludford (eds.), *Preventing Adolescent Drug Abuse: Intervention Strategies.* National Institute on Drug Abuse Research Monograph 47. DHHS Publ. No. (ADM) 83-1280. Washington, DC: Government Printing Office, 1983.
9. Branch, C. H. H., and Eurman, L. J. Social attitudes towards patients with anorexia nervosa. *Am. J. Psychiatr.* 137:631, 1980.
10. Bruch, H. *Eating Disorders: Obesity, Anorexia Nervosa, and the Person Within.* New York: Basic, 1973.
11. Bruch, H. *The Golden Cage: The Enigma of Anorexia Nervosa.* New York: Vintage, 1979.
12. Bry, B. H. Empirical Foundations of Family-Based Approaches to Adolescent Substance Abuse. In T. J. Glynn, C. C. Leukefeld, and J. P. Ludford (eds.), *Preventing Adolescent Drug Abuse: Intervention Strategies.* National Institute on Drug Abuse Research Monograph 47. DHHS Publ. No. (ADM) 83-1280. Washington, DC: Government Printing Office, 1983.
13. Carr, E. G. Contingency Management. In A. P. Goldstein, E. G. Carr, W. S. Davidson, II, et al (eds.), *In Response to Aggression: Methods of Control and Prosocial Alternatives.* New York: Pergamon, 1981.
14. Casper, R. C., and Davis, J. M. On the course of anorexia nervosa. *Am. J. Psychiatry* 134:974, 1977.
15. Chamberlain, C., and Steinhauer, P. D. Conduct Disorders and Delinquency. In P. D. Steinhauer and Q. Rae-Grant (eds.), *Psychological Problems of the Child in the Family* (2nd ed.). New York: Basic, 1983. Pp. 204, 206.
16. Chein, I. Psychological, Social, and Epidemiological Factors in Juvenile Drug Use. In D. J. Lettieri, M. Sayers, and H. W. Wallenstein (eds.), *Theories on Drug Abuse: Selected Contemporary Perspectives.* National Institute on Drug Abuse Research Monograph 30. DHHS Publ. No. (ADM) 80-967. Washington, DC: Government Printing Office, 1980.
17. Chess, S. *An Introduction to Child Psychiatry* (2nd ed.). New York: Grune & Stratton, 1969.
18. Clarizio, H. F., and McCoy, G. F. *Behavior Disorders in Children* (3rd ed.). New York: Harper & Row, 1983.
19. Clay, R. R., and Ritter, C. A developmental perspective on adolescent drug abuse. *Adv. Alcohol Subst. Abuse* 4:69–97, 1985. P. 23.
20. Cohen, S. Adolescents and Drug Abuse. In D. J. Lettieri and J. P. Ludford (eds.), *Drug Abuse and the American Adolescent.* National Institute on Drug Abuse Research Monograph 38. DHHS Publ. No. (ADM) 81-1166. Washington, DC: Government Printing Office, 1981.
21. Coleman, J. C., Butcher, J. N., and Carson, R. C. *Abnormal Psychology and Modern Life* (7th ed.). Glenville, Ill.: Scott, Foresman, 1984.
22. Coleman, S. B. Incomplete Mourning and Addict/Family Transactions: A Theory for Understanding Heroin Abuse. In D. J. Lettieri, M. Sayers, and H. W. Pearson (eds.), *Theories on Drug Abuse: Selected Contemporary Perspectives.* National Institute on Drug Abuse Research Monograph 30. DHHS Publ. No. (ADM) 80-967. Washington, DC: Government Printing Office, 1980.
23. Crisp, A. H., Hsu, L. K. G., Harding, B. et al. Clinical features of anorexia nervosa: A study of 102 female patients. *J. Psychosom. Res.* 24:179, 1980.
24. Densen-Gerber, J. *We Mainline Dreams: The Odyssey House Story.* Garden City, N.J.: Doubleday, 1973. P. 96.
25. Dodge, K. A., and Murphy, R. R. The Assess-

ment of Social Competence in Adolescents. In P. Karoly and J. J. Steffen (eds.), *Adolescent Behavior Disorders: Foundations and Contemporary Concerns: Advances in Child Behavioral Analysis and Therapy,* Vol. 3. Lexington, MA: Lexington Books, 1984.

26. Donovan, J. E., and Jessor, R. Problem drinking and the dimension of involvement with drugs: A Guttman scalogram analysis of adolescent drug use. *Am. J. Public Health* 73:543–552, 1983.

27. Filstead, W. J., and Anderson, C. L. Conceptual and Clinical Issues in the Treatment of Adolescent Alcohol and Substance Misusers. In R. Isralowitz and M. Singer (eds.), *Adolescent Substance Abuse: A Guide to Prevention and Treatment.* New York: Haworth, 1983.

28. Fishman, C., Stanton, M. D., and Rosman, B. L. Treating Families of Adolescent Drug Abusers. In M. D. Stanton and T. C. Todd (eds.), *The Family Therapy of Drug Abuse and Addiction.* New York: Guilford, 1982. P. 354.

29. Flay, B. R., and Sobel, J. L. The Role of Mass Media in Preventing Adolescent Substance Abuse. In T. J. Glynn, C. G. Leukefeld, and J. P. Ludford (eds.), *Preventing Adolescent Drug Abuse: Intervention Strategies.* National Institute on Drug Abuse Research Monograph 47. DHHS Publ. No. (ADM) 83-1280. Washington, DC: Government Printing Office, 1983.

30. Freudenberger, H. J., and Carbone, J. The reentry process of adolescents. *J. Psychoactive Drugs* 16:95–99, 1984.

31. Gardner, R. A. Helping Children Cooperate in Therapy. In S. I. Harrison and J. D. Noshpitz (eds.), *Basic Handbook of Child Psychiatry III: Therapeutic Interventions.* New York: Basic, 1979.

32. Gersick, K. E., Grady, K., Sexton, E., et al. In D. J. Lettieri and J. P. Ludford (eds.), *Drug Abuse and the American Adolescent.* National Institute on Drug Abuse Research Monograph 38. DHHS Publ. No. (ADM) 81-1166. Washington, DC: Government Printing Office, 1981.

33. Giles, G. M. Anorexia nervosa and bulimia: An activity-oriented approach. *Am. J. Occup. Ther.* 39:510, 1985.

34. Giles, G. M., and Allen, M. E. Occupational therapy in the rehabilitation of the patient with anorexia nervosa. *Occup. Ther. Ment. Health* 6:47, 1986.

35. Glynn, T. J. From Family to Peer: Transitions of Influence Among Drug-Using Youth. In D. J. Lettieri and J. P. Ludford (eds.), *Drug Abuse and the American Adolescent.* National Institute

on Drug Abuse Research Monograph 38. DHHS Publ. No. (ADM) 81-1166. Washington, DC: Government Printing Office, 1981.

36. Goldstein, A. P. Problem Solving Training. In A. P. Goldstein, E. G. Carr, W. S. Davidson, II, et al. (eds.), *In Response To Aggression: Methods of Control and Prosocial Alternatives.* New York: Pergamon, 1981.

37. Goldstein, A. P. Social Skill Training. In A. P. Goldstein, E. G. Carr, W. S. Davidson, II, et al. (eds.), *In Response To Aggression: Methods of Control and Prosocial Alternatives.* New York: Pergamon, 1981. P. 162.

38. Graziano, A. M., De Giovanni, I. S., and Garcia, K. A. Behavioral treatment of children's fears: A review. *Psychol. Bull.* 86:1352, 1978.

39. Hatzenbuehler, L. C., and Schroeder, H. E. Desensitization procedures in the treatment of childhood disorders. *Psychol. Bull.* 85:831, 1978.

40. Hendin, H. Psychosocial Theory of Drug Abuse: A Psychodynamic Approach. In D. J. Lettieri, M. Sayers, and H. W. Pearson (eds.), *Theories on Drug Abuse: Selected Contemporary Perspectives.* National Institute on Drug Abuse Research Monograph 30. DHHS Publ. No. (ADM) 80-967. Washington, DC: Government Printing Office, 1980.

41. Hofmann, F. G. *A Handbook on Drug and Alcohol Abuse: The Biomedical Aspects* (2nd ed.). New York: Oxford University Press, 1983.

42. Horney, K. *The Neurotic Personality of Our Time.* New York: Norton, 1937. Pp. 80–81.

43. Johnston, L. D., Bachman, J. G., and O'Malley, P. M. *Highlights from Student Drug Use in America 1975–1981.* National Institute on Drug Abuse. DHHS Publ. No. (ADM) 82-1208. Washington, DC: Government Printing Office, 1981.

44. Johnston, L. D., O'Malley, P. M., and Bachman, J. G. *Use of Licit and Illicit Drugs by America's High School Students 1975–1984.* National Institute on Drug Abuse. DHHS Publ. No. (ADM) 85-1394. Washington, DC: Government Printing Office, 1985.

45. Kalucy, R. S., Crisp, A. H., and Harding, B. A study of 56 families with anorexia nervosa. *Br. J. Med. Psychol.* 50(4):381, 1977.

46. Kandel, D. B. Developmental Stages in Adolescent Drug Involvement. In D. J. Lettieri, M. Sayers, and H. W. Pearson (eds.), *Theories on Drug Abuse: Selected Contemporary Perspectives.* National Institute on Drug Abuse Research Monograph 30. DHHS Publ. No. (ADM) 80-

967. Washington, DC: Government Printing Office, 1980. P. 126.

47. Kandel, D. B. On processes of peer influences in adolescent drug use: A developmental perspective. *Adv. Alcohol Sust. Abuse* 4:139–163, 1985.

48. Kanner, L. *Child Psychiatry* (4th ed.). Springfield: Thomas, 1972.

49. Kennedy, R. E. Cognitive-behavioral approaches to the modification of aggressive behavior in children. *School Psychol. Rev.* 11:1, 1982.

50. Leukefeld, C. G., and Moskowitz, J. M. Discussion and Recommendations. In T. J. Glynn, C. G. Leukefeld, and J. P. Ludford (eds.), *Preventing Adolescent Drug Abuse: Intervention Strategies*. National Institute on Drug Abuse Research Monograph 47. DHHS Publ. No. (ADM) 83-1280. Washington, DC: Government Printing Office, 1983.

51. Liebman, R., Minuchin, S., and Baker, L. An integrated treatment program for anorexia nervosa. *Am. J. Psychiatry* 131:432, 1974.

52. Lukoff, I. F. Toward a Sociology of Drug Use. In D. J. Lettieri, M. Sayers, and H. W. Wallenstein (eds.), *Theories on Drug Abuse: Selected Contemporary Perspectives*. National Institute on Drug Abuse Research Monograph 30. DHHS Publ. No. (ADM) 80-967. Washington, DC: Government Printing Office, 1980.

53. Maloney, M. J., and Farrel, M. K. Treatment of severe weight loss in anorexia nervosa with hyperalimentation and psychotherapy. *Am. J. Psychiatry* 137:310, 1980.

54. Mavisskalian, M. Anorexia nervosa treated with response prevention and prolonged exposure. *Behav. Res. Ther.* 20:27, 1982.

55. McColl, M. A., Friedland, J., and Kerr, A. When doing is not enough: The relationship between activity and effectiveness in anorexia nervosa. *Occup. Ther. Ment. Health* 6:137, 1986. P. 139.

56. Melamed, B. G., and Siegel, L. J. Reduction of Anxiety in Children Facing Hospitalization and Surgery by Use of Filmed Modeling. In C. M. Franks and G. T. Wilson (eds.), *Annual Review of Behavior Therapy Theory and Practice*. New York: Brunner/Mazel, 1976.

57. Mikulas, W. L. *Behavior Modification: An Overview*. New York: Harper & Row, 1972.

58. Mosey, A. C. *Three Frames of Reference for Mental Health*. Thorofare, NJ: Slack, 1970.

59. Moskowitz, J. M. Preventing Adolescent Substance Abuse Through Drug Education. In T. J. Glynn, C. G. Leukefeld, and J. P. Ludford (eds.), *Preventing Adolescent Drug Abuse: Intervention Strategies*. National Institute on Drug Abuse Research Monograph 47. DHHS Publ. No. (ADM) 83-1280. Washington, DC: Government Printing Office, 1983.

60. Moustakas, C. E. *Psychotherapy with Children: The Living Relationship*. New York: Ballantine, 1959. P. 3.

61. Mushin, D. N. General Principles of Treatment in Child Psychiatry. In P. D. Steinhauer and Q. Rae-Grant (eds.), *Psychological Problems of the Child in the Family*. New York: Basic Books, 1983.

62. National Institute on Alcohol Abuse and Alcoholism. *Prevention Plus: Involving Schools, Parents, and the Community in Alcohol and Drug Education*. DHHS Publ. No. (ADM) 83-1256. Washington, DC: Government Printing Office, 1983.

63. Palmer, R. L. *Anorexia Nervosa: A Guide for Sufferers and Their Families*. New York: Penguin, 1980.

64. Patterson, G. R., Reid, J. B., Jones, R. R., et al. *A Social Learning Approach To Family Intervention: Vol. I, Families With Aggressive Children*. Eugene, OR: Castalia, 1975.

65. Pillay, M., and Crisp, A. H. Some psychological characteristics of patients with anorexia nervosa whose weight has been newly restored. *Br. J. Med. Psychol.* 50(4):375, 1977.

66. Rampling, D. Anorexia nervosa: Reflections on theory and practice. *Psychiatry* 41:269, 1978.

67. Roth, D. Treatment of the hospitalized eating disorder patient. *Occup. Ther. Ment. Health* 6:67, 1986.

68. Shamsie, S. J. Antisocial adolescents: Our treatments do not work—Where do we go from here? *Can. J. Psychiatry* 26:5, 1981.

69. Smart, R. G. An Availability-Proneness Theory of Illicit Drug Abuse. In D. J. Lettieri, M. Sayers, and H. W. Wallenstein (eds.), *Theories on Drug Abuse: Selected Contemporary Perspectives*. National Institute on Drug Abuse Research Monograph 30. DHHS Publ. No. (ADM) 80-967. Washington, DC: Government Printing Office, 1980.

70. Smith, G. M. Perceived Effects of Substance Use: A General Theory. In D. J. Lettieri, M. Sayers, and H. W. Wallenstein (eds.), *Theories on Drug Abuse: Selected Contemporary Perspectives*. National Institute on Drug Abuse Research Monograph 30. DHHS Publ. No. (ADM) 80-967. Washington, DC: Government Printing Office, 1980. P. 53.

11. Psychosocial Disorders 313

71. Stanton, M. D. A Family Theory of Drug Abuse. In D. J. Lettieri, M. Sayers, and H. W. Wallenstein (eds.), *Theories on Drug Abuse: Selected Contemporary Perspectives.* National Institute on Drug Abuse Research Monograph 30. DHHS Publ. No. (ADM) 80-967. Washington, DC: Government Printing Office, 1980.

72. Steffenhagen, R. A. Self-Esteem Theory of Drug Abuse. In D. J. Lettieri, M. Sayers, and H. W. Wallenstein (eds.), *Theories on Drug Abuse: Selected Contemporary Perspectives.* National Institute on Drug Abuse Research Monograph 30. DHHS Publ. No. (ADM) 80-967. Washington, DC: Government Printing Office, 1980.

73. Steinhauer, P. D., and Berman, G. Anxiety, Neurotic, and Personality Disorders in Children. In P. D. Steinhauer and Q. Rae-Grant (eds.), *Psychological Problems of the Child in the Family.* New York: Basic Books, 1983.

74. Stonehill, E., and Crisp, A. H. Psychoneurotic characteristics of patients with anorexia nervosa before and after treatment and at follow-up 4–7 years later. *J. Psychosom. Res.* 21:187, 1977.

75. Thomas, A., Chess, S., and Birch, H. G. *Temperament and Behavior Disorders in Children.* New York: New York University Press, 1968.

76. Todd, T. C. A Contingency Analysis of Family Treatment and Drug Abuse. In J. Grabowski, M. L. Stitzer, and J. E. Henningfield (eds.), *Behavioral Intervention Techniques in Drug Abuse Treatment.* National Institute on Drug Abuse Research Monograph 46. DHHS Publ. No. (ADM) 84-1282. Washington, DC: Government Printing Office, 1984.

77. Weathers, L., and Liberman, R. P. Contingency Contracting with Families of Delinquent Adolescents. In C. M. Franks and G. T. Wilson (eds.), *Annual Review of Behavior Therapy Theory and Practice.* New York: Brunner/Mazel, 1976.

78. Zeller, C. L. Treatment of ego deficits in anorexia nervosa. *Am. J. Orthopsychiatry* 52:356, 1982.

ASSOCIATIONS

Alcoholics Anonymous World Services, P.O. Box 459, Grand Central Station, New York, NY 10163
Phone: (212) 686-1100

Alcohol Education for Youth and Community, 362 State St., Albany, NY 12210
Phone: (518) 436-9319

American Academy of Child and Adolescent Psychiatry, 3615 Wisconson Ave., N.W., Washington, D.C. 20016
Phone: (202) 966-7300

American Anorexia/Bulimia Association, 133 Cedar Ln., Teaneck, NJ 07666
Phone: (201) 836 1800

American Counsel for Drug Education, 5820 Hubbard Dr., Rockville, MD 20852
Phone: (301) 984-5700

ANAD—National Association of Anorexia Nervosa and Associated Eating Disorders, Box 7, Highland Park, IL 60035
Phone: (312) 831-3438

Families in Action National Drug Information Center, 3845 N. Druid Hills Rd., Suite 300, Decatur, GA 30033
Phone: (404) 325-5799

National Alliance for the Mentally Ill, 1901 N. Fort Myer Dr., Suite 500, Arlington, VA 22209
Phone: (703) 524-7600

Directory of North American Suppliers

GENERAL
A and B Products
255 University Blvd.
Berrian Springs, MI 49103

A Bec
20803 Higgins Ct.
Torrance, CA 90501

Abbey Medical
3216 El Segundo Blvd.
Hawthorne, CA 90250

Able Child
154 Chambers St.
New York, NY 10007

Accumec Corp.
32 Race St.
San Jose, CA 95126

Achievement Products, Inc.
P.O. Box 547
Mineola, NY 11501

Adaptive Aids
3721 East Technical Dr.
No. 7
Tucson, AZ 85713

Adaptive Communication
Systems, Inc.
P.O. Box 12440
Pittsburgh, PA 15231

Adaptive Enterprises
P.O. Box 2019B
1120 Main
Standpoint, ID 83864

Adco Hearing Conservation
1558 California St.
Denver, CO 80202

Adler Royal Business Machines
1600 Route 22
Union, NJ 07083

Adlib Orthotics
P.O. Box 905
Lakewood, CA 90714

Advanced Mobility Systems, Inc.
P.O. Box 548
Troy, MT 59935

AFW of North America
Bank of New York Building
Olean, NY 14760

American Bio Medics
P.O. Box 530
Old Bethpage, NY 01608

American Communication Corp.
180 Roberts St.
East Hartford, CT 06108

American Foundation for the Blind
15 W. 16 St.
New York, NY 10011

American Printing House
for the Blind
1839 Frankfort Ave.
P.O. Box 6085
Louisville, KY 40206

American Stair Glide Corp.
4001 East 138 St.
Grandview, MO 64030

Amigo Mobility Center, Inc.
7500 Bluewater N.W.
Albuquerque, NM 87105

Andrews Maclaren
P.O. Box 2004
New York, NY 10017

Apollo Electronic
Visual Aids
P.O. Box 7455
Mountain View, CA 94039

Apollo Lazers
20932 Lassen St.
Chatsworth, CA 91311

Aristera Machines
Renovators Old Mill
Miller Falls, MA 01349

Automated Data Systems, Inc.
P.O. Box 4062
Madison, WI 53711

Basic Telecommunications Corp.
4414 East Haramony Rd.
Fort Collins, CO 80525

Bema U.S.A., Inc.
2015 Weaver Park Dr.
P.O. Box 4280
Clearwater, FL 33518

Beneficial Designs, Inc.
5858 Empire Grade
Santa Cruz, CA 95060

Benjamin Michael Industries
65 E. Palatine Rd.
Suite 105
Prospect Heights, IL 60070

Bernina Co.
534 W. Chestnut
Pacific Palisades, CA 90272

Best Visual Products
65 Earle Ave.
Lynbrook, NY 11563

BIM
P.O. Box 3413
Terre Haute, IN 11563

Blackburn Research Products
830 Traverse du lac Sergent
Co Portneuf PQ, GOA 2JO
Canada

Brookstone Company
11 Brookstone Building
127 Vose Farm Rd.
Peterborough, NH 03458

California Retyping
Data Display Systems
2240 Colby Ave.
Los Angeles, CA 90064

Carnac Industries
P.O. Box 7010
353 Bridgeport Dr.
Port St. Lucie, FL 53085

Camp International
P.O. Box 89
Jackson, MI 49204

Canadian Hearing Society
60 Bedford Rd.
Toronto M5R 2K2
Canada

Childsafe
P.O. Box 633
Pacific Palisades, CA 90272

Cleo Living Aids
3957 Mayfield Rd.
Cleveland, OH 44121

Clothing for Handicapped People
The President's Committee
on Employment of the Handicapped
Washington, DC 20210

Coastline Controls
414 East Inman Ave.
P.O. Box A
Rahway, NJ 07065

Columbia Medical Manufacturing
P.O. Box 633
Hinsdale, IL 60521

Com Tek Communication Technology
375 Bridgeport Dr.
Port St. Lucie, FL 33485

Comfortably Yours
52 W. Hunter Ave.
Maywood, NJ 07607

Commetrics, Ltd.
P.O. Box 278
St. Lambert
Canada J4P 3N8

Community Playthings
Rifton Equipment for the Handicapped
Route 213
Rifton, NY 12471

Computers for the
Physically Handicapped
7602 Talbert Ave.
Huntington Beach, CA 92647

Computers to Help People
1221 West Johnson St.
Madison, WI 53715

Consumer Care Products, Inc.
6405 Paradise Ln.
Sheboygan Falls, WI 53085

Controlonics Corp.
Five Lyberty Way
Westford, MA 01886

Cooper Canada, Ltd.
501 Alliance Ave.
Toronto, Ontario M6N 2J3
Canada

C. P. Wainman Chapter
Northwestern Bell Telephone Co.
224 South 5th St., Rm. 1300
Minneapolis, MN 53204

C. R. Bard, Inc.
731 Central Ave.
Murray Hill, NJ 07974

Crestwood Co.
331 South Third St.
P.O. Box 04513
Milwaukee, WI 53204

Cyberon
1175 Wendy Rd.
Ann Arbor, MI 48103

Danmar Products, Inc.
2390 Winewood
Ann Arbor, MI 83651

Dean Rosecrans
P.O. Box 710
Nampa, ID 83651

Delta Faucet Co.
Div. of Masco Group of IN
P.O. Box 40980
Greensburg, IN 47240

Desmond J. Carron
10541 Farnham Drive
Bethesda, MD 20014

Don Johnston Developmental Equipment
981 Winnetka Terrace
Lake Zurich, IL 60047

Dufco
2410 Broad St.
San Luis Obispo, CA 93401

Earmark
1125 Dixwell Ave.
Hamden, CT 06514

Educational Teaching Aids
159 West Kinzie St.
Chicago, IL 60610

Elayo Americas
P.O. Box 23927
Fort Lauderdale, FL 33307

Electrolurgy
1121 Duryea Ave.
Irvine, CA 92714

Electronic Handicapped
Equipment, Ltd.
1299 Portland Ave.
Rochester, NY 14621

Engle Enterprises, Inc.
530 E. 9th St. No. 1
Azusa, CA 91702

Equipment Shop
P.O. Box 33
Bedford, MA 01730

Everest and Jennings, Inc.
3233 East Mission Oaks Blvd.
Camarillo, CA 93010

Exceptionally Yours
The Salk Co., Inc.
P.O. Box 452
Boston, MA 24014

Executive Distributors of America
15055 32 Mile Rd.
Romeo, MI 48065

Extensions for Independence
635-5 N. Twin Oaks Valley Rd.
San Marcos, CA 02134

Eyetronics
P.O. Box 693
Lenox, MA 01240

Face Guards, Inc.
P.O. Box 8425
Roanoke, VA 24014

Fairway King
3 East Main St.
Oklahoma City, OK 73104

FashionAble
P.O. Box 3
Rocky Hill, NJ 08553

Flaghouse
18 W. 18 St.
New York, NY 10011

Frank B. Jewett Chapter
Bell Laboratories, Inc.
150 John F. Kennedy Parkway
Rm. 3L-218
Short Hills, NJ 07078

Fred Sammons, Inc.
Brookfield, IL 60513

Frost Co.
6523 14 Ave.
Kenosha, WI 53141

Gandy Co.
528 Gandrud Rd.
Owatonna, MN 55060

G. E. Miller
484 South Broadway
Yonkers, NY 10705

GEG Pool Lift
P.O. Box 282
King of Prussia, PA 19406

Gladys E. Loeb Foundation, Inc.
2002 Forest Hill Dr.
Silver Spring, MD 20903

Graham Field Surgical
415 Second Ave.
New Hyde Park, NY 11040

Grayline Housewares
1616 Berkeley St.
Elsin, IL 60120

Grizzly Peak Stables
Berkeley Outreach Program
271 Lomas Cantadas
2539 Telegraph Ave.
Berkeley, CA 94704

Hal Hen Co.
36-14 Eleventh St.
Long Island City, NY 11106

Hammacher Schlemmer
147 E. 57 St.
New York, NY 10022

Handi Aid Co.
2907 W. Warner Ave.
Santa Ana, CA 92704

Harper
3125 West Hampton Ave.
Englewood, CO 80110

Harriet Carter
Stump Rd.
Montgomeryville, PA 19836

Hausmann Industries, Inc.
130 Union St.
Northvale, NJ 07647

Hein A. Ken Corp.
102 Fosse Ct.
Thief River Falls, MN 56701

Help Me to Help Myself
324 Acre Ave.
Brownsburg, IN 46112

Help Yourself Aids
P.O. Box 192
Hinsdale, IL 60512

H. G. McCully Upstate Chapter
New Jersey Bell Telephone Co.
540 Broad St. Rm. 1300
E. Newark, NJ 07107

Hillan Creative Playstructures
1750 Courtwood Crescent
Suite 109
Ottawa, Ontario K2C 2B5
Canada

Howe Press of Perkins School for the Blind
175 North Beacon St.
Watertown, MA 02172

Independence Factory, The
P.O. Box C
Middletown, OH 45042

Independent Living Aids, Inc.
111 Commercial Ct.
Plainview, NY 11803

Industrial Research and Engineering
2409 North Kerby
Portland, OR 97227

IPAS International Corp.
1440 Broadway
Suite 2250
New York, NY 10018

JAL Co., The
2046 Banlet Rd.
Royal Oak, MI 48073

J. A. Preston Corp.
60 Page Rd.
Clifton, NJ 07012

Jay L. Warren
P.O. Box 25413
Chicago, IL 60625

J. E. Nolan and Co., Inc.
1826 Laser Ln.
Louisville, KY 40299

Julian A. McDermott
1639 Stephen St.
Ridgewood, NY 11227

KE Series Electronic
Devices for the Deaf
2801 Berry St.
Sioux City, IA 51103

Kentucky Industries
for the Blind
1900 Brownsboro Rd.
Louisville, KY 40206-2199

Kilgour Chapter
Cincinnati Bell, Inc.
209 West Seventh St., Rm. 107
Cincinnati, OH 45202

Knightsbridge Medical
236 East Castle Harbour
Friendswood, TX 77546

Kristen Wear
127 Nutley Ave.
Nutley, NJ 07110

Lakeshore Curriculum Materials
2695 E. Dominguez St.
P.O. Box 6261
Carson, CA 90749

Laurel Designs
5 Laurel Ave., No. 1
Belvedere, CA 94920

Leonard's Health Care Products
65 19th St.
Brooklyn, NY 11232

Linda J. Burkhart
8503 Rhode Island Ave.
College Park, MD 20740

Lo Rich Enterprises, Inc.
Corner 1st St. and Central Ave.
Suite 112
Miamisburg, OH 45342

Lozanov Learning Institute
1315 Apple Ave.
Silver Spring, MD 20910

Luminaud, Inc.
8688 Tyler Blvd.
P.O. Box 268
Mentor, OH 44060

Maddak, Inc.
6 Industrial Rd.
Pequannock, NJ 07440

Magnistitch
P.O. Box 2424
Birmingham, AL 35201

Mailhawk Mfg. Co.
Warm Springs, GA 31830

Manhattan Empire Chapter
New York Telephone Co.
1095 Avenue of the Americas
New York, NY 10036

Maple Leaf Chapter
Bell Canada
393 University Ave.
F8, Toronto, Ontario M5G 1W9
Canada

Maryland Chapter
The Chesapeake and Potomac
Telephone Co. of Maryland
320 St. Paul Place
11 Fl.
Baltimore, MD 21202

Maxi-Signal Products, Inc.
5 E. 49 St.
P.O. Box 398
LaGrange, IL 60525

Mechanicaids Aquanaids, Inc.
P.O. Box 405
Olean, NY 14760

Medi Sport Corp.
2545 E. 64 St.
New York, NY 11234

Medical Equipment Distributors
1701 South First Ave.
Maywood, IL 60153

Minnesota Mining and Manufacturing
3M Company Medical Products
3M Center
St. Paul, MN 55101

Mobility Plus
P.O. Box 391
Santa Paula, CA 93060

Modern Education Corp.
P.O. Box 721
Tulsa, OK 74101

Modular Medical Corp.
1558 Hutchinson River
Parkway East
Bronx, NY 10461

Motor Development Corp.
P.O. Box 4054
Downey, CA 93041

Mountain Man
720 Front St.
Bozeman, MT 59715

Mountainsmith
12790 W. 6 Place
Golden, CO 80401

Nationwide Flashing Signal Systems
8120 Fenton St.
Silver Spring, MD 20910

Nelson Medical Products
5690 Sarah Ave.
Sarasota, FL 33583

New England Handcycles
228 Winchester St.
Brookline, MA 02146

Northern Plastics Corp.
6733 Myers Rd.
East Syracuse, NY 13057

Northern Telecom
304 E. Mall Islington
Ontario, M9B 2E4
Canada

Nuday Creations
712 Wagonwheel Dr.
Fort Collins, CO 80526

On the Rise
171 Grandview Rd.
Nepean, Ontario K2H 8B9
Canada

One Eighty Nine Systems
101 Fox St.
Harrisburg, PA 17109

One to One
P.O. Box 235
Olathe, KS 66061

Orthopedia GmbH
Inter. Med. Equipment
11000 Rush St. No. 4
South El Monte, CA 91733

PCA Industries
2298 Grissom Dr.
St. Louis, MO 63141

Pelco Industries
351 E. Alondra Blvd.
Gardena, CA 90248

Playlearn Products
Majistic Supply Co.
1100 Turnpike St.
Canton, MA 02021

Phone TTY, Inc.
202 Lexington Ave.
Hackensack, NJ 07601

Phonic Ear Phonic Mirror
250 Camino Alto
Mill Valley, CA 94941

Prentke-Romich Co.
8769 Township Rd. 513
Shreve, OH 44676

Preston Special Education
60 Page Rd.
Clifton, NJ 07012

Proctor and Associates
15050 N.E. 36
Redmond, WA 98052

PSI, Pauls Sports
125 Columbia Ct.
Chasko, MN 55318

PTL Designs
Route 3, Box 745
Perkins, OR 74059

Radio Shack International
(Tandy)
500 One Tandy Center
Fort Worth, TX 76102

Rajowalt Co.
Carters Rehabilitation Div.
Atwood, IN 46502

Recreational Mobility, Inc.
P.O. Box 147
Elmira, OR 97437

Rehab Technology
C/O George Zuriene
Box 185
Aviston, IL 62216

Research Plus, Inc.
P.O. Box 324
Bayonne, NJ 07002

Richards Manufacturing Co., Inc.
1450 Brooks Rd.
Memphis, TN 38116

Rifton Equipment for the Handicapped
Route 213
Rifton, NY 12471

Rocky Mountain Software, Inc.
214–131 Water St.
Vancouver, B.C. V6B 4M3
Canada

Roloke Co.
8919 Sunset Blvd.
Los Angeles, CA 90069

Ronnie Lee, Inc.
P.O. Box 315
Winter Park, CO 80482

Royal Doulton
700 Cottontail Ln.
Somerset, NJ 08873

Science Products
P.O. Box A
Southeastern, PA 19399

Scitronics
523 S. Clewell St.
Bethlehem, PA 18015

SCM Corp.
Smith Corona
65 Locust St.
New Canaan, CT 06840

Sears, Roebuck & Co.
Home Health Department (608)
Sears Tower
Chicago, IL 60684

Selwyn, Mr. Don
N.I.R.E.
97 Decker Rd.
Butler, NJ 07405

Sensory Aids Corp.
Suite 110, White Pines Office
205 W. Grand Ave.
Bensenville, IL 60106

Sensory Interface Equipment
4442 Kasson Rd.
Syracuse, NY 13215

Sharp Electronics
10 Keystone Place
Paramus, NJ 07652

Shea Products
P.O. Box 184
Clawson, MI 48017

Siemens Hearing Instruments
685 Liberty Ave.
Union, NJ 07083

Sitting Pretty, Sitting Proud
2112 Eastman Ave. No. 115
Ventura, CA 93003

Snitz Manufacturing Co.
2096 S. Church St.
East Troy, WI 53120

Sock On
P.O. Box 4174
Palm Springs, CA 92263

Sola, Inc.
242 W. 27 St.
New York, NY 10001

Sonic Alert
209 Voorheis
Pontiac, MI 48053

Sound Barrier, Inc.
401–417 Fayette Ave.
Springfield, IL 62704

Southpaw Enterprise
800 W. Third St.
Dayton, OH 45407

Sparr Telephone Arm Co.
P.O. Box 143
Allamuchy, NJ 07820

Special Clothes
P.O. Box 4220
Alexandria, VA 22303

Special Friends
P.O. Box 1262
Lowell, MA 08153

Specialized Audio Engineering
Suite K, 6240 Church Ln.
Baltimore, MD 21207

Stall and Dean
95 Church St.
Brockton, MA 02403

Susquehanna Rehabilitation Products
RD 2 Box 41
9 Overlook Dr.
Wrightsville, PA 17368

Teachers Institute for
Special Education
2947 Bayside Ct.
Wantagh, NY 11793

Techni Flair Corp.
P.O. Box 40
Cotter, AR 77626

Ted Hoyer and Co.
2222 Minnesota St.
Oshkosh, WI 11793

Telegraphics, Inc.
P.O. Box 1061
Carrollton, TX 75006

Telephone Pioneers of America
Oregon Chapter No. 31
421 S.W. Oak St., Rm. 114
Portland, OR 97204

Telesensory Systems, Inc.
455 North Bernado Ave.
P.O. Box 7455
Mountain View, CA 94043

Telex Communications
9600 Aldrich Ave. So.
Minneapolis, MN 55420

Texas Instruments
P.O. Box 6448
Midland, TX 79701

Texas Technical University
Textile Research Center
P.O. Box 5888
Lubbock, TX 79417

Textile Research Center
Texas Technical University
P.O. Box 5217
Lubbock, TX 79417

Theodore N. Vail State Chapter
Illinois Bell Telephone Co.
406 East Monroe St., 3E
Springfield, IL 62721

Therafin Corp.
3800 Union Ave.
Steger, IL 60475

Therapeutic Recreation Systems
1280 28 St., Suite 3
Boulder, CO 80303

Toys for Special Children
101 Lefurgy Ave.
Hastings-on-Hudson, NY

Trans Aid Corp.
13130 Normandie Ave.
Gardena, CA 90249

Triformation Systems
3132 S.E. Jay St.
Stuart, FL 33494

Trujillo Industries
5040 Firestone Blvd.
South Gate, CA 90280

Tufts Biomedical Engineering Center
171 Harrison Ave.
Boston, MA 02111

Typewriting Institute
for the Handicapped
3102 W. Augusta Ave.
Phoenix, AZ 85021

Ultratec
P.O. Box 4062
Madison, WI 53711

Vermont-New Hampshire Chapter
New England Telephone and
Telegraph Co.
1228 Elm St.
Manchester, NH 03101

Visualtek
1610 26 St., Dept. C
Santa Monica Springs, CA 90404

Wal Jan Surgical Products, Inc.
Drawer H, 25 Buena Vista Ave.
Lawrence, NY 11559

Water Sport Industries
10230 Freeman Ave.
Santa Fe Springs, CA 90670

Weitbrecht Communication, Inc.
652 Bair Island Rd., Suite 104
Redwood, CA 94063

Williams Sound Corp.
6844 Washington Ave.
South Eden Prairie, MN 55344

Wings of VGRS
2239 E. 55 St.
Cleveland, OH 44103

Wolverine Chapter
Michigan Bell Telephone Co.
444 Michigan Ave.
Room 1110
Detroit, MI 48226

Wooden Environments
1890 Evergreen Ave.
Speonk, NY 11972

Words +
1125 Stewart Ct.
Suite D
Sunnyvale, CA 94086

Wormald International Sensory Aids
Suite 110
Bensenville, IL 60106

YLI Corp.
742 Geneviene
Solana Beach, CA 92075

Zygo Industries, Inc.
P.O. Box 1008
Portland, OR 97207

WHEELCHAIRS SUPPLIERS
A Bec
20803 Higgins Ct.
Torrance, CA 90501
(Wheelchairs)

Abbey Medical
3216 Segundo Blvd.
San Jose, CA 90250
(Strollers)

ABS Plastic Insert Seat
Little Rock Orthotics
1010 South Taylor
Little Rock, AR 72207
(Seating for neurologically handicapped)

Accumec Corp.
32 Race St.
San Jose, CA 95126
(Wheelchairs)

Achievement Products
P.O. Box 547
Mineola, NY 11501
(Strollers)

American Stair Glide Corp.
4001 E. 138 St.
Grandview, MO 64030
(Wheelchairs)

Amigo Mobility Center, Inc.
7500 Bluewater NW
Albuquerque, NM 87105
(Wheelchairs)

Andrews Maclaren
P.O. Box 2004
New York, NY 10017
(Strollers)

Cleo Living Aids
3857 Mayfield Rd.
Cleveland, OH 44121
(Strollers)

Columbia Medical Mfg.
P.O. Box 2731
Pacific Palisades, CA 90272
(Strollers)

Convaid
P.O. Box 2731
Palos Verdes, CA 90274
(Wheelchairs)

Desemo Seat
Desemo Project
P.O. Box 313
University Station
Birmingham, AL 35294
(Custom-molded foam module)

E & J Canadian Ltd.
111 Snidercroft Rd.
Concord, Ontario L4K 1B6
Canada
(Wheelchairs)

Educational Teaching Aids
159 W. Kinzie St.
Chicago, IL 60610

Electric Mobility
591 Mantua Blvd.
Sewell, NJ 08080
(Wheelchairs)

Electrolurgy
1121 Duryea Ave.
Irvine, CA 92714
(Wheelchairs)

Equipment Shop
P.O. Box 33
Bedford, MA 01730
(Wheelchairs)

Everest & Jennings
3233 E. Mission Oaks Blvd.
Camarillo, CA 93010
(Wheelchairs)

Executive Distributors of America
15055 32 Mile Rd.
Romeo, MI 48065
(Wheelchairs)

Flaghouse
18 W. 18 St.
New York, NY 10011
(Strollers)

Foam-In-Place
University of Tennessee
Rehabilitation
Engineering Center
1248 La Paloma St.
Memphis, TN 38114
(Custom-molded seat)

Gorham Products
189 Lake St.
Brooklyn, NY 11223

Invacare Corp.
1200 Taylor St.
Elyria, OH 44035
(Wheelchairs)

Jung Products
5801 Mariemont Ave.
Cincinnati, OH 45227
(Wheelchairs)

Magnum International
2930 W. Central
Santa Ana, CA 92704
(Wheelchairs)

Mastercraft Metal
P.O. Box 591
Santa Cruz, CA 95061
(Wheelchairs)

Mobility Plus
P.O. Box 391
215 N. 12 St.
Santa Paula, CA 93060
(Wheelchairs)

Modular Medical
1558 Hutchinson River
Parkway E
(Strollers/wheelchairs)

Motion Designs
1075 Cole
Clovis, CA 93612
(Wheelchairs)

Mulholland Corp.
1563 Los Angeles Ave.
Ventura, CA 93003
(Mulholland Growth Guidance Chair)

Northside Surgical Supply
1165 Portland Ave.
Bronx, NY 10461
(Strollers/wheelchairs)

Ortho-Kinetics, Inc.
P.O. Box 436
Waukesha, WI 53187
(Orthokinetic Travel Chair)

Palmco Engineering Co.
12005 Rivera Rd.
Santa Fe Springs, CA 90670
(Strollers)

Pin Dot Products
P.O. Box 642
Northbrook, IL 60062
(Standing wheelchair)

Quadra Wheelchair, Inc.
31125 Via Colinas No. 903
Westlake Village, CA 91361
(Wheelchairs)

Safety Travel Chairs, Inc.
147 Eady Ct.
Elyria, OH 44035
(Strollers/wheelchairs)

Stainless Medical Products
9386 Dowdy Dr.
San Diego, CA 92126
(Strollers/wheelchairs)

Theradyne Corp.
21730 Hanover St.
Lakeville, MN 55044
(Wheelchairs)

Wheel Ring, Inc.
175 Pine St.
Manchester, CT 06040
(Wheelchairs)

XL Wheelchairs
2003 Palm Ave.
Chico, CA 95926
(Wheelchairs)

Source: Adapted from The Nordic Committee on Disability. *The More We Do Together.* New York: The World Rehabilitation Fund, 1985.

B Special Equipment Available from North American Suppliers*

CHILD'S ROOM

CHAIR LEG EXTENDER
  Abbey Medical
  Camp International
  Comfortably Yours
  Cleo Living Aids
  Fred Sammons, Inc.
  Graham Field Surgical
  Help Yourself Aids
  Jan Surgical
  Roloke Co.

BABY CRY SIGNAL
  American Communications Corp.
  Bell Telephone Co. with Telecommunication
    Centers for Disabled Persons
  Canadian Hearing Society
  Hal Hen Co.
  KE Series Electronic Devices
  Nationwide Flashing Signal Systems, Inc.
  Phone TTY, Inc.
  Sonic Alert
  Sound Barrier
  Ultratec
  Weitbrecht Communications, Inc.

*Adapted from: *The More We Do Together*. The Nordic Committee on Disability in cooperation with the World Rehabilitation Fund, 1985.

BED VIBRATOR
  Nationwide Flashing Signal Systems, Inc.
  Phone TTY, Inc.
  Hal Hen Co., Inc.

SPEECH-TRAINING TOYS (SOUND-ACTIVATED
SPEECH THERAPY AID)
  Knightsbridge Medical
  Manhattan Empire Chapter, NY Telephone
    Co.
  Theodore N. Vail State Chapter, Illinois Bell
    Telephone Co.
  Wolverine Chapter, Michigan Bell Telephone
    Co.

FLASHING LIGHT SIGNALS
Telephone signals
  Nationwide Flashing Signal Systems, Inc.
  Phone TTY, Inc.

Wake-Up alarm converter
  Nationwide Flashing Signal Systems, Inc.

Smoke alarm
  Maryland Chapter, The Chesapeake and Po-
    tomac Telephone Co.

Flashing alarms
  Telephone Pioneers of America

Doorbell signals
  Phone TTY, Inc.

Flashing light remote-control transmitter
  Weitbrecht Communication, Inc.
  (Hal Hen Co., Inc. carries all types of flashing
    signals)

BATHROOM
SHOWER TABLE/STRETCHER/COMMODE
  Mobility Plus
  Trujillo Industries

BATH SLINGS AND SUPPORT RINGS
  Abbey Medical
  Achievement Products, Inc.

  Carnac Industries
  Columbia Medical Manufacturing
  G. E. Miller
  J. A. Preston
  Modular Medical Corp.

ANTISCALD GUARD (THERMOSTAT FAUCET)
  Delta Faucet Co.

SOAP BAG AND WASH MITT
  American Bio Medics
  Fred Sammons, Inc.
  Hammacher Schlemmer
  Maddak, Inc.
  NuDay Creations

POTTIE/COMMODES/SEAT REDUCER/SHOWER
CHAIR/AIDS
  Abbey Medical
  Childsafe
  Cleo Living Aids
  Fred Sammons, Inc.
  G. E. Miller
  J. A. Preston
  Lakeshore Curriculum Materials
  Motor Development Corp.
  Ortho-Kinetics, Inc.
  Rifton Equipment for the Handicapped

**ADAPTED CLOTHING FOR CHILDREN
(DRESSING AIDS/SEWING AIDS)**
CLOTHING
  On the Rise (all kinds of clothing)
  PTL Designs (jumpsuits, trousers, skirts, robes,
    nightgowns)
  Sitting Pretty, Sitting Proud (jeans)
  Techni Flair Corp. (warm-up suits, trousers)
  Clothing for Handicapped People (annotated
    bibliography and resource list)
  Exceptionally Yours (casual wear)
  Kristen Wear (all kinds of clothing)
  Laurel Designs (vests, skirts, T-shirts, rain pon-
    chos)
  Natural Creations, The (Texas Tech Univer-
    sity) (pattern designs for handicapped)
  Special Clothes (all kinds of clothing)

330

SHOE FASTENERS (ZIPPERS, FASTENERS, ELASTIC SHOE LACES)
  Cleo Living Aids
  FashionAble
  Fred Sammons, Inc.
  Help Yourself Aids
  J. A. Preston Corp.
  Maddak, Inc.
  Medi Sport Corp.

DRESSING AIDS
  Adaptive Enterprises

STOCKING AIDS
  Adlib Orthotics
  American Bio Medics
  Comfortably Yours
  Eagle Enterprises, Inc.
  Fred Sammons, Inc.
  Handi Aid Co.
  Help Yourself Aids
  J. A. Preston
  Rajowalt Co.
  Sears, Roebuck & Co.
  Sock-On
  Susquehana Rehab. Products

LABELING FOR CLOTHING
  American Foundation for the Blind
  Kentucky Industries for the Blind

SEWING AIDS

SCISSORS
  Aristera Machines (left hand)
  Comfortably Yours (Scissor with flexible handle)
  FashionAble
  Fred Sammons, Inc.
  Nelson Medical Products
  Maddak, Inc.

MAGNIFYING LENS WITH NECK STRAP
  American Foundation for the Blind
  Comfortably Yours
  Maddak, Inc.
  Magnistitch

NEEDLE THREADERS
  American Foundation for the Blind
  FashionAble
  Maddak, Inc.

PATTERNS MANUAL
  Textile Research Center (Texas Technical University)

KITCHEN AND DINING AREA

NONSLIP PLACEMATS AND MOLDED PADS
  Abbey Medical
  Cleo Living Aids
  Fred Sammons, Inc.
  G. E. Miller
  Help Yourself Aids
  Maddak, Inc.
  Medical Equipment Distributors

DRINKING CUP
  Abbey Medical (with spout)
  Fred Sammons, Inc. (with holder)
  G. E. Miller (with spout, two handles)
  J. A. Preston (twin handle)
  Maddak, Inc. (clip-on drink holder, nonslip base, etc.)
  Sola, Inc. (glass)

DRINKING STRAW
  Cleo Living Aids
  Fairway King
  Fred Sammons, Inc.
  Help Yourself Aids
  Maddak, Inc.
  Medical Equipment Distributors
  Nelson Medical Products

FOOD WARMER DISH
  Fred Sammons, Inc.
  Maddak, Inc.

FOOD GUARD
  American Bio Medics
  Fairway King
  FashionAble
  Fred Sammons, Inc.

Handi Aid Co.
Sears, Roebuck & Co.

Some other items for the kitchen and dining area available at the above-named suppliers include scoop dishes, bowls, and wheelchair drink holders.

MILK CARTON OPENER, CARRIER
Abbey Medical
American Bio Medics
Comfortably Yours
Grayline Housewares
Independence Factory, The
Maddak, Inc.

PLAY, HOBBY, AND RECREATION

TOYS
Battery-operated toys
Benjamin Michael Industries
Electronic Handicapped Equipment, Ltd.
Linda J. Burkhart (homemade)
Telegraphics, Inc.
Toys for Special Children
Visualtek
Zygo Industries, Inc.

Foam rubber toys
Able Child
J. A. Preston (Tumble Forms)
Rifton Equipment for the Handicapped
Southpaw Enterprises

Child life-size dolls
Abbey Medical
Adaptive Enterprises (dressing doll)
Ronnie Lee, Inc. (Best Friends)

Stuffed animals
Special Friends (animals with disabilities)

Rocking Friends (Animals with Safety Seat)
Able Child
Community Playthings

Talking toy kit
H. G. McCully Upstate Chapter—N.J. Bell Telephone Co.

Battery interface control
Prentke-Romich Co.

STROLLERS AND SPORTS WHEELCHAIRS
Cycles (specially equipped)
Abbey Medical
Cleo Living Aids
Community Playthings
Consumer Care Products
Educational Teaching Aids
Gandy Co. (tandem bicycle)
G. E. Miller
Harper
Hillan Creative Play Structures
J. A. Preston
Maddak, Inc.
Playlearn Products
Recreational Mobility, Inc.
Rifton Equipment for the Handicapped

SANDBOXES AND PLAYGROUND EQUIPMENT
Abbey Medical
Wooden Environments

ADAPTIVE EQUIPMENT FOR WINTER AND SUMMER SPORTS ACTIVITIES
Skiing, skating, sledding
Beneficial Designs, Inc. (ski, sled)
Hein A. Ken Corp. (skate aids)
Mountain Man (ski, sled)
Mountainsmith (sleds)
PSI Pauls Sports (ski aids)
Quadra Wheelchair (snow wheelchair)

Swimming (pool lifts, bars, and transfer aids)
Advanced Mobility Systems, Inc.
AFW of North America
Frost Co.
GEG Pool Lift
G. E. Miller

Industrial Research and Engineering
J. A. Preston
J. E. Nolan and Co., Inc.
Lo Rich Enterprises, Inc.
Mechanicaids Aquanaids
Northern Plastics Corp.
Trans Aid Corp.
Water Sport Industries

MISCELLANEOUS: CORNER SEATS
Abbey Medical
Community Playthings
Equipment Shop
G. E. Miller
J. A. Preston
Maddak, Inc.

SWIMMING AND FLOATING AIDS
Bema U.S.A., Inc.
Danmar Products, Inc.

RIDING SADDLE (ADAPTED)
Grizzly Peak Stables

BOWLING BALL HOLDER
Snitz Manufacturing Co.

PROTECTIVE HELMETS
Cleo Living Aids
Cooper Canada, Ltd.
Danmar Products, Inc.
Face Guards, Inc.
Fred Sammons, Inc.
G. E. Miller
J. A. Preston
Maddak, Inc.
Medical Equipment Distributors
Modular Medical Corp.
Preston Special Education
Stall and Dean

PHOTOGRAPHY (ADAPTIVE EQUIPMENT)
Beneficial Designs, Inc.
Therapeutic Recreation Systems

COMMUNICATION-SCHOOL (See also CHILD'S ROOM, baby cry signal)
PORTABLE COMMUNICATORS
Adaptive Aids
Automated Data Systems, Inc.
Commetrics, Ltd.
Computers for the Physically Handicapped
Crestwood Co.
Don Johnston Developmental Equipment (also has Bliss Symbolics Technology)
Dufco
Northern Telecom
Phonic Ear Phonic Mirror
Prentke-Romich Co.
Radio Shack International
Rehab Technology
Sharp Electronics
Shea Products
Telesensory Systems, Inc.
Texas Instruments
Triformation Systems
Words +
Zygo Industries, Inc.

COMMUNICATION BOARDS
Crestwood Co.
Don Johnston Developmental Equipment
Fred Sammons, Inc.
Help Me to Help Myself
Modern Education Corp.
Research Plus, Inc.
Tufts Biomedical Engineering Center

HOLDER FOR TELEPHONE RECEIVER
Abbey Medical
Basic Telecommunications Corp.
Cleo Living Aids
Coastline Controls
Extensions for Independence
FashionAble
Help Yourself Aids
Jal Co., The
Maddak, Inc.
Medical Equipment Distributors
Sparr Telephone Arm Co.
Zygo Industries, Inc.

PHONE RECEIVER WITH AMPLIFIER
  Adco Hearing Conservation
  Basic Telecommunications Corp.
  Bell Telephone Co. with Telecommunications
    Centers
  Comfortably Yours
  Desmond J. Carron
  Hammacher Schlemmer
  Harriet Carter
  Leonard's Health Care Products
  Maddak, Inc.
  Phonic Ear Phonic Mirror
  Radio Shack International
  Telephone Pioneers of America

TV AMPLIFIERS
  Adaptive Communications Systems, Inc.
  Comfortably Yours

OPTACON
  Telesensory Systems, Inc.

PENCIL HOLDERS
  Abbey Medical
  American Bio Medics
  Blackburn Research Products
  Cleo Living Aids
  Fairway King
  Fred Sammons, Inc.
  Help Yourself Aids
  Independence Factory, The
  Maddak, Inc.
  Medical Equipment Distributors
  Richards Manufacturing Co., Inc.

CHILD'S DESK
  Abbey Medical
  Cleo Living Aids
  G. E. Miller
  J. A. Preston
  Medical Equipment Distributors

LOW VISION READING SYSTEMS
  Adaptive Communications Systems, Inc.
  Apollo Electronic Visual Aids
  Best Visual Products

  Elayo Americas
  Eyetronics
  Howe Press of Perkins School for the Blind
  Pelco Industries
  Sensory Aids Corp.
  Visualtek
  Wormald International Sensory Aids

TYPING AIDS, TYPEWRITERS, TYPING INSTRUCTION
Instruction
  Cleo Living Aids
  Teachers Institute for Special Education

Computer typewriter programs
  Computers to Help People
  Cyberon
  Rocky Mountain Software, Inc.

Remote-control typing units
  C. R. Bard, Inc.

Large-print typewriters and aids
  Apollo Lazers
  California Retyping, Data Display Systems
  Lozanov Learning Institutes
  SCM Corp.
  Typewriting Institute for the Handicapped

Other typing aids
  Adler Royal Business Machines
  Cleo Living Aids
  Executive Distributors of America
  Fred Sammons, Inc.
  Medical Equipment Distributors
  SCM Corp.

TALKING CALCULATOR
  American Printing House for the Blind
  Sensory Interface Equipment
  Visualtek

TALKING CLOCKS
  American Foundation for the Blind
  Crestwood Co.
  Sears, Roebuck & Co.
  Sharp Electronics

Index

RD
797
.P42
1989

RD
797
.P42

1989

$20.98